Residency Programs Thriving

Letter dated December 17, 1964:

I feel it is significant that all but one of the present interns are staying for residencies at this hospital, and have confidence in our training programs after their association [as an intern] since July. It is too early to predict, but we also expect a larger complement of interns for July, 1965.

Z

Letter dated June 10, 1965, to the US Selective Service System in reply to the letter above:

We have just been informed that Dr. Glenn VanRoekel has received an "Order to Report for Induction." We respectfully request that Dr. VanRoekel's case be reconsidered.

Dr. VanRoekel is under contract with this hospital for a three-year Radiology Residency, commencing July 1, 1965. Since most doctors have signed contracts by this time of year, it would be impossible to replace Dr. VanRoekel in our residency program. The loss of Dr. VanRoekel would place a serious burden on our program, not only during the 1965-66 academic year but for the duration of the three year residency.

It is felt that Dr. VanRockel could greater serve the Armed Forces after completion of his radiology residency. We will very much appreciate any consideration you can give our request for the postponement of Dr. VanRoekel's induction orders.

Sincerely,
Milton Sacks, Director

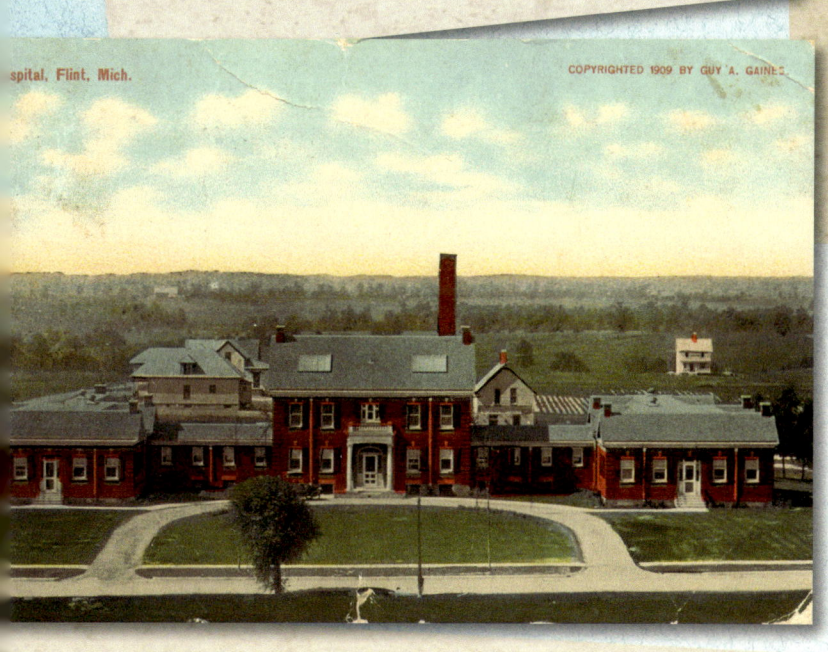

...these last few days. ...e night by crawling ...ghtened to move. We keep moving on in -- could go on for hours about the horrible trip across, and the beachhead experiences since our arrival, but would only be deleted. Six of us in this group are the first American nurses as near as we can find out, to be here, or were at that time. The country is really beautiful but all the buildings and towns have been pulverized. Our men are to be commended for their bravery and work, only wish that we could do more for them.

Letter #2:

Since you read the article of our crossing on the LST . . . there are a few experiences I do not wish to remind myself of. Our position is in actual combat behind the front lines and we are most mobile. May I brag a bit and say we do have an excellent setup and a well-trained unit: at least we have received considerable praise from the Ninth Air Force to which we are attached. Our hospital is under one tentage and we are able to accommodate one hundred casualties at a time. We administer emergency treatment and hospitalize until conditions permit transfer by air to a general hospital. I have seen days when cots were so thick in the area with soldiers waiting to be taken care of that we could hardly get around. I wonder how many barrels of plasma and whole blood we have poured into our men. It has proven wonders and saved many lives that couldn't possibly have been saved otherwise. Most casualties are due to mines and booby-traps that the ******* so thoughtfully and carefully left behind. Of course gun shot and flak wounds are numerous but nothing like those caused from the petty pranks. Surgery is very extensive. I owe a great deal to Hurley Hospital for my past experience enabling me to do the type of work that I have been most interested in. Amputations are common. It has gotten so we can set up for any type of brain surgery and have it complete without several trips back to the instrument case and autoclave.

I have my operating room tent lined with sheets and divided into rooms which adds greatly to the lighting system, and allows more space for and privacy for patients. The ward tents circle the OR with admission and X-ray directly in front. The personnel is scattered throughout the field and we try to disperse as much as possible. We are atop a hill surrounded with trees and overlooking a very picturesque valley. The remains of the small village. Lie at the foot of the hill and each day a few French people with carts loaded with what odds and ends they may have been able to save, return to the ruins and start rebuilding for the winter months. Its most pathetic to see the frightful expressions on their faces of these people and also see the reaction of the children at any false move by a stranger. This has been a wonderful experience. I would never have been satisfied if not a part of this great invasion. However, let it be the last. I marvel at what our young men have gone through and also at the excellent work in planning and preparing for this day and how our soldiers were ever able to capture this territory so quickly is indeed a miracle. They are to be commended and all praise can't sufficiently cover their bravery and efficient work.

Letter dated February 4, 1929:

To Business Manager of the Hurley Hosp. Flint Mich.

Dear Sir:

Is there a young intern there by the name of Leslie Lambert, and is he very, very busy or is he sick, we have had no word from him, except a parcel at Christmas since about 1 week after Thanksgiving? Will you just answer this question please. I am sending you an envelope and wish you would be as kind as to answer, please.

Respectfully, Mrs. R.L. Lambert.

P.S. If he's not there do you know where he is.

Reply dated February 12, 1929:

Dear Madam: Replying to yours of the 4th relative to Leslie Lambert, will say that he has been very busy, is enjoying the best of health, and is as happy as interns are. Very truly yours, HURLEY HOSPITAL

Frank D. King
Superintendent

...ters dated July 21, 1952, regarding an intern application request sent to the chairman of ...Michigan Volunteer Advisory Committee, Detroit, Michigan:

...ley Hospital is a large city hospital in a highly industrialized area, a good part of whose ...ities are devoted to defense production. An acute general hospital of this type is subject to ...rge number of admissions as a result of industrial accidents. The intern in this hospital ...s the Emergency Room on a 24-hour basis, and the intern who covers the hospital night ...day for medical emergencies and the immediate medical care. Our resident staff has ...decimated by the demands of the armed services, and we have become more and more ...ndent upon the interns for medical coverage. It is our considered opinion, therefore, ...this man is extremely essential not only to the operation of the hospital, but to the ...tenance of the working population in the interests of defense production.

HURLEY
MEDICAL CENTER
THE BEACON ON THE HILL

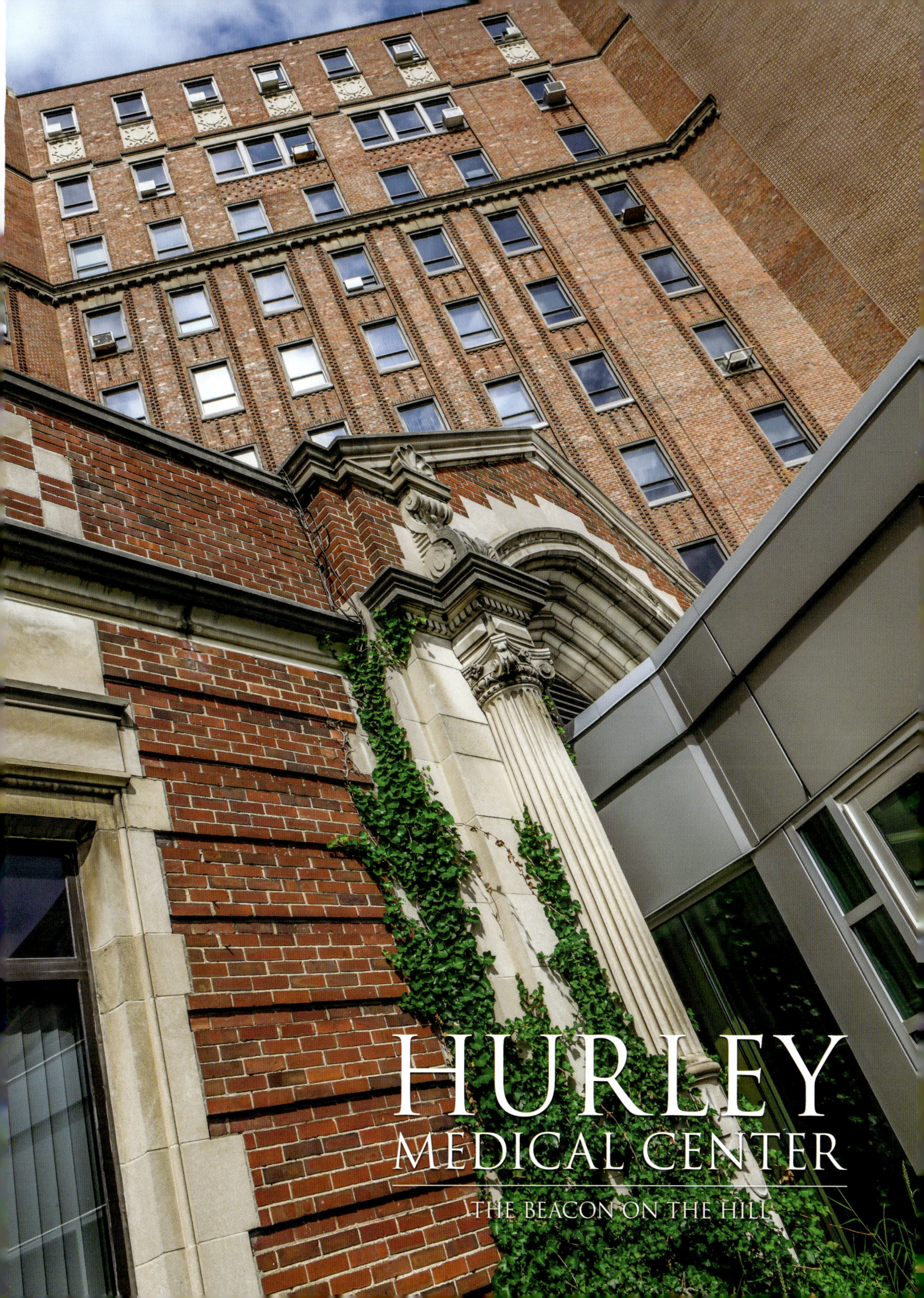

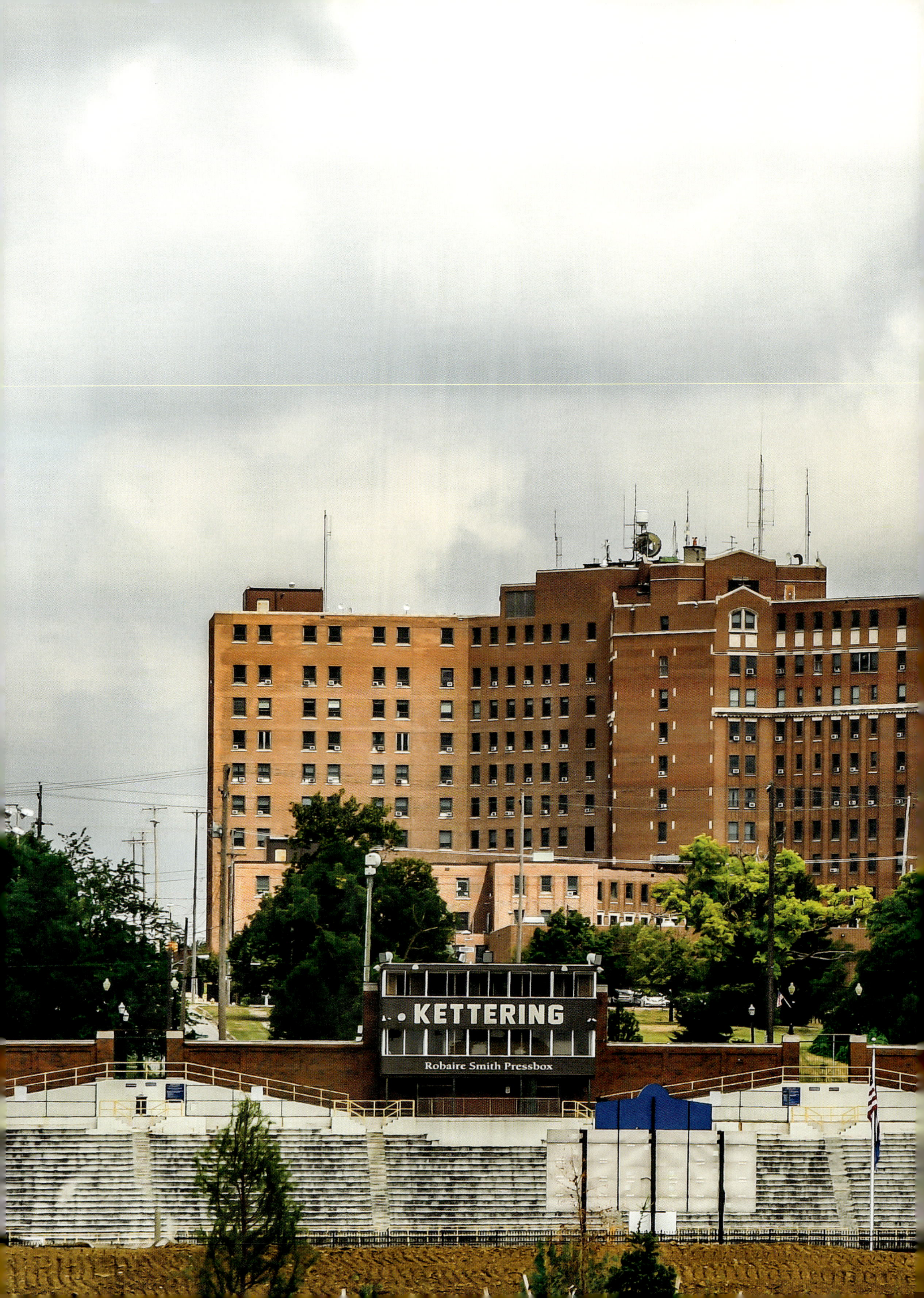
KETTERING
Robaire Smith Pressbox

HURLEY
MEDICAL CENTER

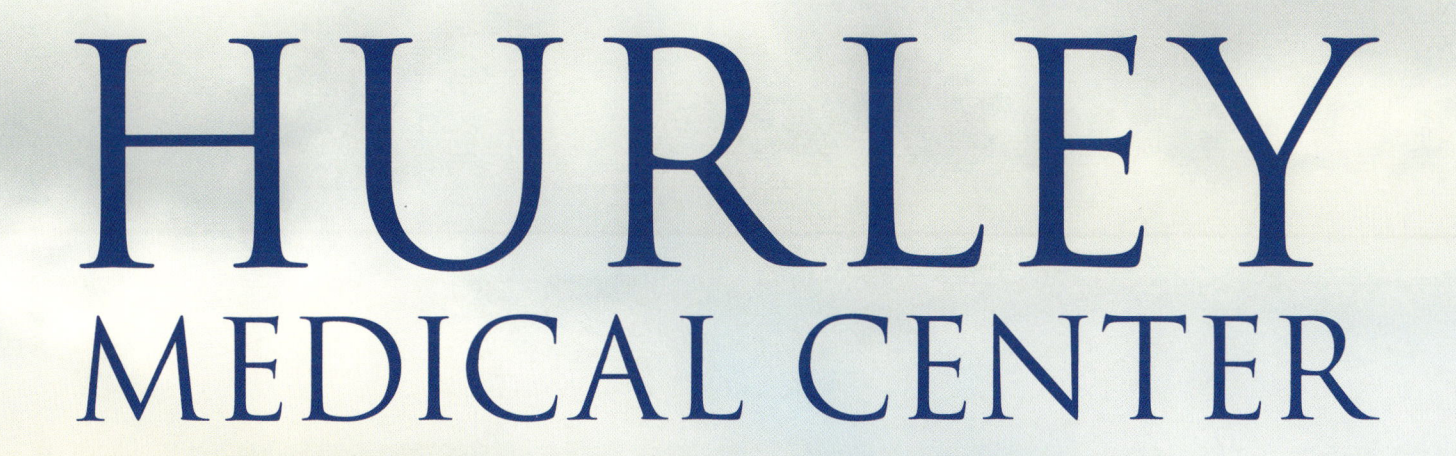

THE BEACON ON THE HILL

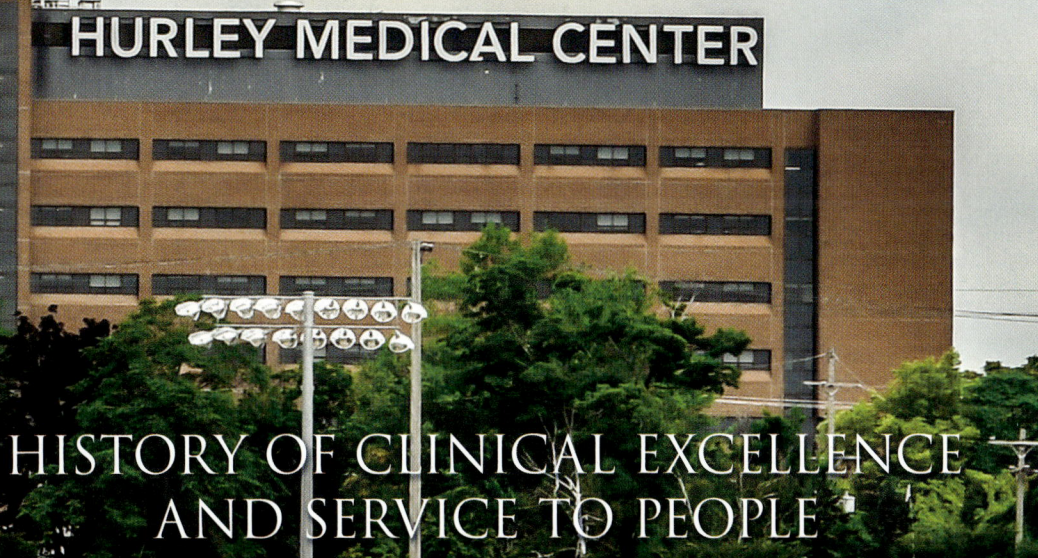

HISTORY OF CLINICAL EXCELLENCE
AND SERVICE TO PEOPLE

1905–2020

BY
JULIE M. WALKE

Copyright © 2022 by Hurley Foundation

All rights reserved, including the right to reproduce this work in any form whatsoever without permission in writing from the publisher, except for brief passages in connection with a review. For information, please write:

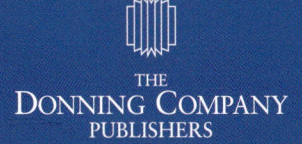

THE DONNING COMPANY PUBLISHERS

The Donning Company Publishers
731 South Brunswick Street
Brookfield, MO 64628

Lex Cavanah, *General Manager*
Nathan Stufflebean, *Production Supervisor*
Philip Briscoe, *Editor*
Stephanie L. Danko, *Graphic Designer*
Katie Gardner, *Marketing and Project Coordinator*
Alyssa Niemeier, *Project Research Coordinator*

George Nikolovski, *Project Director*

Library of Congress Cataloging-in-Publication Data
Names: Walke, Julie M., 1958- author.
Title: Hurley Medical Center - the beacon on the hill : history of clinical excellence and service to people, 1905-2020 / by Julie M. Walke.
Description: Brookfield : The Donning Company Publishers, 2021. | Summary: "A pictorial history of Hurley Medical Center, located in Flint, Michigan"— Provided by publisher.
Identifiers: LCCN 2021039061 | ISBN 9781681843087 (hardcover)
Subjects: LCSH: Hospitals—Michigan—Flint. | Hospitals—Michigan—History—20th century. | Hospitals—Michigan—History—21th century. | Hurley Medical Center.
Classification: LCC RA981.M5 W35 2021 | DDC 362.1109774/37—dc23/eng/20211007
LC record available at https://lccn.loc.gov/2021039061

Printed in the United States of America at Walsworth

Contents

- 6 Foreword
- 7 Acknowledgements
- 8 **CHAPTER ONE: A LANDMARK INSTITUTION**
  - 9 James J. Hurley
  - 11 Hurley's Hospital
  - 12 The First Ten Years
  - 13 The Second Decade – Expansion and Reputation
  - 16 Hurley Hospital – Fifty Years of Stability and Growth, 1930s–1970s
  - 21 Health Care and the Auto Industry
- 22 **CHAPTER TWO: A REGIONAL LEADER IN ADVANCED MEDICAL CARE**
  - 22 HMC – Advancing Medical Care
  - 25 Emergency Medicine
  - 27 Trauma Medicine
  - 31 Emergency Department
  - 32 Breaking the Cycle of Violence
  - 36 Traumatic Events with HMC at the Front Line
  - 37 Regional Burn Center – Medical Department of Excellence
  - 40 Pharmacological Medicine
  - 41 Embracing Information Technology and Epic
- 52 **CHAPTER THREE: FROM BUMP TO BABY – WOMEN AND CHILDREN**
  - 52 Obstetrics and Gynecology
  - 57 The Early Years
  - 60 Pediatric Hematology and Oncology
  - 62 Hurley Children's Hospital – A Children's Miracle Network Hospital
  - 66 Level II Pediatric Trauma Center
  - 73 Pediatric Public Health Initiative
- 76 **CHAPTER FOUR: AN EDUCATION LEADER**
  - 78 Graduate Medical Education – Medical Residency Programs
  - 86 Wars and Their Impact on Graduate Medical Education
  - 89 Hurley School of Nursing – 86 Years of Excellence
  - 97 Hurley School of Radiologic Technology
  - 98 Hurley School of Medical Technology
  - 99 Hurley School of Anesthesia
  - 100 Teaching Special Operations Combat Medics
- 102 **CHAPTER FIVE: THOSE WHO SERVE – HONORING EXCELLENCE**
  - 103 Leadership at the Top
  - 106 Hurley Medical Center Board of Managers
  - 108 Leadership at Its Best
  - 110 Medical Excellence
  - 115 Multiple Generations at HMC
  - 117 Dedicated Spaces
  - 121 A Great Place to Work
- 124 **CHAPTER SIX: THE FOUNDATION – A FOUNTAIN OF SUPPORT**
  - 129 Foundation Leadership Remains Strong
  - 130 History of the Hurley Medical Center Auxiliary and Volunteer Corps
  - 137 Honoring Longtime Volunteers
  - 138 Staff Who Return as Volunteers
  - 139 Fundraising and the Community at Large
  - 140 Breast Health Nurse Navigator
  - 141 Annual Hurley Trauma Center Fall Golf Classic
  - 142 The James J. Hurley Society
- 144 **CHAPTER SEVEN: TRANSFORMING HEALTH**
  - 144 Reaching into Neighboring Communities
  - 148 Food FARMacy
  - 150 Senior Services
  - 152 Palliative Care and Hospice
  - 153 Behavioral Medicine
  - 154 Hurley Wellness Services – Community Programs

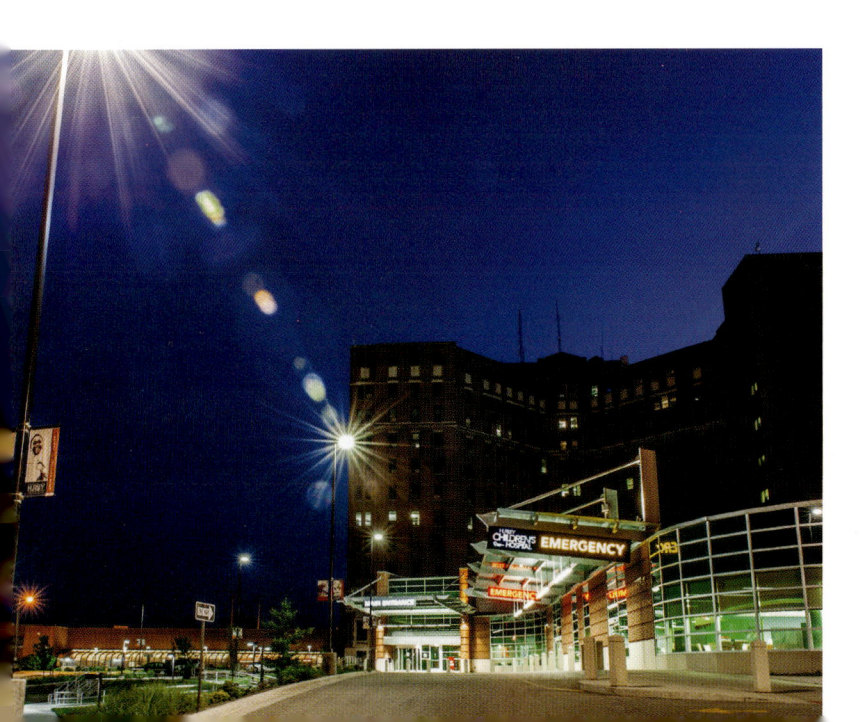

Foreword

Hurley opened its doors in Flint, Michigan, on December 19, 1908, and has operated around the clock every minute of every day since then. Within those days, weeks, and years are countless hours of service from many individuals dedicated to providing "Clinical Excellence and Service to People." While not everyone is a bedside caregiver, those working in any capacity for Hurley Medical Center all recognize the privilege we are given when a patient chooses Hurley for their care.

This compilation of Hurley's history features many individuals, events, and accomplishments that were assembled with the full knowledge that the medical center stands on a foundation of so much more than these highlights. For that reason, we dedicate this book to those individuals, teams, and support systems that may not stand out in the following pages, yet their service is critical to Hurley's ongoing excellence. Gratitude and appreciation go out to each of our support service areas, our labor union partners, our community partners, and donors for all you do as part of our health care family.

As you read through the following chapters, we hope you are amazed by Hurley firsts and the degree to which we have dedicated the work of the medical center outward, back to our patients, community, and supporters. As impressive as you could find this, we hope you recognize that behind each staff member you may encounter on a Hurley visit, there are thousands of others working to help care for you as well. This was James J. Hurley's wish, and this is the history of our promise to fulfill it.

HURLEY FOUNDATION

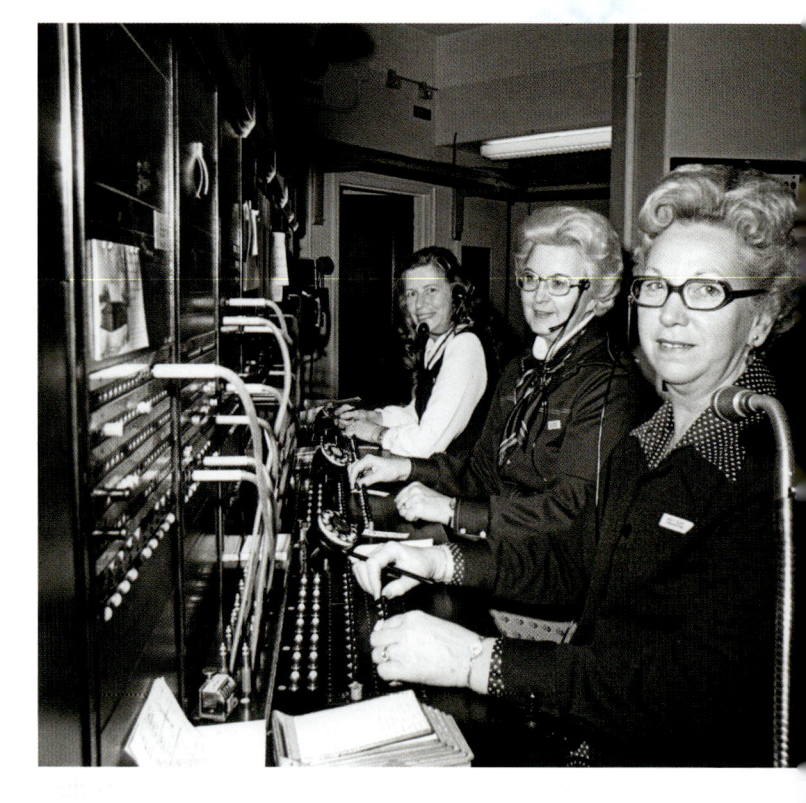

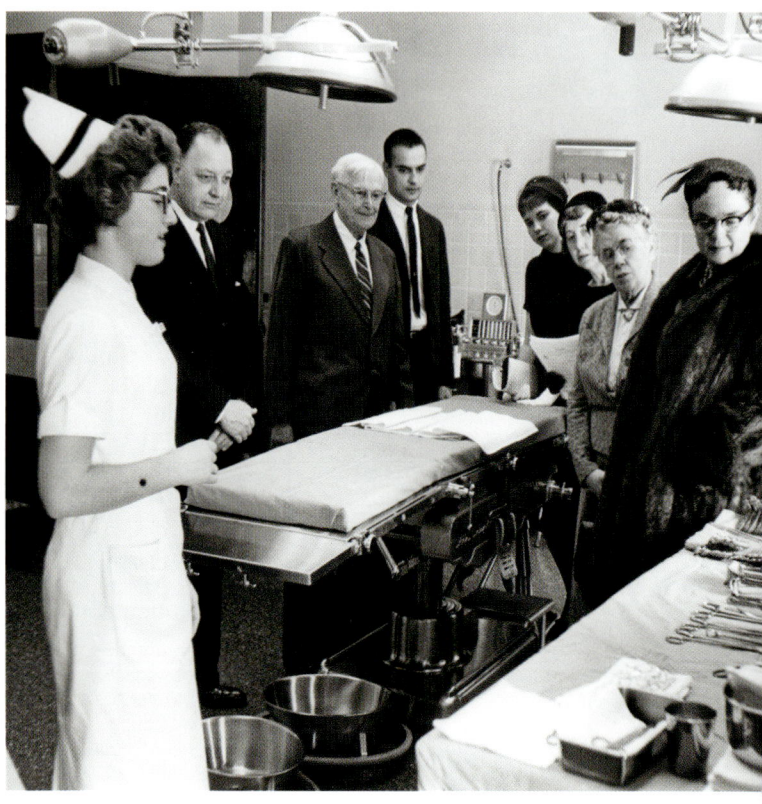

Acknowledgements

Whenever I begin to write a history book, I know that I will learn about a place and a world that will both surprise and captivate me. It is with fresh eyes that I see Hurley Medical Center and have come to realize that it is so much more than a building—it is a culture of people who have a singular mission of helping those in need. This philosophy was started by founder James J. Hurley and is currently guided by President and CEO Melany Gavulic, RN, MBA, who has been at the helm since 2012. With their mission of "Clinical Excellence and Service to People," it seems to me that the guiding principles are safe for decades to come.

I have enjoyed this journey in learning about both the place and the people of Hurley Medical Center, as well as The Hurley Foundation. Everyone has been extremely gracious in giving access and support through the completion of this work. First, I would like to thank Melany Gavulic for taking the time in her busy schedule to be an active participant. I am appreciative of Foundation President Mike Burnett and Jordan Brown, director of Volunteer and Community Engagement, both of whom initially saw the value of having a book written and have guided me well.

There are people without whom this project would not have come to fruition. Most notably, Jordan Brown, MBA, and Jennifer Godlesky, MLIS library manager, Hamady Health Sciences Library, who were my partners in the research, writing, and editing process. I could always rely on Jordan's steady direction. I appreciate Jeni's responsiveness and loyalty to the project. She allowed me to spend incalculable hours in the library conference room. Together, we searched through countless boxes looking for treasure. Doug Pike, Hurley staff photographer, has been invaluable in shaping the overall look of the book. Doug handled a mountain of requests with great enthusiasm, always giving more pictures than I asked for so that I could make good choices. Then there are key staff members whom I counted on to help clarify facts and give an opinion. They are as follows:

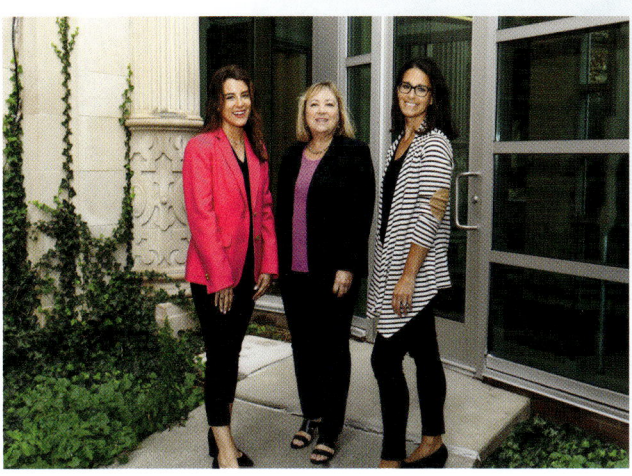

Hurley History Book Team (left to right): Jordan Brown, Julie Walke, and Jennifer Godlesky

Linda Tracy-Stephens, John Stewart, F. Michael Jaggi, DO, Elizabeth Wenstrom-Williams, and Debi Wright. My favorite interviews were with Samuel Dismond Jr., MD; Susumu Inoue, MD, FAAP; Brian Nolan, MD, FAAP; Raouf Mikhail, MD, FACS, FRCS; John Hebert, MD; Phillip C. Dutcher; Frankie Perry; V. Mitra Tewari; Diane Welker; Alisa Stewart; and Margie Murray-Wright. I will stop short of thanking individual departments, but I would like to acknowledge the Marketing Department for their assistance whenever asked.

My final thanks also to the many Hurley history-team members who initially met for several brainstorming sessions. They are the ones who helped provide a preliminary outline of what was considered important or noteworthy. Finally, to all the medical staff, administrative staff, former staff, and community leaders whom I interviewed and/or met who are not mentioned here: I am thankful to have spent time in your world, if only for a short while. Hurley Medical Center is a special place. I hope that you enjoy reading this history as much as I did when writing about it.

JULIE M. WALKE
Author

A LANDMARK
Institution
CHAPTER ONE

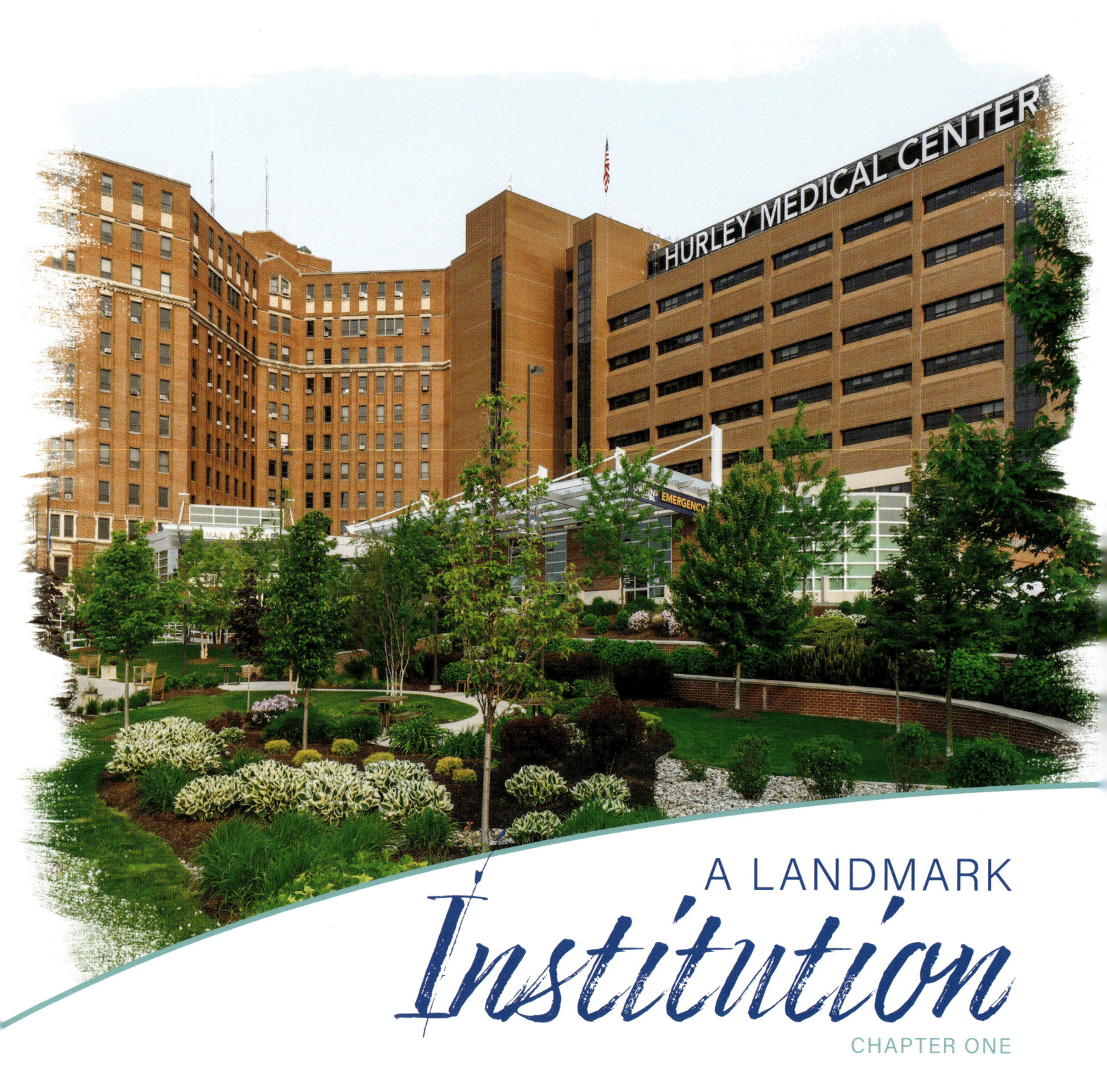

Situated in America's heartland and located in Michigan's seventh-largest city is a thriving medical center that has stood the test of time. This landmark institution is known as Hurley Medical Center (HMC)—a 443-bed, premier public-teaching hospital recognized throughout the state as a trailblazer in advanced specialized health care. Throughout its continual evolution, HMC has held fast to founder James J. Hurley's dream of offering clinical excellence and service to people in the city of Flint.

HMC hails as the region's only Level I Trauma Center with an Emergency Department (ED) that handles more than 90,000 emergency cases a year, along with an extraordinary capacity to save lives with the area's only Burn Unit, Neonatal Intensive Care Unit, Pediatric Intensive Care Unit, and Pediatric Emergency Department. HMC staff not only honor the commitment to provide the highest level of critical care to those in need, but they also go the extra mile by offering follow-through care beyond the hospital stay in support of more than 20,000 people annually who choose HMC for their inpatient hospital care.

HMC has a decades-long legacy of high standards of excellence and exceptional clinical care delivery, utilizing advanced diagnostic and treatment technology alongside highly trained medical staff who are dedicated to caring for every patient who comes through the doors. There is no doubt that there is a high demand for HMC's educational and employment opportunities.

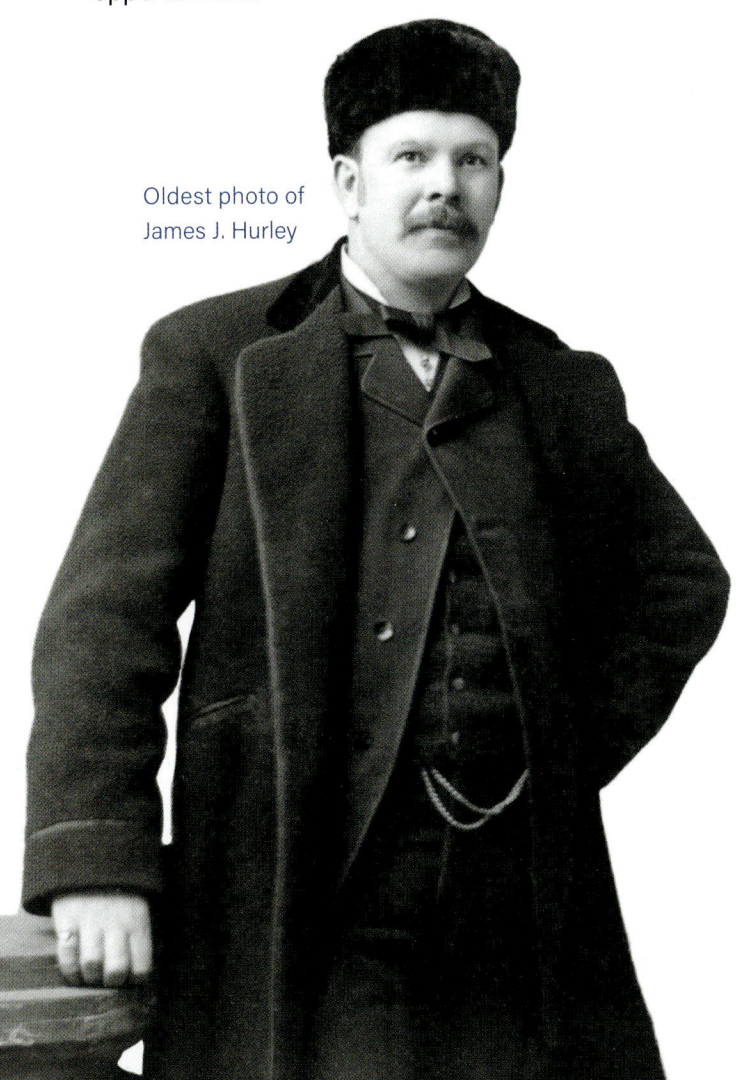

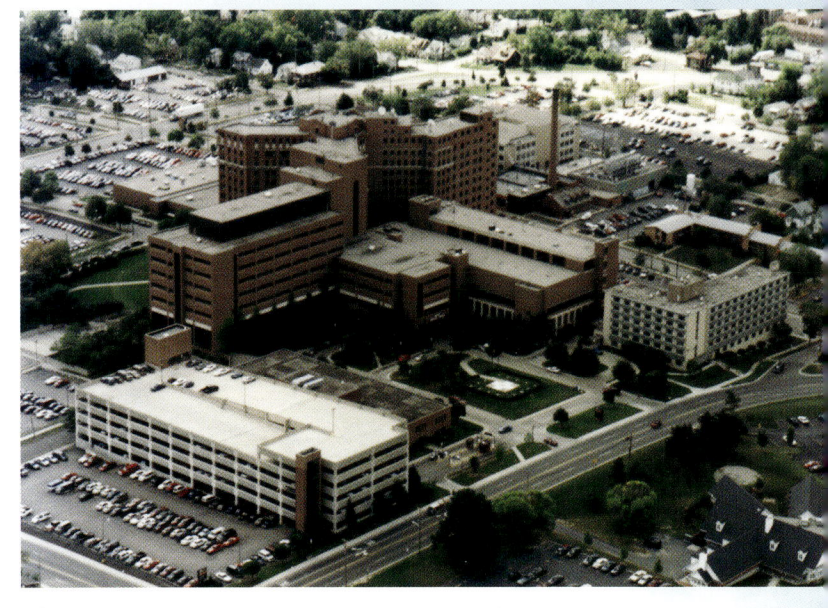

Circa 1998

Oldest photo of James J. Hurley

This book illustrates how HMC has not only been the heartbeat of a community from its early launch in 1908 through decades of leadership in medical care, but how it also continues to inspire a culture of trust, compassion, and respect as "the beacon on the hill" for many generations.

James J. Hurley

James J. Hurley's vision of a hospital that would be available to every citizen of Flint remains strong 113 years later. During his time, Flint was a small town of 15,000 residents. Today, Flint has 96,000 residents within Genesee County's population of 405,813 people (2019).

An English immigrant, Hurley came to Genesee County and persuaded a farmer to hire him for whatever he was worth. "He quickly learned, however, that farming was not to be his forte, when, after two weeks, the farmer fired him. Carrying the one dollar that the farmer gave him to start over, the dauntless Mr. Hurley walked from Grand Blanc to Flint where he became a porter at the Sherman Hotel; he stayed a number of years. "[1]

CHAPTER ONE A LANDMARK INSTITUTION

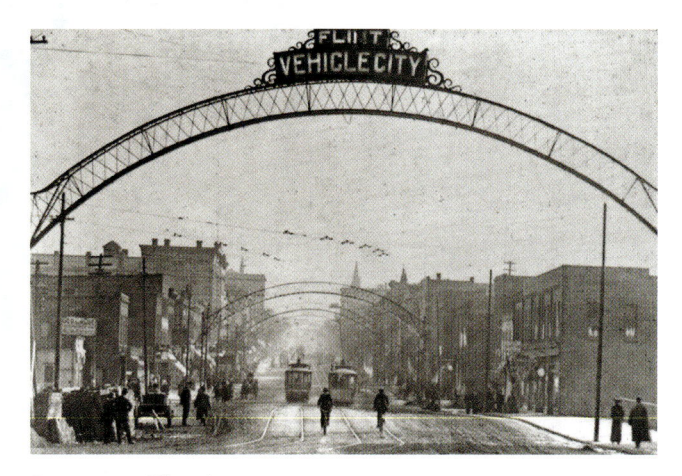

Downtown Flint circa 1900

He married Mary Flinn, and together, they commenced housekeeping with little or no means, and what little they had was expended on doctors' bills to care for his wife during a severe illness.

Hurley's reputation was that of a shrewd, sharp businessman. He became interested in working with Flint P. Smith in the sawmill, and together, they built 20 or more houses in the city. Hurley was one of the earliest stockholders in the W. A. Paterson Carriage Factory. He later invested capital in the organization of the Union Trust and Savings Bank and, as such, served as a director on the bank's first board of directors. Along with his shrewd business acumen, he was also known to be kindhearted, and he liberally gave to the poor in a quiet and reserved manner. His life was characteristic of the manner in which he disposed of all of his property at the time of his death, wherein he not only remembered the city, but also all of the churches, many of the poor, and his old employees.[2]

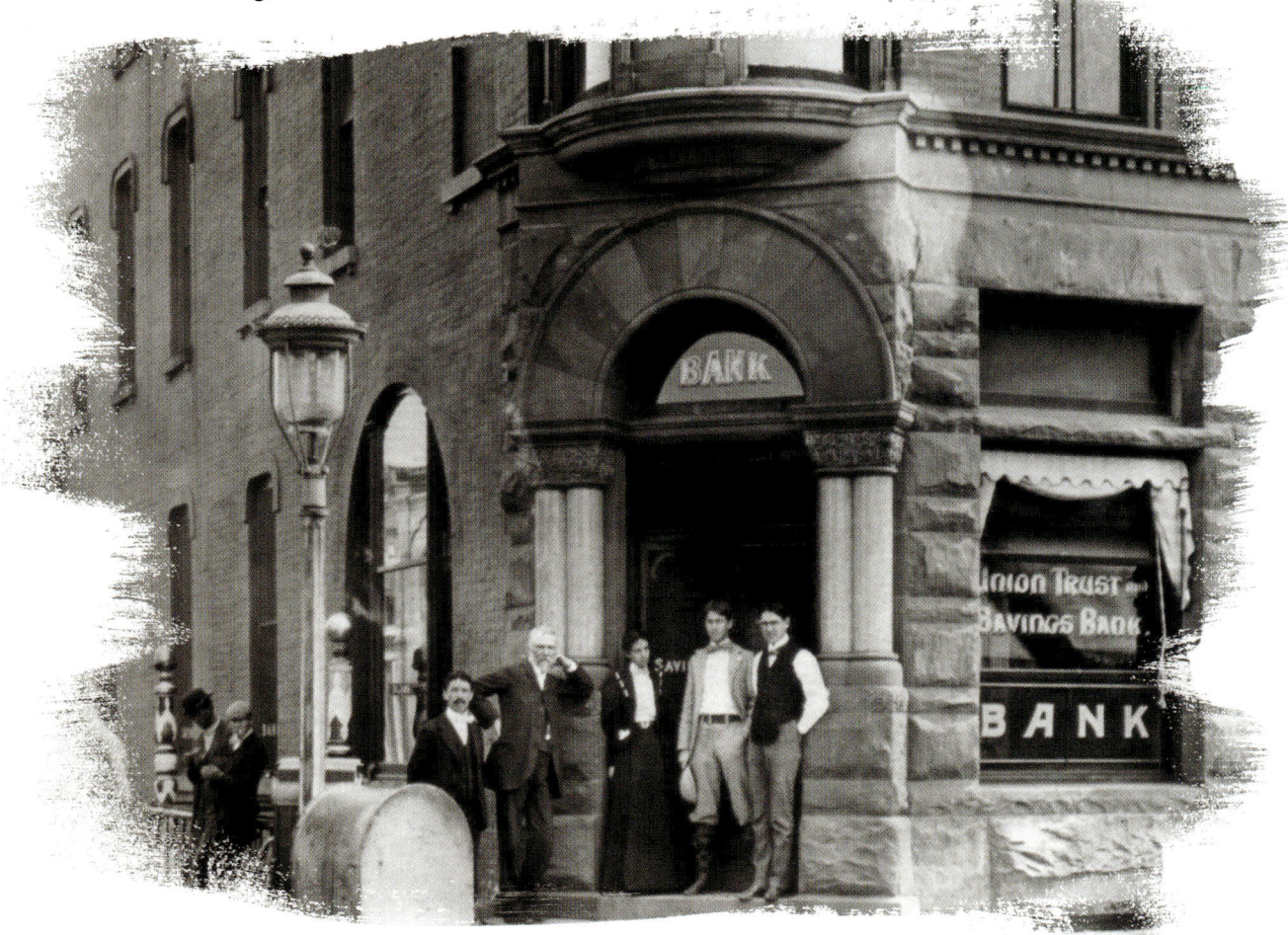

Union Trust and Savings Bank, where James J. Hurley was a founder

James J. Hurley Papers

The Hurley Papers, a collection of 16 letters from 1900 to 1908, document the life of a blue-collar worker, an underrepresented figure in historical manuscript collections. James Hurley proudly defined himself as a father, a husband, an Irish Catholic, and a member of the working class: "A working man has as much pride and spirit about him as any rich man." The Hurley Papers are located at the William L. Clements Library, University of Michigan.

Hurley's Hospital

To express his gratitude to the people of Flint who had treated him with generosity along the way, Hurley bequeathed to the City of Flint the acreage of real estate on Begole Street between Sixth and Seventh Avenues, the site where the current medical center stands, along with what amounted to $55,000 "for the purpose of establishing and building on said land, a free hospital to be non-sectarian . . . said hospital is to be called Hurley's Hospital."[3]

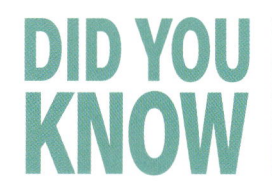

DID YOU KNOW | . . . the cost of a private room at Hurley Hospital in 1908 was $15 to $25 a week, ward beds cost $7 per week, and operating room charges ranged from $3 to $5.

By the time of his death in April 1905, Hurley, the versatile entrepreneur with a stock portfolio of mining, copper, and bank stocks, had become one of the most influential men in the area—the founder and director of the Union Trust and Savings Bank and the Flint Light & Power Company, a major stockholder in the W. A. Patterson Carriage Factory, and, ironically, the owner of the Sherman Hotel, the place where he had started his career.

This history began with the presentation of the James J. Hurley bequest, July 18, 1905, by Frances O'Hare, executrix of the will of Mr. Hurley to the Common Council of Flint;[4] the council accepted Mr. Hurley's gift. During that meeting, Mayor D. D. Aitken also made the first appointments to the Hurley Hospital Board of Managers. They were George L. Walker, W. E. Martin, E. D. Black, J. Dallas Dort, and C. A. Lippincott.[5]

The Wolverine Citizen newspaper, December 9, 1908 – "New Hurley Hospital Formally Opened . . ."

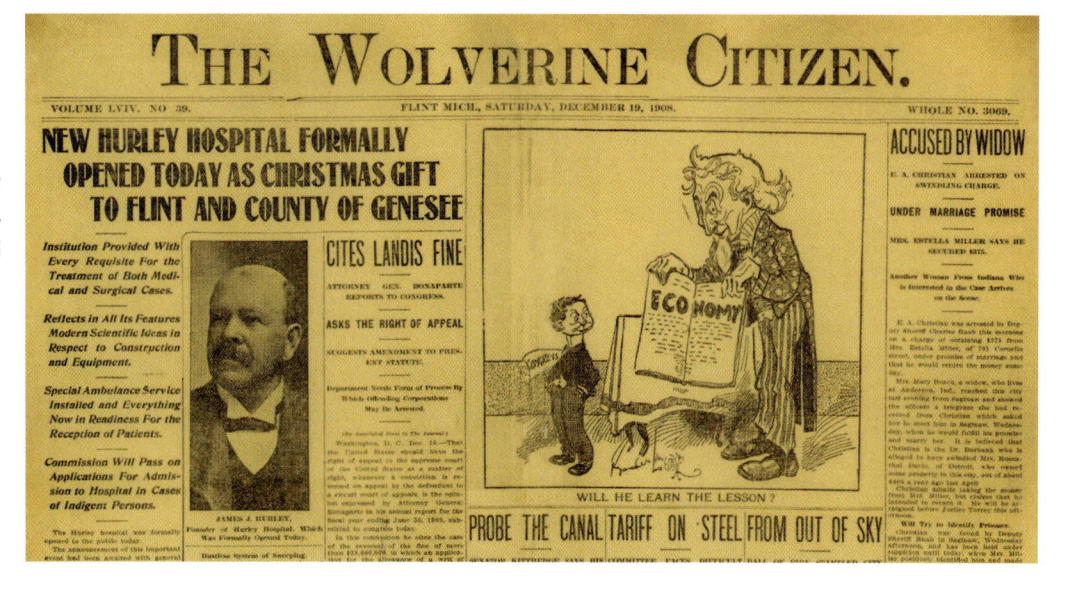

The board first met on September 23, 1905, to elect officers, formulate bylaws, procure a suitable record book for recording the proceedings of the board, take various steps to receive Hurley's bequest, and begin to establish the city's first hospital. Construction began on October 24, 1907, on the highest point in the city. The original building was of colonial design, with a two-story administration building and three ground-level wings, to the north, south, and west of the main building.

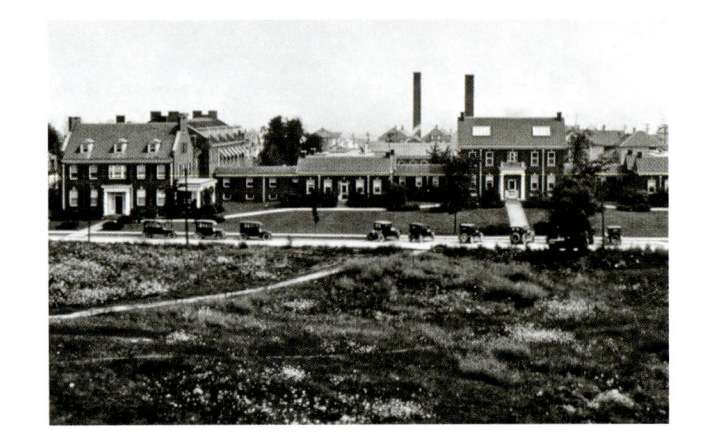

Hurley Hospital officially opened on December 19, 1908, with 40 beds, six bassinets, and a staff of eight nurses. The northern wing featured the women's ward, with a solarium, seven private rooms, and the nursery. Probationary nurses and other employees were housed in the western wing. The kitchens, dining rooms, laundry, storage, and boiler room were located in the basement. In May 1909, Hurley Hospital Training School of Nurses began a diploma program. Over the next 87 and a half years, more than 3,800 registered nurses graduated from Hurley's program.

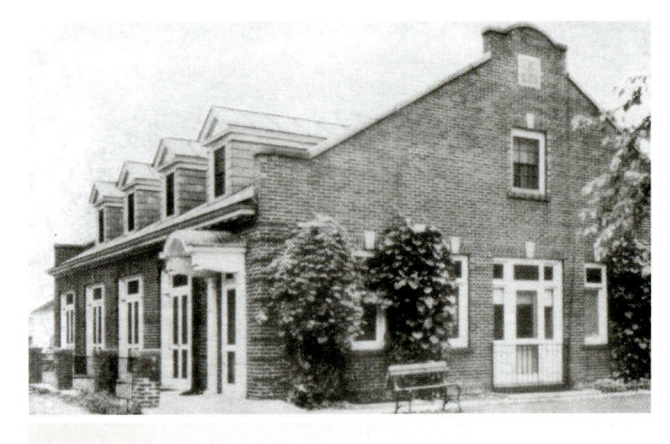

The First Ten Years

Hurley Hospital opened as Flint's first modern health care institution. This new type of hospital was centrally located and capable of handling patients with

Original Hurley Hospital circa 1908

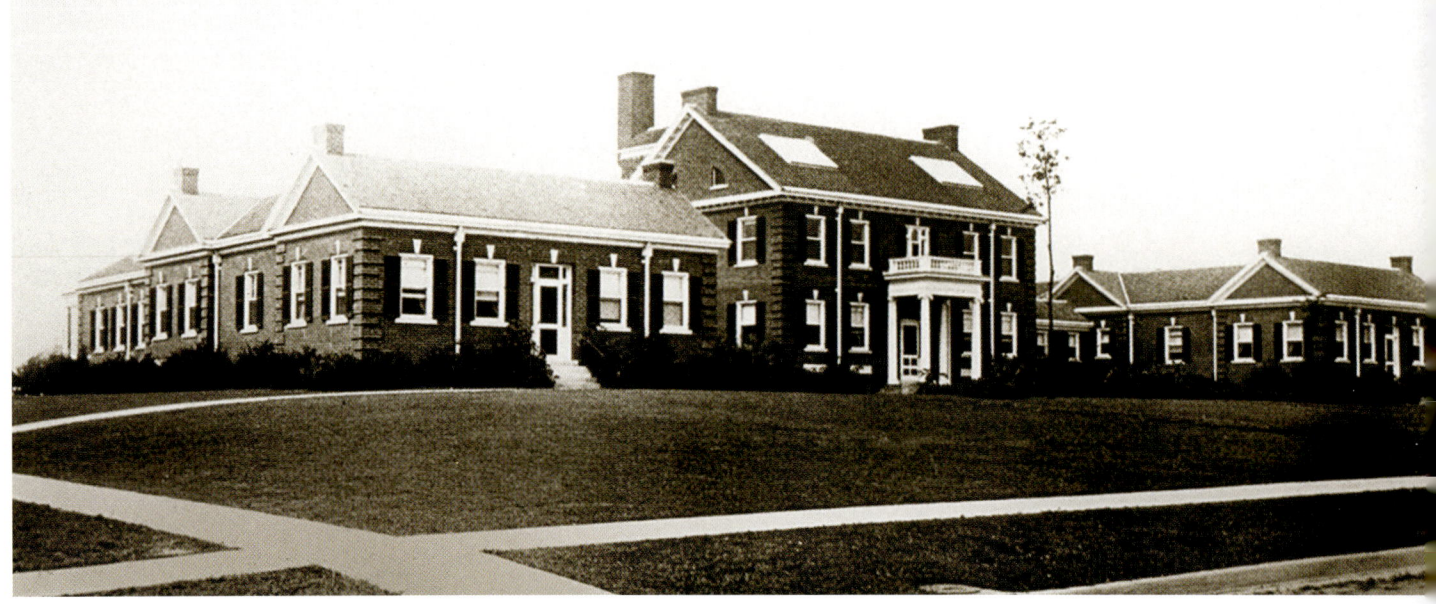

12 • HURLEY MEDICAL CENTER

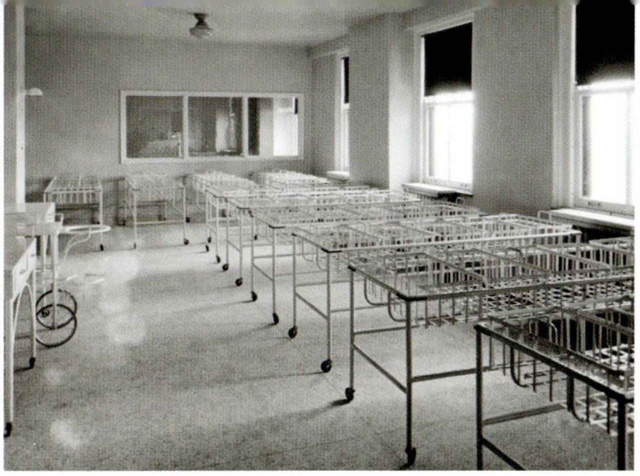

Original baby isolettes

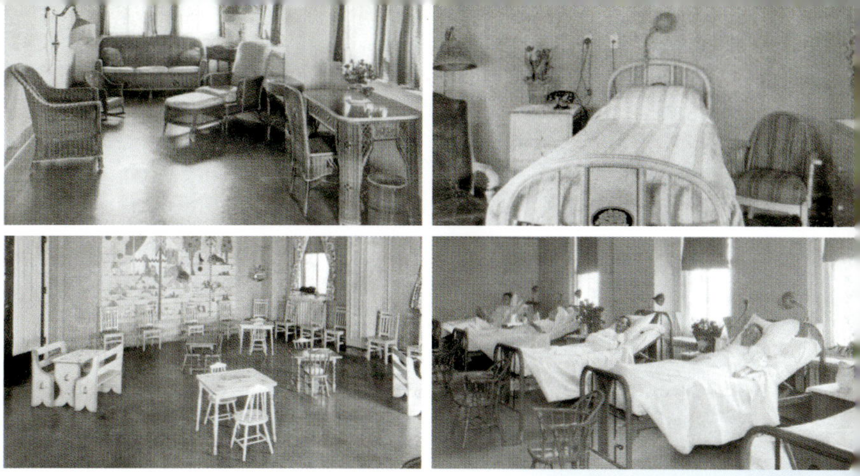

Original interior; patient ward and children's ward

influenza, pneumonia, diphtheria, measles, meningitis, and tuberculosis, all major illnesses of the time. Along with common ailments, such as goiters and rickets, nutrition and metabolism were yet to be fully understood. Prior to this, doctors made house calls or treated small groups of patients in remodeled homes that also served as the doctor's residence; the doctor's wife was both nurse and cook.[6]

Within the first 10 years, Hurley Hospital was under construction again, this time to create a larger campus that offered more services to accommodate Flint's expanding auto industry. In 1911, a second story was built over the western wing to provide seven private rooms and two small, five-patient wards. The architect connected this addition to the second floor of the main building, where three operating rooms and surgical facilities were housed. In October 1912, the first nurses' home was completed to house 21 nurses.

In 1915, additional construction took place along Patrick Street at the back of the hospital grounds. This complex included a power plant, a laundry, and an 18-bed, one-and-a-half-story Isolation Unit, which was a gift from General Motors co-founder Charles Stewart Mott. In 1916, Carl Chapell, MD, who specialized in radiology, radium therapy, and X-rays, started the Radiology Department. A small detention hospital, built by the city in 1910 to take care of contagious diseases, was abandoned and sold in 1916 when a new isolation cottage opened. Between the opening in 1908 and 1919, the hospital had expanded its capacity from 40 beds to 125 beds.

The Second Decade – Expansion and Reputation

During this time, the city of Flint was experiencing rapid growth that resulted in overcrowding conditions at many public institutions, including Hurley Hospital. Priorities for the common council (city council) were stretched thin. Even though the hospital's board worked heroically to meet each situation, followed by the communication of their needs, they had to work hard for support.

Enter local factory worker Merliss Brown, who was first appointed to the board of managers on May 1, 1920, as a direct result of his efforts to expand the hospital. He became deeply interested in Flint's health needs during the 1918 influenza pandemic when, as he recalls, "people were dying like flies for a lack of sufficient hospital facilities." He

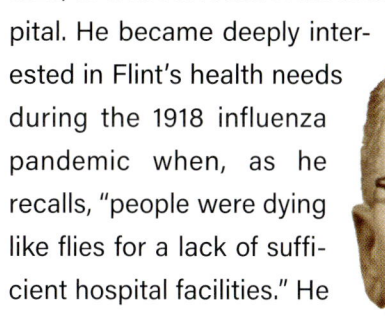

Merliss Brown

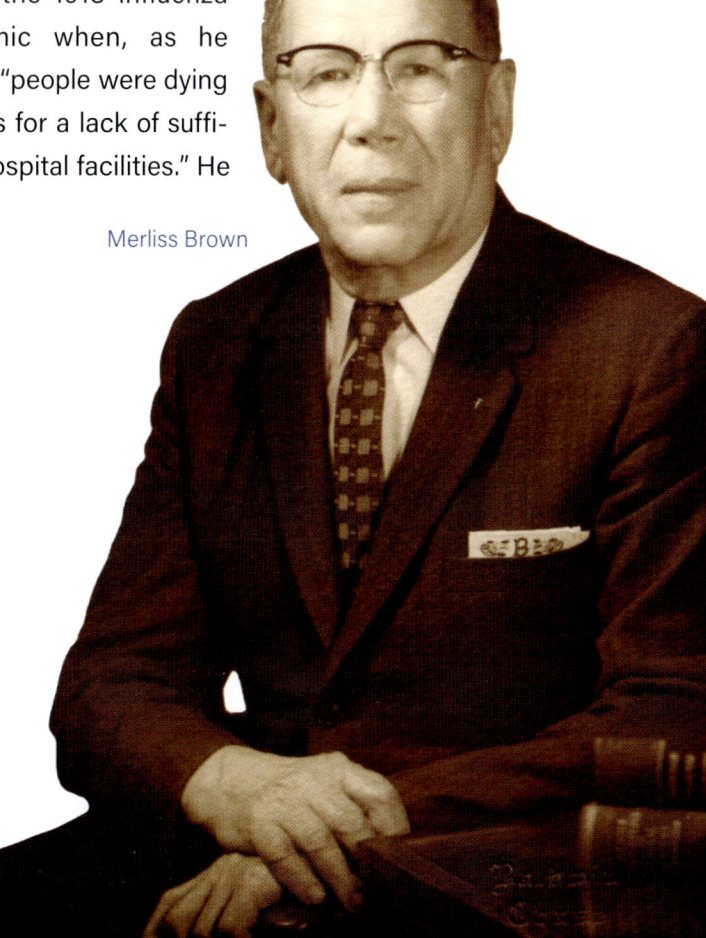

The Foundation of Hospital Care

The American Medical Association (founded 1847) and the American College of Surgeons (established 1913) set standards that included education and practice and created a structure from a system of hospitals, with early roots from a network of marine hospitals. Medical practices were greatly influenced by lessons learned on the battlefield of World War I, with blood transfusions and X-rays. Radium treatments and radiation therapy were the first methods to be used to treat cancer. Aseptic and antiseptic techniques made surgery safer and controlled infection. Best practices and new medical techniques continued to shape an emerging medical field, along with technological advancements, such as anesthesia and X-rays. A new field of study, bacteriology, made laboratories a key part of health.[7]

approached fellow workers at the Buick Motor Division to rally support. He pleaded with the city council without success, until E. W. Atwood promised cooperation if he were to be elected mayor. Brown dived into politics and Atwood was elected mayor of Flint in 1920. Atwood named Brown to the hospital's board, and a bond was submitted to the voters. Brown put his effort behind the campaign, and the $1.5 million bond passed. The hospital would be enlarged to 10 floors, and a nurses' home would be added. Brown received permanent recognition with the construction of the Merliss Brown Auditorium.[8] The original Hurley building was razed, and the total patient capacity was increased to 432 beds when it opened on April 20, 1928.

Along with the physical building expansion, Hurley's educational programs grew. The first intern joined Hurley's staff in 1919; one year later, other interns joined.

The new nurses' home was a catalyst of Hurley becoming a center of medical education. In February 1924, construction began on a 150-person, five-story nurses' home at the corner of Patrick Street and Sixth Avenue. Its completion in 1926 allowed the original nurses' quarters to be used solely for interns.

The following quote is from an archived letter in a past intern's personnel file, dated February 19, 1927: "At the present time, Hurley Hospital has about two hundred twenty-five beds, but is built on the cottage plan. Just a few days ago ground was broken here for the erection of a ten-story hospital building, upon which will be spent one million dollars without equipment. This is to be ready for occupancy January 1st, 1928. The capacity will then be some over three hundred beds. This building is to be especially equipped, and is supposed to be the last work in hospital construction for a community like Flint."

Hurley Hospital Board of Managers, 1922

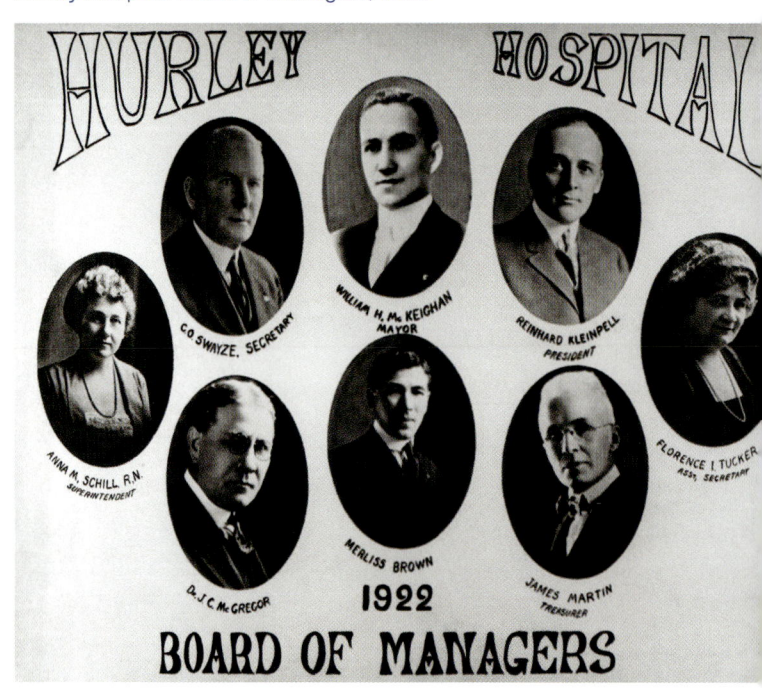

Hurley Hospital as described in the *Hurley Tower* publication, 1928

"On the highest point of Flint stands its tallest building—Hurley Hospital—which can be sighted from any direction for miles around. As one approaches from any of the distant points, it can be seen as a sentinel, guarding all who are under a square block, which will be made into a park set with arrays of flowers and shrubs thus arranging a wonderful setting for allowing every room its full share of God's glorious light and sunshine—healer of all ills. Its architecture is a symbol of powerful simplicity, representing an institution founded on the Rock of Progress, made possible by the people of Flint who well appreciate the result of their own efforts. The front entrance of the hospital, one of the most picturesque revelations of architecture, is indeed an inspiration. Portals of sublime beauty open the way to an institution visited by hundreds of men, women, and children daily. Stepping inside, what a spectacle greets the eye!—Colossal, marble pillars, cathedral-like structure, chandeliers of palatine beauty, type of art never before carried out in a like institution. Archways on either side form an aisle which leads to the main waiting room, and just above the entrance to the rotunda is a beautiful bronze clock, a special type of workmanship set in a colorful background."[9]

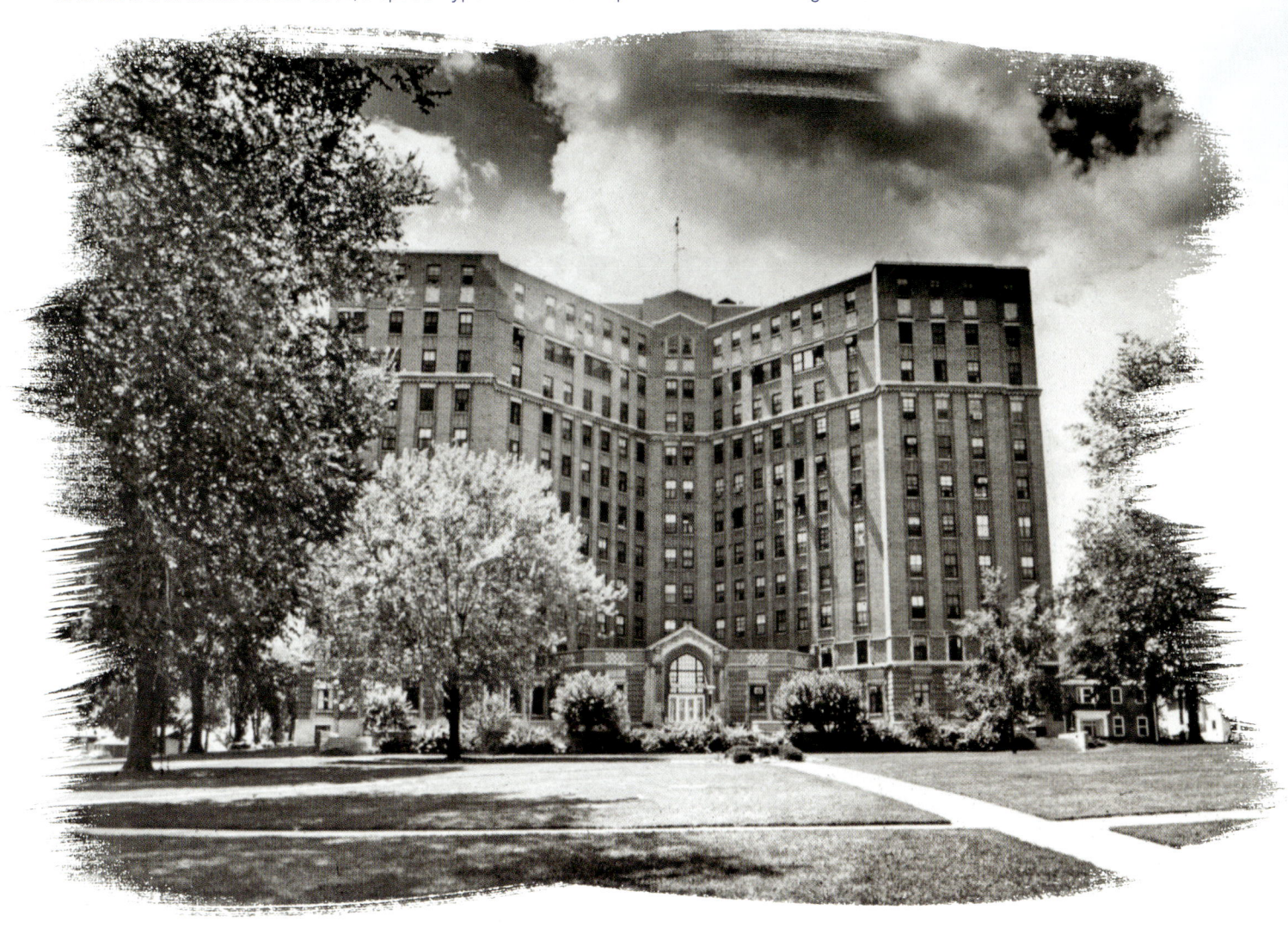

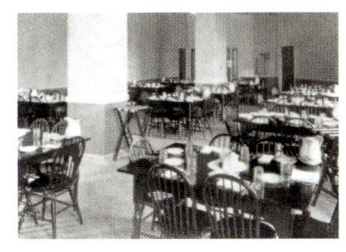

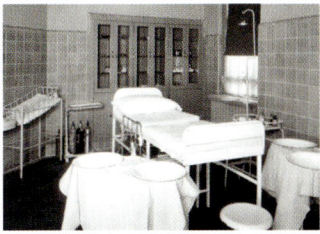

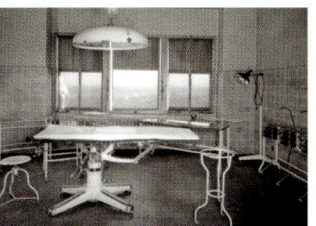

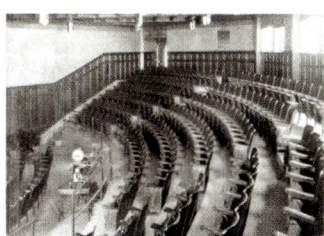

CHAPTER ONE A LANDMARK INSTITUTION

Hurley Hospital – Fifty Years of Stability and Growth, 1930s–1970s

During the 1930s, the federal government's role in health care expanded as the Great Depression negatively impacted public health. A national health survey showed the great need for the coordination of services and equal concern over how to pay for medical care, research, and education. Medical insurance was limited at that time and only available through lodges, religious institutions, and other organizations, until Blue Cross organized hospitalization insurance in 1933.

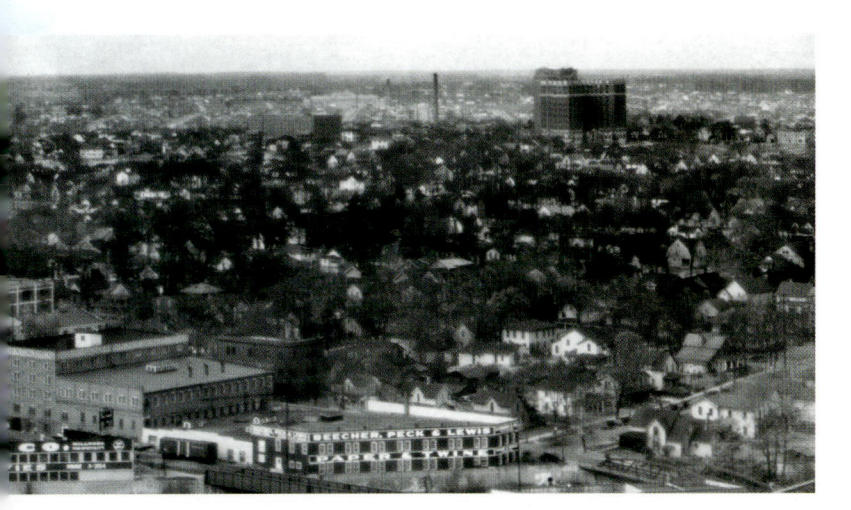

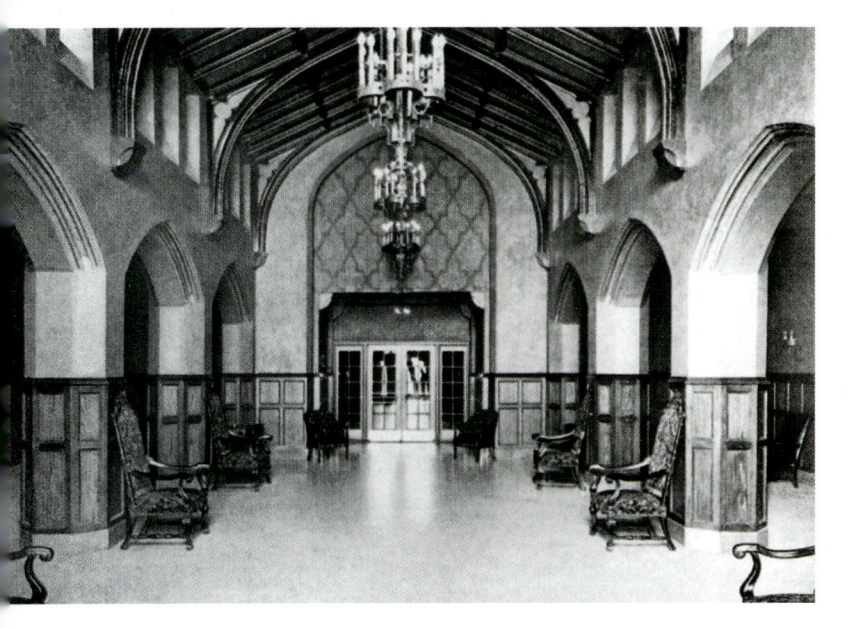

DID YOU KNOW | . . . the slogan adopted for Hurley Hospital's 50th anniversary was "The Golden Dream – Yesterday's Heritage, Today's Humility and Tomorrow's Hope."

The 1930s and 1940s were a time of unprecedented changes in public health policy, as well as in medical advances and innovations as a result of World War II. The war hastened many medical advances; for the first time ever, battlefield wounds did not necessarily result in infection, amputation, or a soldier's death. "The value of immunizations, sanitation and coordinated clinical research was demonstrated. Anti-malarial drugs were developed and large-scale production of penicillin was achieved. More emphasis was put on physical rehabilitation. The need for beds for injured military, forced earlier post-surgery ambulation, which was found to be not only safe, but beneficial."[10]

Hurley Hospital administrators adapted to the community's needs, with the first outpatient clinics opening in the 1930s. In 1941, a basement and a one-story addition were built on the southern side of the main hospital building to correspond in size and shape of

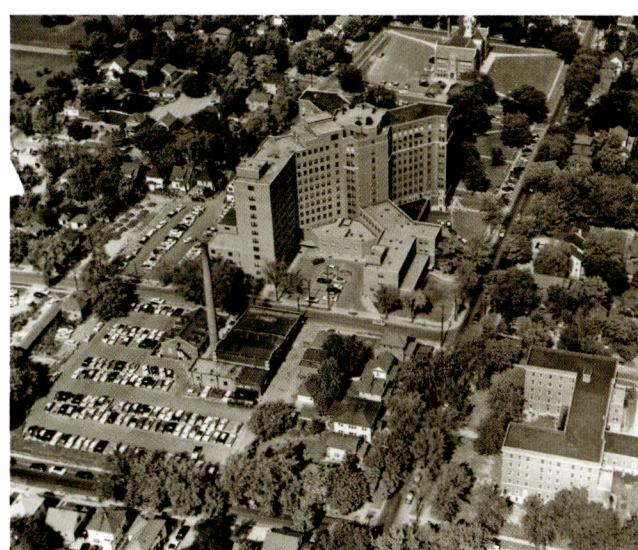

1954

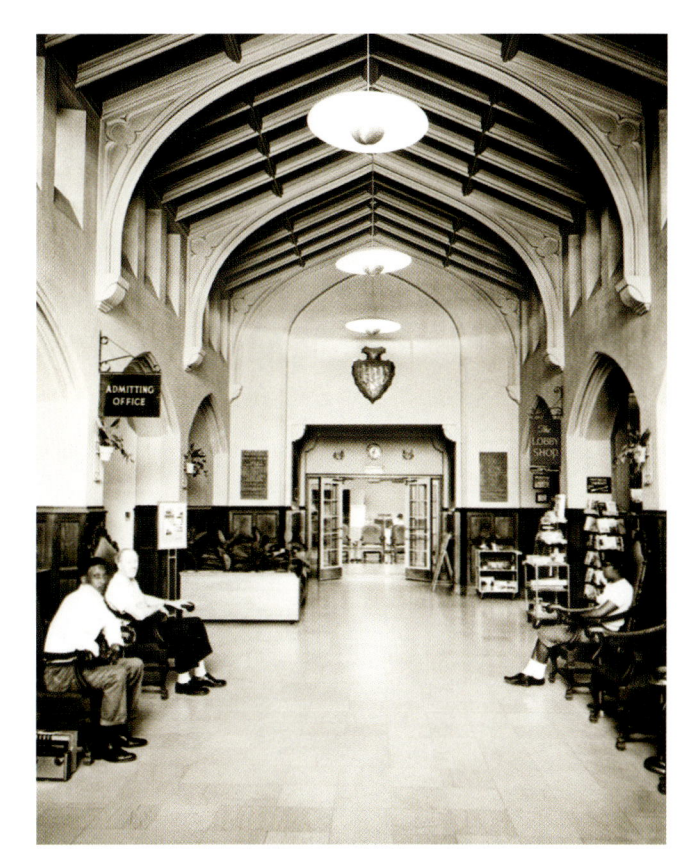

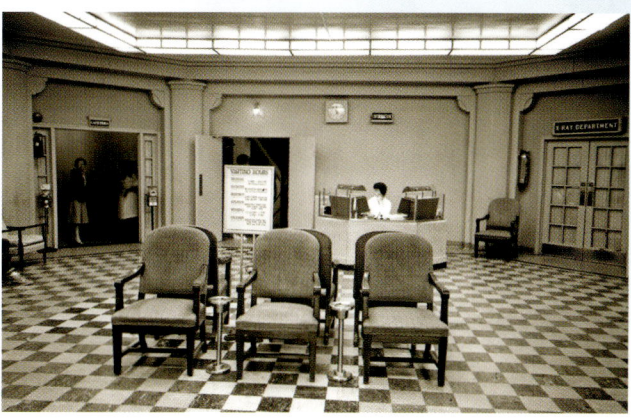

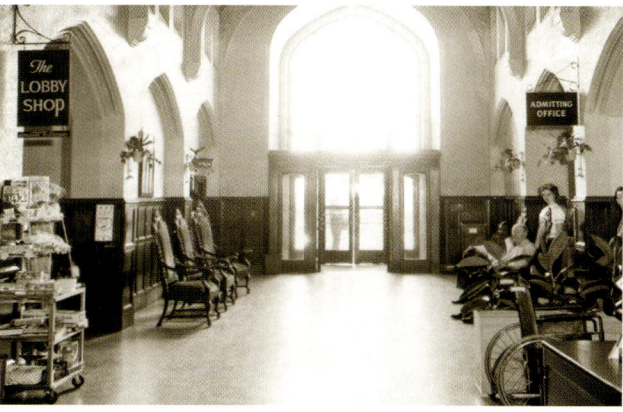

The Hurley Hospital lobby was refurbished in January 1940 through a Work Projects Administration (WPA) government grant. These photos, taken in the 1950s, show the entrance lobby and rotunda walls that were painted a lighter color and given a stone-like finish. The plaster ceiling beams were given a wood effect. The main panel over the passage was adorned with a Flint crest with interlocking *H*s, and floor lamp lighting was changed to wall-mounted lighting.

the auditorium on the northern side. The dining room was enlarged, and the medical library and doctors' conference room were moved. A larger laundry was built in 1942, and in 1943, the 11th floor was added to accommodate another 50 patients.

Additional educational programs were added in the late 1940s and early 1950s with the School of Radiologic Technology, the School of Anesthesia for nurse anesthetists, and a School of Medical Technology. In 1954, a new ED—located on the ground level facing Patrick Street at the rear of the hospital—opened. In 1956, the City of Flint finance committee considered capital improvement funding for the hospital; the measure was passed by voters in July with 2,000 more votes than needed. This expansion allowed for the completion of the 11-story northwestern ("C") wing, having oxygen piped in, adding 135 more beds, replacing old wiring and plumbing, and renovating the old section of the hospital, which was finalized in 1959. This was during a time of great medical advances, such as the first kidney transplant, the first practical pacemaker, open-heart surgery, and the introduction of the Salk polio vaccine. In the late 1950s, Hurley Hospital became one of the first hospitals in the nation to begin an alcoholism therapy program and opened a unit to specifically treat alcoholic patients.[11]

In 1960, Hurley opened the service area's first Intensive Care Unit. In 1964, the service area's first Cobalt Therapy Unit to treat cancer was established from a donation by the Florence Whiting Dalton Foundation. In 1966, a Hemodialysis Unit was opened, followed by a specialized Coronary Care Unit in 1968. Measles and rubella immunizations were widely introduced in the 1960s. Cardiac care took center stage with the dramatic leaps of the development of the artificial heart, the first successful heart transplant, and the first coronary bypass. The passage of the Medicare and Medicaid acts made health care more available to seniors and low-income families.

By 1970, to continue adapting to medical innovation, Hurley Hospital administrators realized that another major renovation would be needed. In 1972, a group of service-area pediatricians formed and opened an after-hours Pediatric Center on-site, which offered non-emergency care on evenings and weekends—the first center of its kind in the nation. Also in 1972, Hurley opened the service area's first and only Burn Unit. In 1973, after a long history of helping premature infants, Hurley opened a Neonatal Intensive Care Unit, followed by a Pediatric Intensive Care Unit in 1974.

Top: Hurley Hospital early construction phases

Right: The 1957 patient care team—representing 27 staff persons—that was necessary during a 24-hour, seven-day period in order for the patient to be fully recovered and discharged, according to the *Hurley News*. The patient is sitting in the chair. First row, left to right: resident, registered nurse, and intern. Second row: student nurse, laboratory technician, practical nurse, and x-ray technician. Third row: ward helper, nurse aide, ward clerk, electroencephalogram (EEG) technician, and orderly. Fourth row: pharmacist, dietician, and physical therapist. Fifth row: social service worker, housemaid, admitting clerk, medical records librarian, account clerk, buyer, and cook. Sixth row: elevator operator, switchboard operator, laundress, stock clerk, and building maintainer.

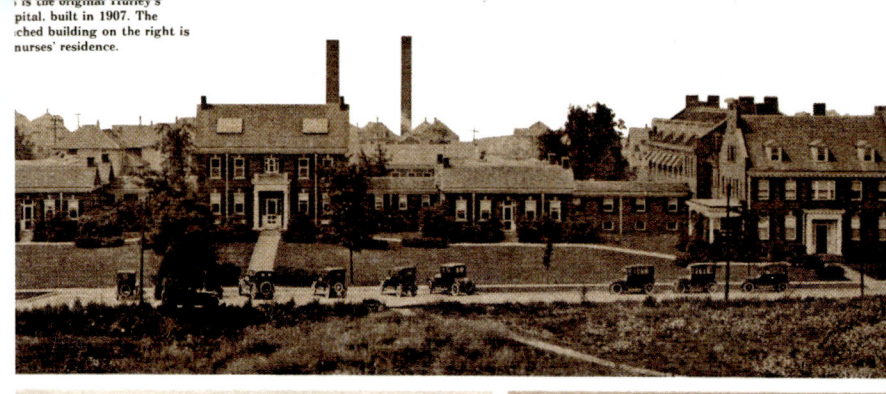

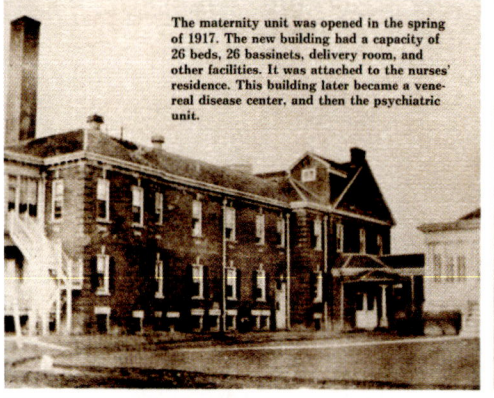

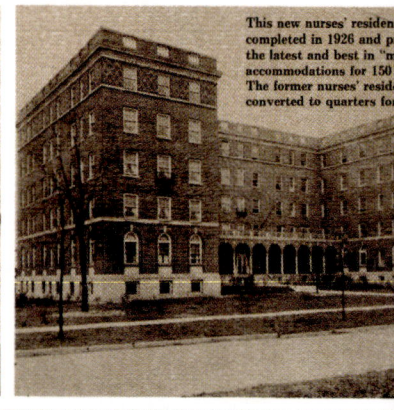

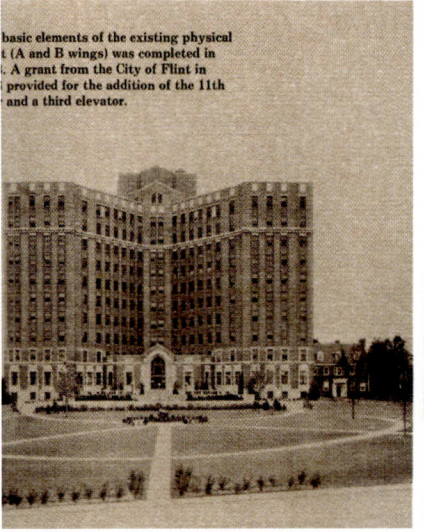

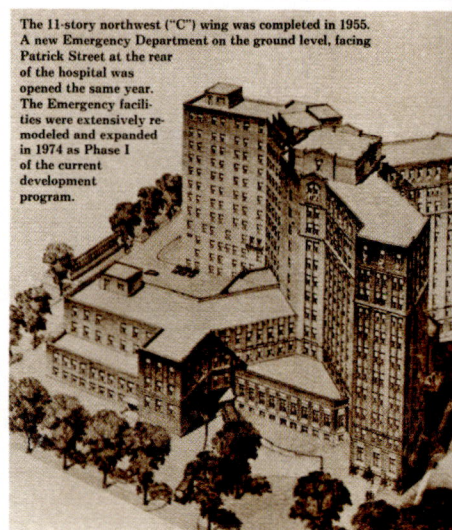

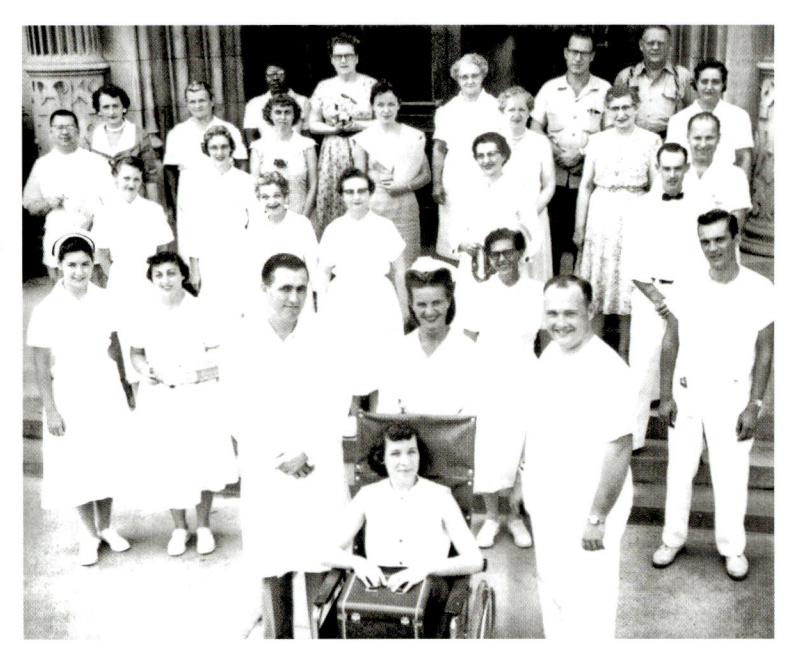

18 • HURLEY MEDICAL CENTER

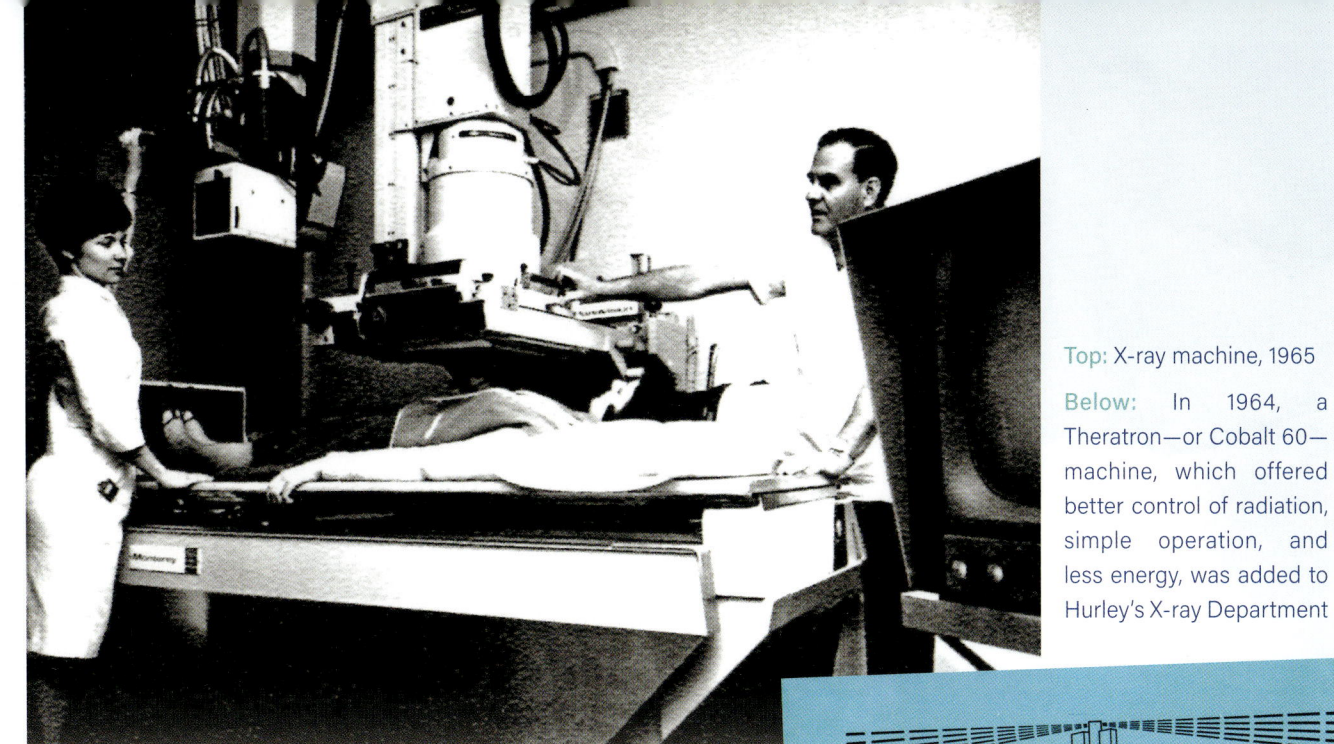

Top: X-ray machine, 1965

Below: In 1964, a Theratron—or Cobalt 60—machine, which offered better control of radiation, simple operation, and less energy, was added to Hurley's X-ray Department

On January 1, 1975, Hurley Hospital officially changed its name to Hurley Medical Center. According to hospital administrators, the new name reflected the wide scope of services being offered.[12]

The year 1976 was a busy one, with the opening of the Neuroscience Unit, the Hemodialysis Satellite Location, and the Family Crisis Center, followed by

Hurley Hospital's name was changed to Hurley Medical Center on January 1, 1975.

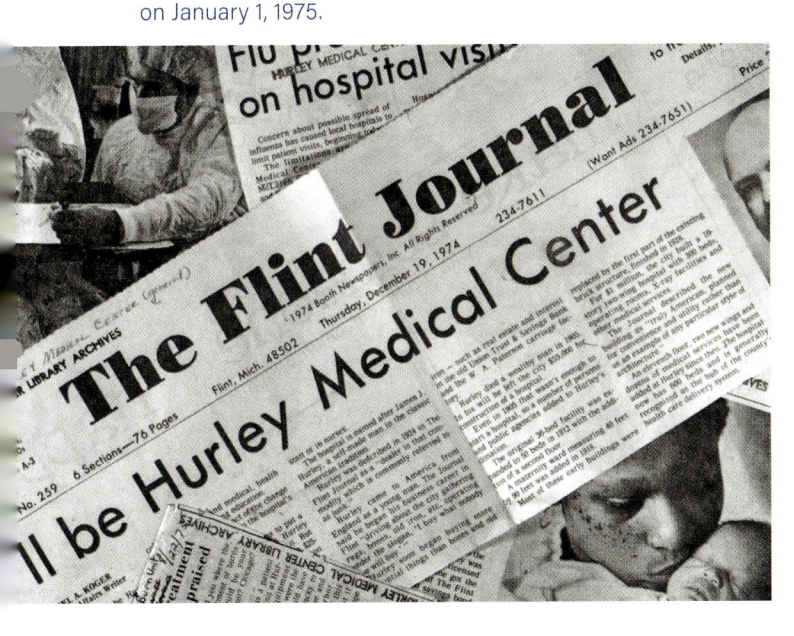

HURLEY TOWER
"The Tower on the Hill" Which Sheds Its Beacon Light to All Who Seek It

Our New Cobalt Unit - May It Benefit Many

the December 5 dedication of the $13 million northern building addition, which would encompass 15 operating suites, 14 emergency treatment rooms, two trauma treatment rooms, an expanded outpatient clinic, a larger medical library, an expansion to the laboratory, physical medicine space, and a modern Obstetrics Unit.

The culmination of a three-year development and fundraising campaign called "The New Face of Hurley"

CHAPTER ONE A LANDMARK INSTITUTION • 19

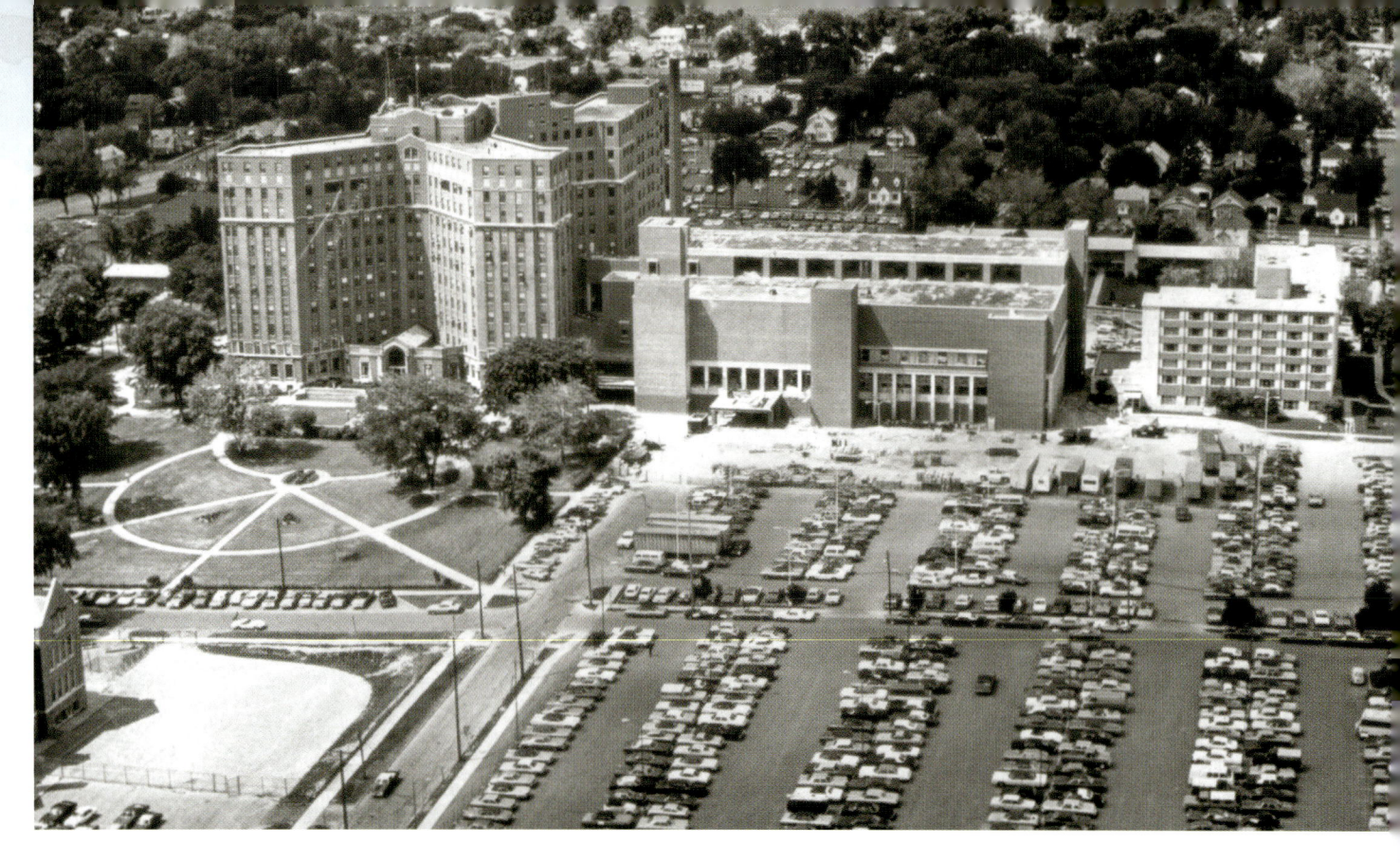

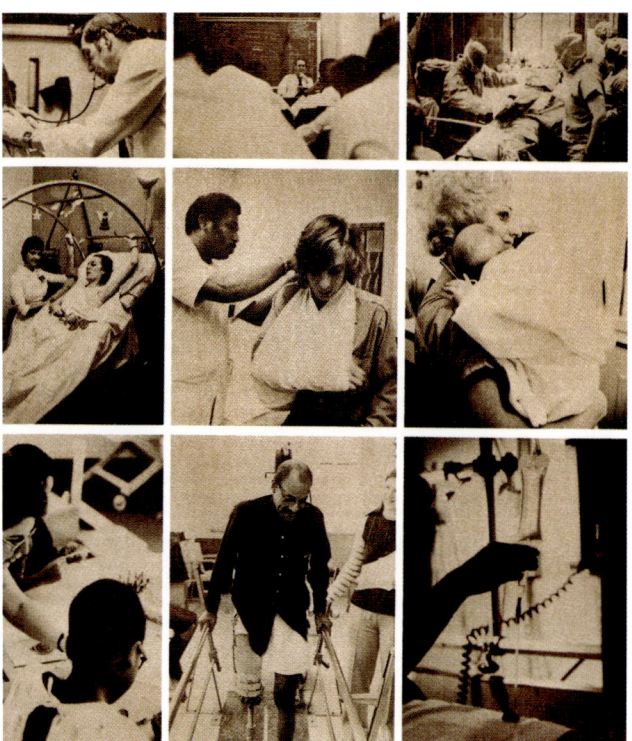

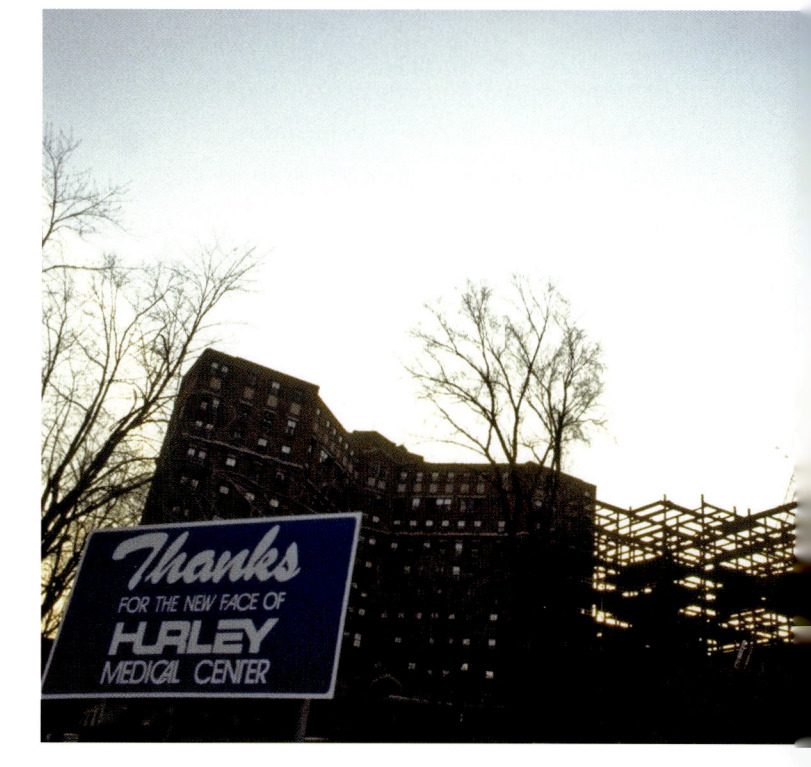

New Face of Hurley campaign and construction, 1977

resulted in the new East Tower building dedication on November 4, 1979. A community campaign led by 70 community volunteers resulted in gifts from community residents and grant funds accounting for $6.7 million of the $21.3 million cost of the new building. Hurley employees gave more than $300,000 toward the building. The East Tower was purposefully designed with the Intensive Care and Coronary Care Units on the same connecting floor as the operating rooms in the North Tower.

20 • HURLEY MEDICAL CENTER

Health Care and the Auto Industry

Located 70 miles north of Detroit, the city of Flint was at one time the national epicenter of automotive forethought and production. Flint, the birthplace of General Motors (GM) in 1908, the home to the auto workers' union (UAW), and the location of the famous Sit-Down Strike of 1936–37, helped to define the modern American auto industry. By 1954, metropolitan Flint—with approximately 80,000 GM workers on the payroll—was home to the largest agglomeration of GM factories and employees anywhere in the world.

In the late 1970s, General Motors' 80,000 workers began shrinking in numbers until by 2010, less than 8,000 workers remained in Flint—approximately 10 percent of what once defined the community's manufacturing and economic base.[13] The economic downturns of the 1970s and 1980s marked the end of the postwar boom and the onset of a new era of mass deindustrialization.

Flint's fortunes being tied to the automotive industry highlight the importance of renewal and reinvention.

Major employers, like Hurley, must be resilient during downturns and thrive during good times. HMC employees, from administrators to those who serve at the bedside, are proud of their work home and consider themselves to be part of Flint's renaissance. They believe in the education, the community outreach, and the future vitality and growth of Flint.

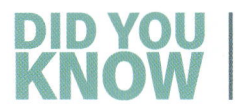

DID YOU KNOW | ... Hurley Hospital became financially independent after a final allocation of $50,000 from the City of Flint in 1973.

NOTES

1. Hurley Foundation, *Inside Report* (Winter 1988), p. 6.
2. Edwin Wood, *History of Genesee County, Michigan: Her People, Industries and Institutions* (Indianapolis: Federal Publishing Company, 1916), p. 804.
3. Hurley Will, File 599, State of Michigan, County of Genesee, May 20, 1905.
4. James J. Hurley bequest, July 18, 1905, by Frances O'Hare, executrix.
5. Wood, *History of Genesee County, Michigan*, p. 802.
6. Hurley Foundation, *Inside Report* (Winter 1988), p. 7.
7. Ibid.
8. *Hurley Tower* Vol. 22, no. 7 (August 1969), p. 7–8.
9. T. Pleger, *Hurley Tower*, 1928. Note: T. Pleger was a student in the Nursing Class of 1929.
10. Hurley Foundation, *Inside Report* (Winter 1988), p. 9.
11. Ibid., p. 4.
12. Ibid., p. 4.
13. Greater Flint Health Coalition, Community Health Needs Assessment report, 2019, p. 5.

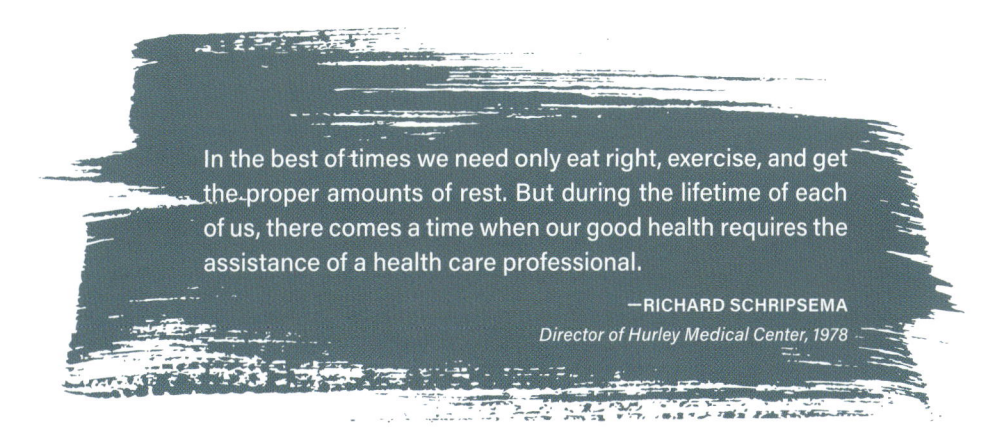

> In the best of times we need only eat right, exercise, and get the proper amounts of rest. But during the lifetime of each of us, there comes a time when our good health requires the assistance of a health care professional.
>
> —RICHARD SCHRIPSEMA
> *Director of Hurley Medical Center, 1978*

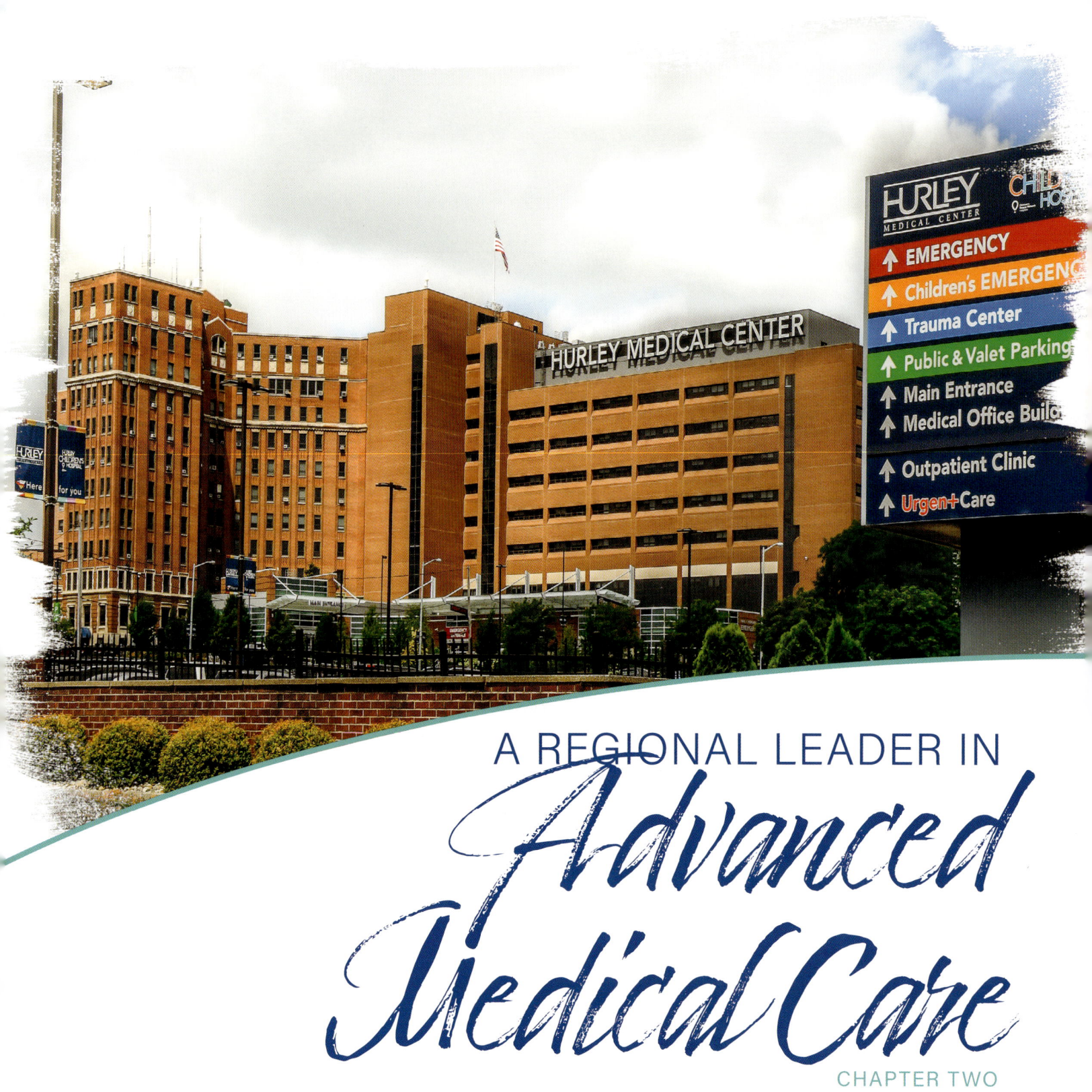

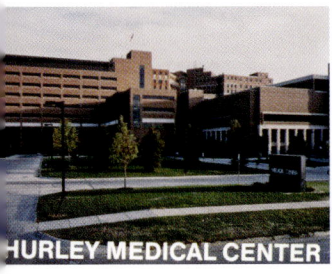

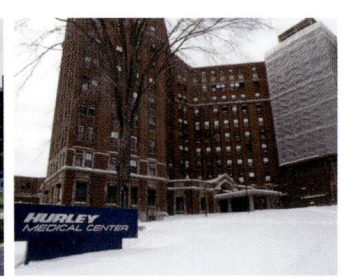

A REGIONAL LEADER IN
Advanced Medical Care
CHAPTER TWO

HMC – Advancing Medical Care

The East Tower opening in 1979 had a profound effect on HMC's capability to advance subspecialties, such as neonatal intensive care and expanded coronary care. It also allowed for an expansion of adult intensive care on the fourth-floor Intensive Care Unit (ICU), Coronary Care Unit (CCU), and Step-Down Units, the sixth-floor

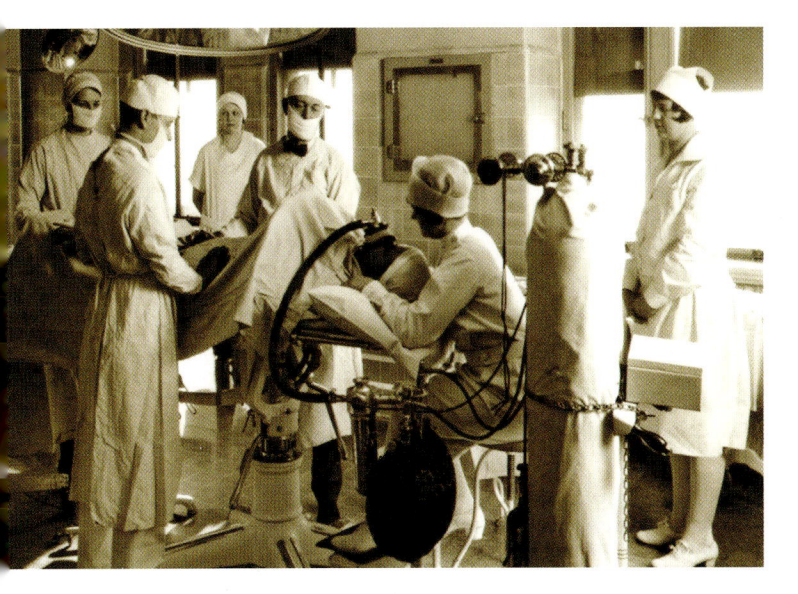

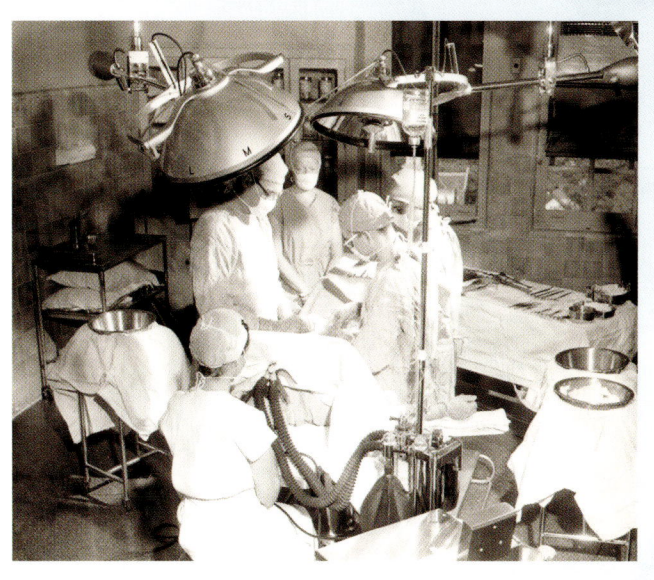

Top left: Circa 1945

Top right: Surgery

Right: Cardiac Care Unit, 1974

Gynecologic Surgical Unit, the seventh-floor Medical-Surgical Unit (with a Rheumatology Unit for patients with joint afflictions ranging from arthritis to lupus erythematous, bursitis, and gout), and the ninth-floor general medical-surgical recovery beds reserved for cancer patients needing specialized therapy and emotional support, along with an interdisciplinary team vital to the Oncology Unit. Alongside hospital construction, plans for a 750-car parking garage and a $2 million physicians' office building—with 110,000 square feet of space to house up to 30 physician offices—completed the new medical campus plan.

In March 1980, the Hurley cardiology team was the first in the service area to successfully use a new "intelligent" heart pacemaker that enabled improved functioning for eight to 12 years. The new device, implanted in a 78-year-old man with a severe heart disorder, generated a more natural heartbeat that provided better performance and an increase in technical and functional capabilities. Though pacemakers had been around since the 1950s, they limited cardiologists in regulating the heartbeat. As the cardiology service became more prominent for Hurley, the new fourth-floor CCU was equipped with similar technology as the ICU, along with telemetry that monitors heart activity.

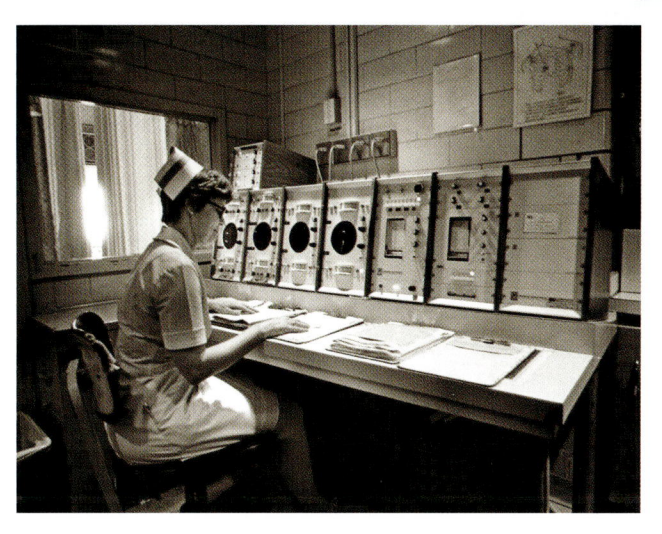

In January 1982, an expanded Renal Medicine Unit located on the fifth floor of the West Tower improved services to further the work of Hurley hemodialysis pioneers from 1966 and also secured HMC as the regional referral center for patients with kidney disease. New within the unit was the capability to purify water for dialysis, and dialyzers were now cleaned and reused for the same hemodialysis patient for

CHAPTER TWO A REGIONAL LEADER IN ADVANCED MEDICAL CARE

DID YOU KNOW

... the worldwide flu pandemic in 1918–1919 influenced the size of Hurley Hospital's design. The architectural plans for the new institution in 1911 were deemed inadequate. In 1928, the new Hurley Hospital opened a larger, two-winged structure featuring 10 stories; Hurley had grown into a 350-bed hospital.

up to seven treatments rather than using a new dialyzer for each session. Hurley also started providing service at a Hemodialysis Satellite Unit on Prospect Street and offered a unique home training unit in the Patrick Street apartments, where patients could learn how to dialyze at home using peritoneal dialysis. Almost 20 years later, HMC expanded their renal services into the community with a 2001 grand opening of the Hurley Northwest Kidney Center, a dialysis and educational center, with 14 state-of-the-art dialysis chairs.

At the time of the 80th anniversary in 1988, new procedures, such as joint replacements, organ transplants, electronic hearing aids, voice synthesizers, CT scans, ultrasound, and laser surgery, were moving the medical field into the next century. This new frontier had no resemblance to the world of medicine in James Hurley's time less than 100 years before.

Revolutionary Orthopedic Surgery First Performed in Michigan at Hurley, 1987

The new orthopedic method, the Ilizarov procedure, offered new treatment hope for patients with limb discrepancies, deformities, bone infections, and severe bone and soft tissue loss. Vladimir Schwartsman, MD, was the first physician to perform this procedure in 1987. Two other Flint Township orthopedic surgeons also learned this technique using a modular system of rings, rods, and wires to create tension stress to hold the bone's position while capitalizing on the bone's ability to regenerate itself without a cast. Gerald Holmes of Flint was one of the first Hurley patients to undergo this procedure. Injured in a work accident in 1979, Holmes was facing his 13th surgery and possible amputation before being referred to Dr. Schwartsman.

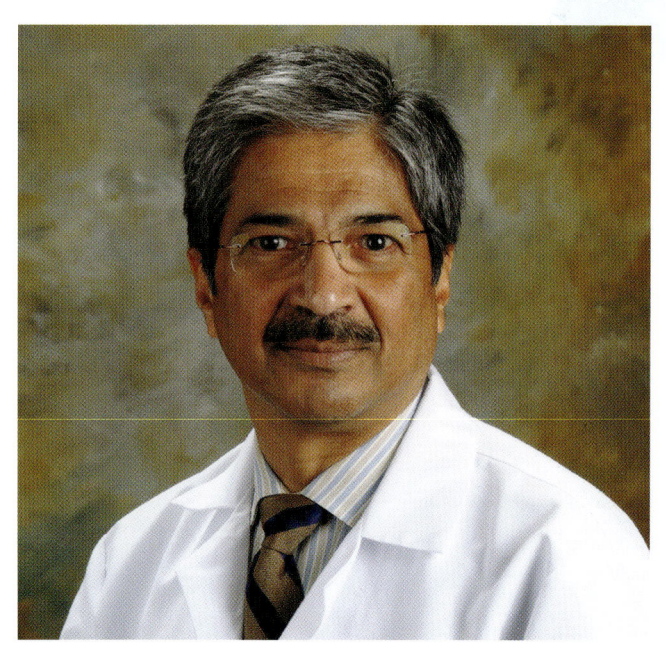

M. Varkey Thomas, MD, pulmonary and critical care medicine and sleep medicine specialist. As a longtime leader and director of Hurley's pulmonology and critical care, Dr. Thomas's expertise in medical education was valued by many with his commitment to bedside clinical teaching. Dr. Thomas received a Pinnacle Award in 1997.

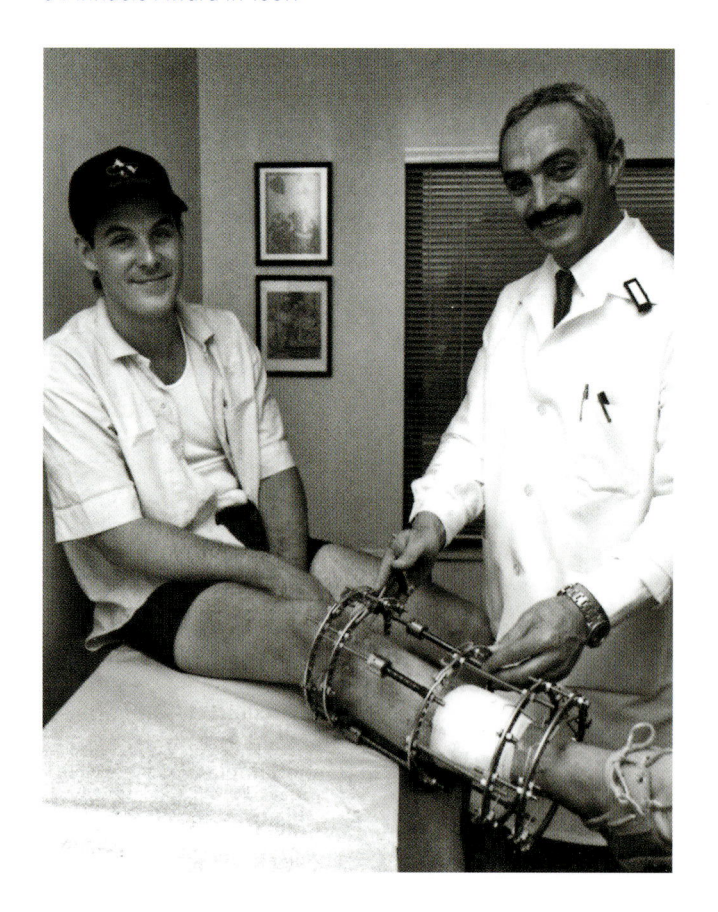

Today, as a Michigan safety net hospital, HMC is fully prepared to handle the complex health needs of the region for decades to come. The vitality of the organization is buoyed by many caring donors and the Hurley Foundation to ensure ongoing medical services, along with dedicated professionals, innovative technology, and advanced facilities.

Emergency Medicine

Emergency medicine (EM) began as a specialty in the 1960s, when Americans began to demand better emergency care. Until that time, emergency departments were staffed by a variety of physicians, mostly interns or residents from differing specialties who worked without supervision.

In 1961, a new concept called the "Alexandria Plan" changed conventional thinking toward using a group of full-time physicians who were focused solely on EM, providing care exclusively in an emergency room that was open 24 hours a day.[1] Dr. James Mills and Dr. John McDade, who founded the specialty of EM, were the first to utilize triage-type services from lessons learned during the Korean War.[2]

In 1965, when Medicare and Medicaid were instituted for those without medical insurance, the number of people with health care coverage in Flint rose exponentially, primarily due to insured auto workers and their families. Many turned to the Emergency Department (ED) for care when doctors' offices and clinics became overwhelmed.

Hurley's first high-tech ED was constructed in 1976 with 13 exam rooms, two cast rooms, an examination/triage area, and four observation beds in 7,025 square feet of space[3] designed to serve 38,000 patients per year.[4] It took almost a decade, until the late 1970s, before EM became a board-certified specialty within the American Board of Medical Specialties.[5] In March of 1980, a new technology known as the "Medical Control Center" for Genesee County was installed and allowed for on-the-scene communication between paramedics at an accident and doctors inside HMC's ED. Vital

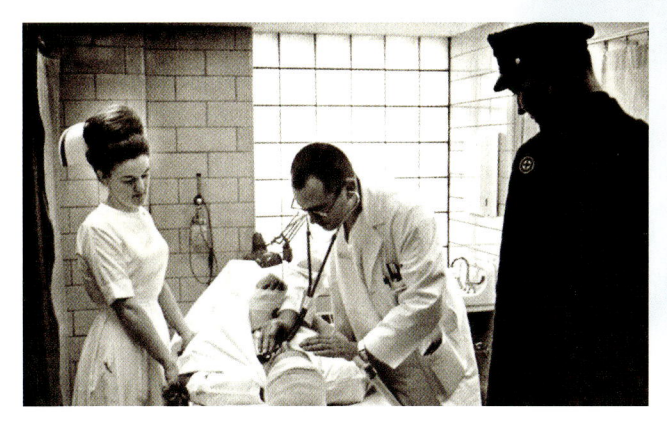

New Year's Eve in the emergency room, 1964

Below: ICU and recovery, February 1965

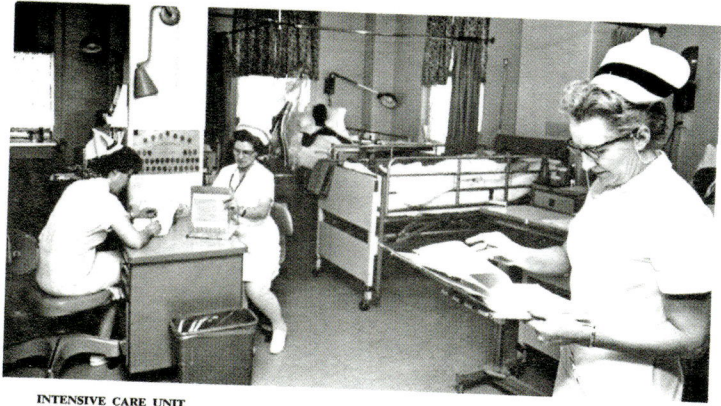

INTENSIVE CARE UNIT
Twenty-four patients can receive care here. This department has all supplies needed to give the finest care for the critically ill patient. The equipment in this department is the finest, newest, and available at all times for immediate usage. The only patients admitted here are the critically ill who require the best care available. The patient who is admitted to this area remains there for a very short time.

CRITICALLY ill patients who require the best possible care are placed in the Intensive Care Unit (above). Immediately following surgery, patients are placed in the Recovery Room (below).

RECOVERY ROOM
This area is located on 10th floor, located between the Laboratory and Surgery. This is where all surgical patients go, immediately following surgery. These patients are kept here until they have satisfactorily reacted from their anesthetic, under the watchful eye of special trained personnel, headed by a Registered Nurse. They are then returned to their room, where their immediate family can see them.

CHAPTER TWO A REGIONAL LEADER IN ADVANCED MEDICAL CARE • 25

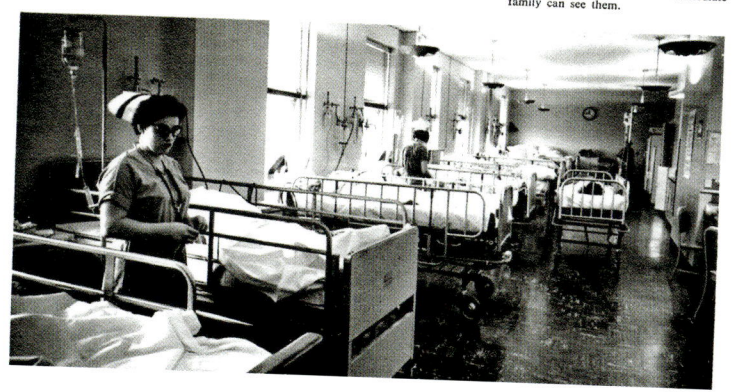

Right and below: First used in the 1970s, the new telemetry system allowed emergency responders to transmit crucial data from an accident scene directly to medical staff at the hospital, who would then prescribe field treatments.

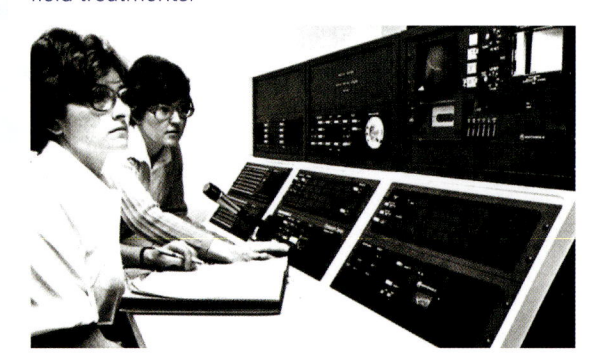

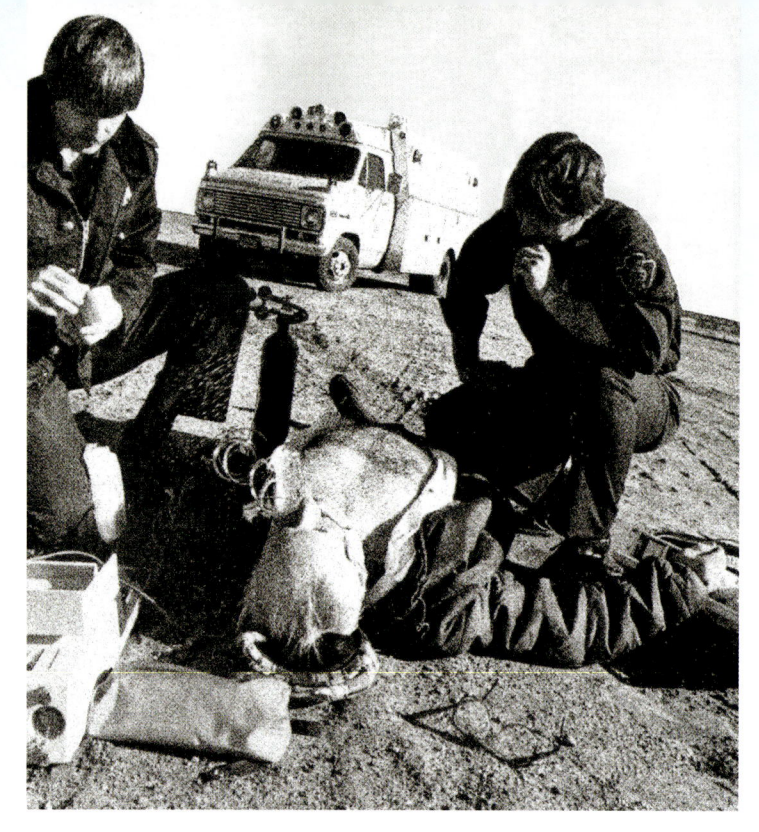

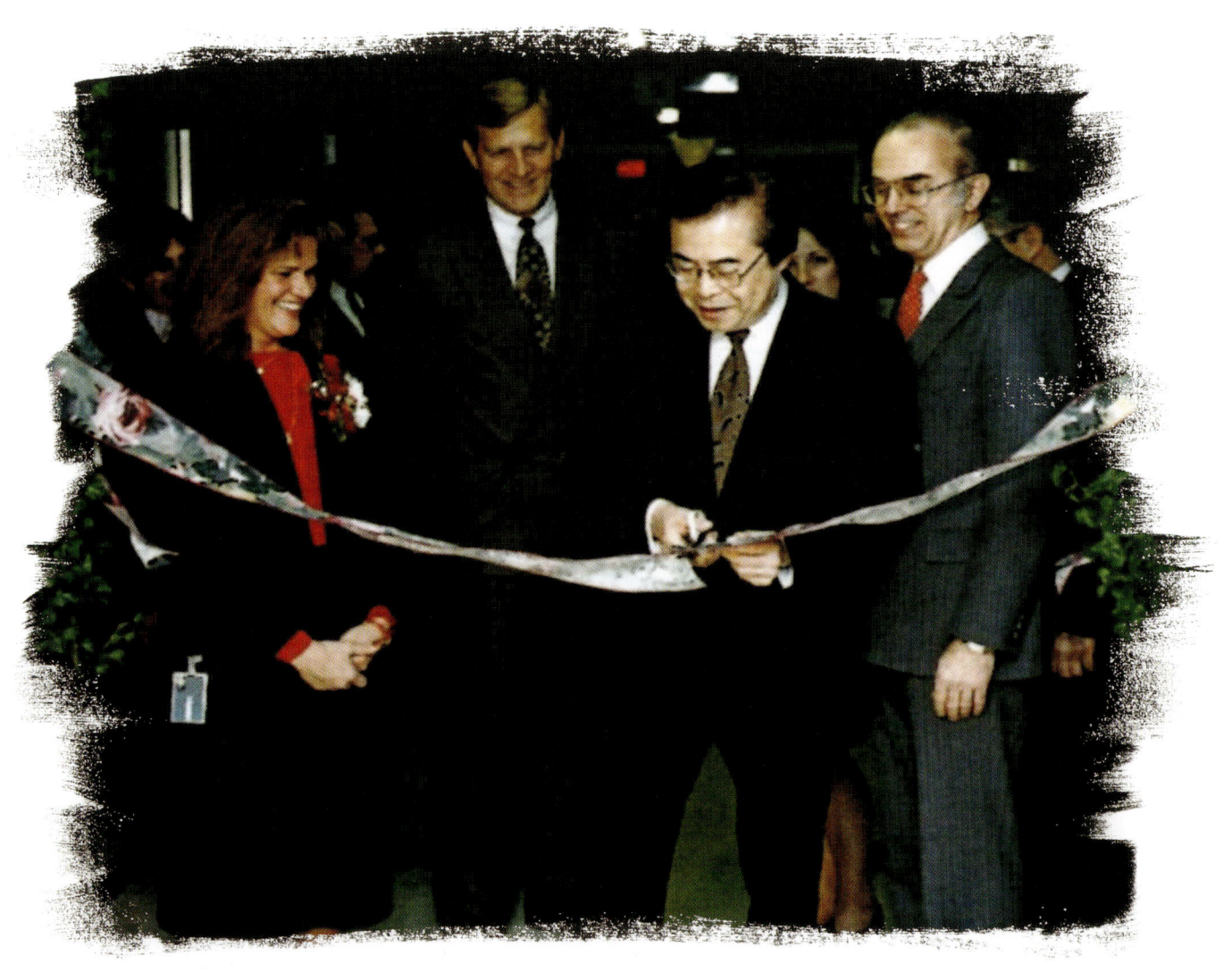

Rodolfo Uy Ham, MD, ribbon cutting for the new 23-bed ortho-surgery-neuro-trauma ICU in 1995. Shown here are Janet Seifferlein, nurse manager, Phillip Dutcher, president and CEO, and Stephen Burton, MD, orthopedic section chief.

information, such as an electrocardiogram (EEG), is transmitted from the victim at the scene to the hospital, allowing doctors at the hospital to assess a heart attack or a trauma patient's condition, or to prescribe field treatments and emergency medications to the off-site patient's emergency medical services (EMS) responder. With this technology, the voice traveled on one channel and heart readings on a separate channel, and they were permanently recorded for later diagnosis and treatment. HMC doctors and technicians could route all paramedic emergency calls into either their own emergency room or to other area hospitals, such as St. Joseph, Flint Osteopathic, and McLaren General.[6]

Trauma Medicine

By 1980, Hurley had all the clinical, technical, and physical capabilities to care for major traumas, including serious burns, head and spinal cord injuries, renal failure, and multiple injuries. Hurley also had the facilities and specialists for coronary, infant, pediatric, and adult intensive care.

In 1981, four HMC physicians were among 37 physicians statewide to complete the Advanced Trauma Life Support course approved by the American

Neuro/Trauma/Surgical/Burn ICU staff, 2020

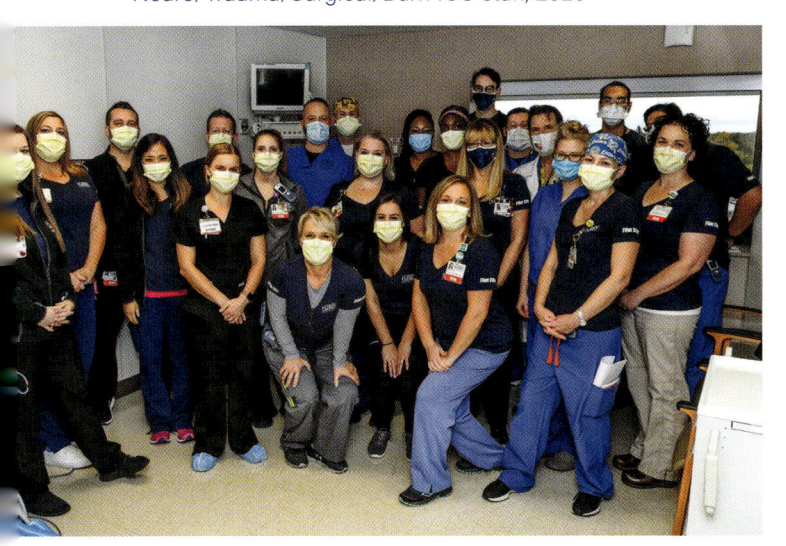

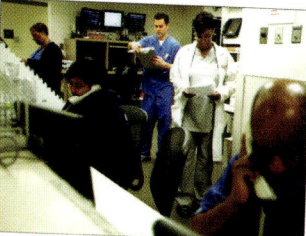

Trauma center construction, 2010

College of Surgeons (ACS), the official training program in the assessment and treatment of seriously injured patients. Franklin Wade, MD, chief of Surgery, Musa Haffajee, MD, Burn Unit director, Alexander Nehme, MD, director of Surgical Education, and L. Scott Ulin, MD, director of Medical Emergency Services, completed the course. The group learned advanced lifesaving techniques, while focusing on stabilizing a patient within the first hour of trauma management. Two Hurley registered nurses, Margie Murray and Thomas Wright, also completed special training as instructors in advanced life-support training. Dr. Wade became the first director of Hurley Trauma Services.

In 1981, at Hurley's request, a team of experts from the ACS assessed the medical center's potential for designation as a Level I or II Trauma Center. "The

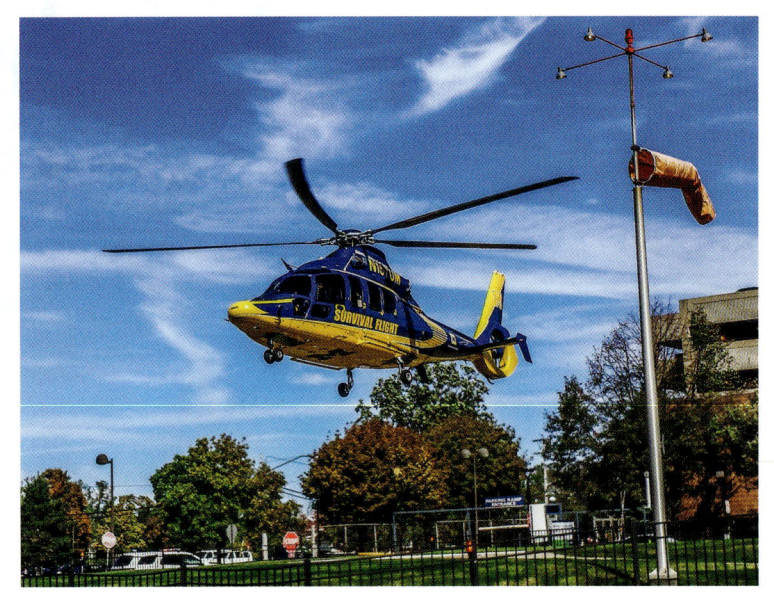

Survival Flight

HMC partners with Michigan Medical Center, University of Michigan (UMMC), helicopter transport services, providing the patient and doctor an additional lifesaving option. The helicopter, staffed by a UMMC critical care nurse, begins treatment at the accident scene and alerts the trauma team of what to expect upon arrival to the hospital. Survival Flight victims from Genesee, Lapeer, and Shiawassee Counties can be treated at HMC's Level I Trauma Center. Hurley's helipad is located near the trauma bay at the northern end of the Emergency Department.

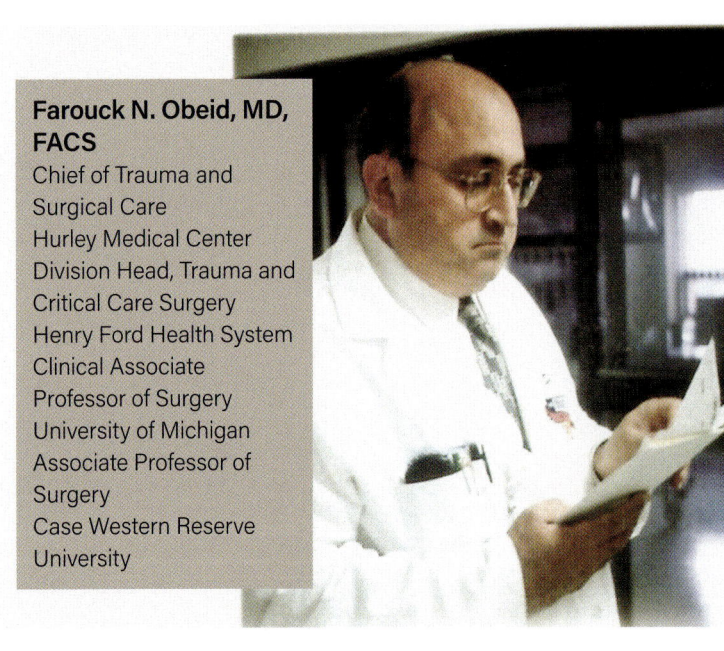

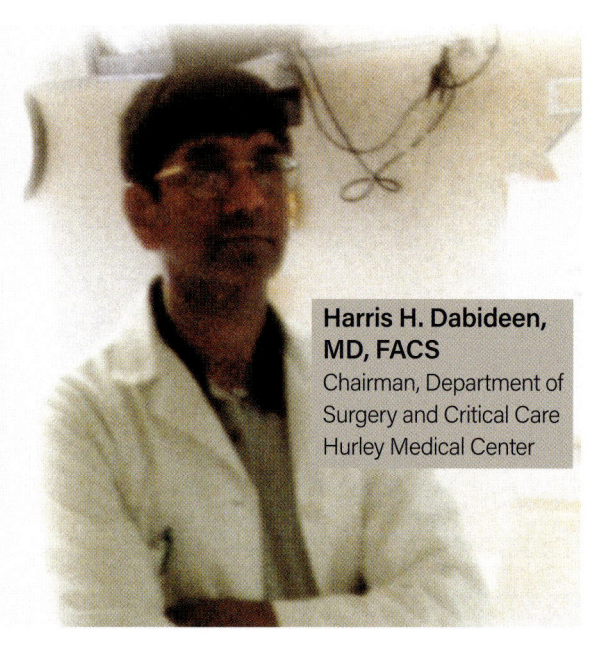

Farouck N. Obeid, MD, FACS
Chief of Trauma and Surgical Care
Hurley Medical Center
Division Head, Trauma and Critical Care Surgery
Henry Ford Health System
Clinical Associate Professor of Surgery
University of Michigan
Associate Professor of Surgery
Case Western Reserve University

Harris H. Dabideen, MD, FACS
Chairman, Department of Surgery and Critical Care
Hurley Medical Center

visit led to several surgical contracts with subspecialists, including cardiothoracic, to ensure that we had full trauma capabilities," said Margie Murray-Wright. Emergency cardiothoracic surgery, also known as open-heart surgery, was introduced in 1982 into Hurley's trauma care, with an emphasis on emergencies involving traumatic penetrating wounds or internal damage precipitated by an accident. "My husband, Tom Wright, Hurley administrator at the time, placed directional signs to the trauma center in Flint." The first step was to develop a board-certified ED group followed by a board-certified surgical group who could take calls. "That process was lengthy and political forces at the local Region V EMS level and state level were complex," adds Murray-Wright. "After a long road to develop a board-certified surgical team, in collaboration with Jorge Rodriguez, MD, at the U of M Department of Surgery, Hurley's ED became the area's first trauma center verified by the ACS as a Level II Trauma Center." The contributions of Dr. Wade and Harris Dabideen, MD, enabled the designation process to be successful. Dr. Dabideen,

DID YOU KNOW | . . . at the time of the 75th anniversary in 1983, Hurley had helped nearly one million patients and was a local employer for 2,500 Flint-area residents.

who trained under Dr. Wade and Max Dodds, MD, for his surgical residency in 1969, became the first medical director during trauma designation. Another person who was essential in the development of HMC's trauma program was neurosurgeon Hugo M. Lopez-Negrete, MD, who served as the neurosurgical liaison for 40 years, until 2018. "Dr. Lopez's legacy within the neuroscience program at Hurley will live on for years to come," said John Stewart, RN, BSN, MSA, Service Line administrator.

In May 1990, construction of a $1.8 million, 11,300-square-foot renovation of the emergency/trauma center began on the ground floor of the North Tower. The project was completed in phases to minimize disruption. Exterior remodeling of the entire triage and waiting areas was performed, and a larger, separate ambulance canopy to lessen congestion was constructed. Interior remodeling included two additional trauma bays located close to the ambulance entrance, 31 exam rooms, a second X-ray room, a six-bed observation area for stable patients being admitted (plus an adjacent isolation room), and an expanded nurses' station to serve 54,000 patients annually. New monitors and Telemetry Units were added. "This new expansion will allow for better patient flow and more consistency of care," said Janet Seifferlein, new ED nurse manager. "In the past, it was not unusual for patients to be moved from room to room, receiving care from several nurses. Now, they will stay in the same exam room and continue to see the same nurse."[7] The project was completed in 1991. Patient volume was driven by an increase in patients using the medical center ED as a primary care site, and also due to its standing as a regional trauma center with air-transport capability, expanded critical care services, trauma services, maternal-child health programs, and renal services. In 1997, Hurley became the area's first trauma center verified by the ACS as a Level II Trauma Center. In 1998, HMC opened the area's only Pediatric Emergency Department and the area's first Chest Pain Center within the ED.

Trauma surgeon Farouck Obeid, MD, and Trauma coordinator Judy Mikhail, RN, MSN, CCNS, testified to legislators in support of 1999 House Bill 4596, which Governor John Engler signed into law, forming the first statewide trauma commission, which started the coordinated trauma system. According to Dr. Obeid, "A Michigan trauma system could reduce mortality by an estimated 1,350 lives and prevent another 15,000 in permanent or long-term disability."

The Hurley trauma center earned the highest verification from the ACS, as a Level I Trauma Center in 2000, the first in the region, joining an elite group of US medical facilities. HMC is the northernmost Level I Trauma Center in the state of Michigan.

Farouck N. Obeid, MD, trauma bay

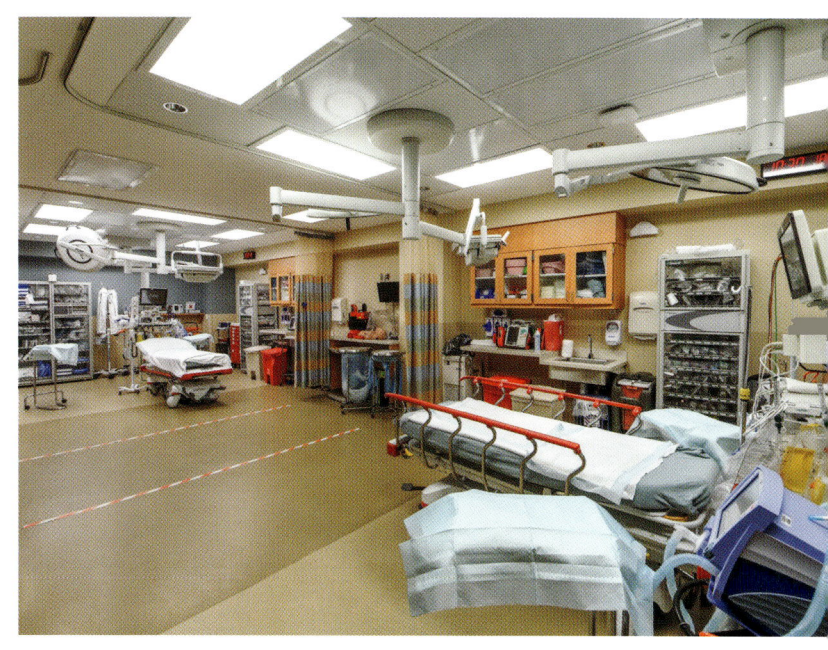

CHAPTER TWO A REGIONAL LEADER IN ADVANCED MEDICAL CARE

Throughout the 2000s, technology drove rapid innovation. In 2010, a ground-breaking ceremony took place for a new high-tech ED to be built from the ground up. A greatly expanded 9,000-square-foot lobby opened as part of the first phase of the project, with a drop-off lane in front of the new, main adult ED and separate Pediatric ED entrances. All ambulance traffic was directed to the back of the hospital off of Mackin Road.

The new Paul F. Reinhart Emergency Trauma Center and Children's Emergency Department opened on March 4, 2012. "We are thrilled to be able to open this modern, advanced emergency trauma center that basically doubles the size of the facility. Hurley Medical Center is investing in the future, allowing us to better serve the needs of our patients and the greater Genesee County community as a whole," said Melany Gavulic, RN, MBA, president, chief operating officer. The new ED was named after the late Paul F. Reinhart, who had been dedicated to ensuring adequate and fair distribution of Medicaid funding for hospitals throughout Michigan. Hospital administrators pushed for the trauma bay to be named in honor of Farouck Obeid, MD, since he was instrumental in HMC getting its initial Level I trauma status.

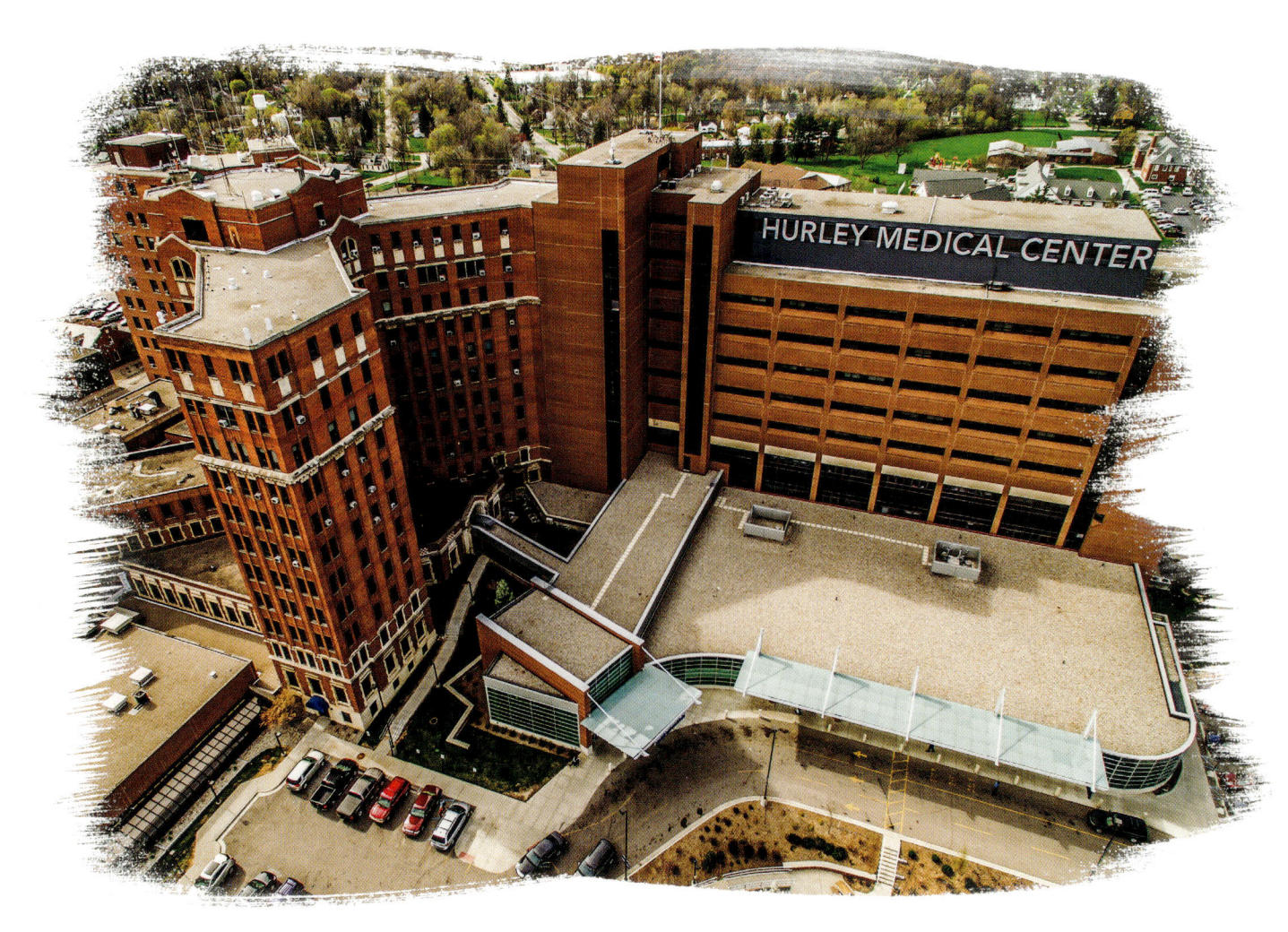

Paul F. Reinhart Emergency Trauma Center, 2020

Margie Murray-Wright
Administrator for Hurley's Trauma and Critical Care Services

Experienced and dynamic leader. Resourceful catalyst dedicated to facilitating the seamless integration of our trauma team's efforts. Energetic champion with a "can-do" attitude. Enthusiastic family devotee.

Margie Murray-Wright, RN, MSN

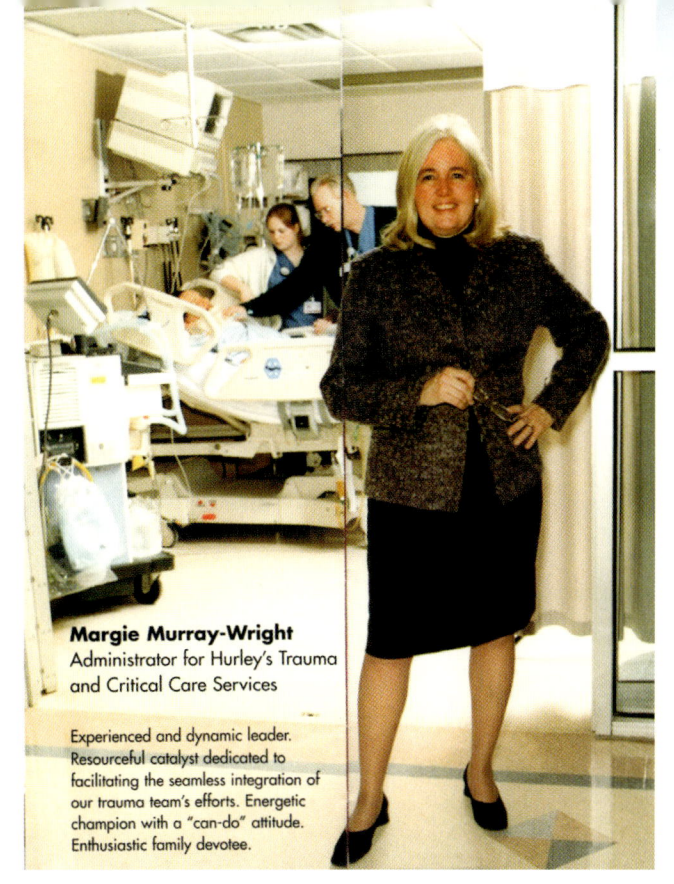

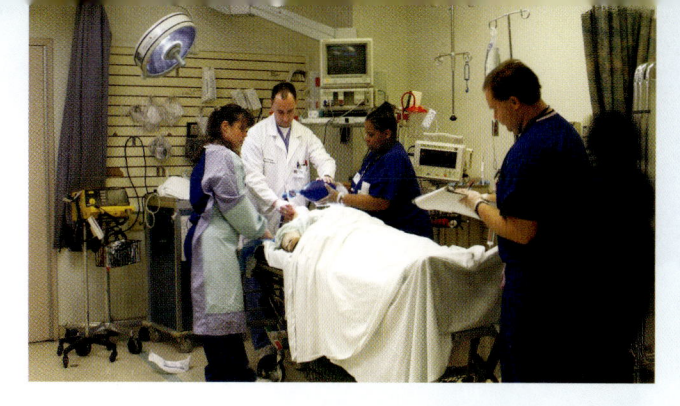

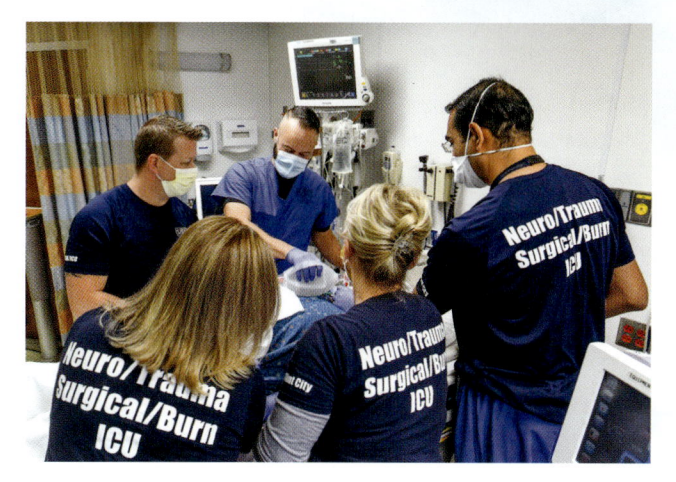

Top: Trauma image, 2008

Bottom: Neuro/Trauma/Surgical/Burn ICU staff, 2020

Emergency Department

As a Level I Trauma Center, when a patient comes into the ED immediately following a traumatic injury, it does not matter what time of day it is—there is always a trauma team on-site waiting for the patient's arrival. This team—a trauma surgeon and an emergency medicine physician, a trauma physician assistant, two dedicated trauma nurses, a respiratory therapist, an anesthesia provider, an X-ray technician, and a social worker—reports immediately to the highly specialized trauma bay and awaits the patient's arrival.

"The shift from ER to trauma is really an acknowledgment of what takes place behind the scenes," said Murray-Wright. "When the emergency room issues a trauma alert, it sets off a signal that is sent simultaneously to the trauma surgeons, the operating room, the blood bank, radiology, Critical Care Units, and any staff that might be needed to help. For instance, if we have an alert where an injured eight-year-old was incoming, then the pediatrics team would also be notified. Knowing that an expert interdisciplinary team is prepared to meet every trauma offers great peace of mind to everyone involved."

"Minutes matter when you have someone's life in your hands and it's common for a patient to be in our operating room within minutes of arrival to the hospital,"

Emergency medicine physicians Michael Tupper, MD, Michael Roebuck, MD, F. Michael Jaggi, DO, and James Weber, DO, in the Farouck N. Obeid Trauma Bay

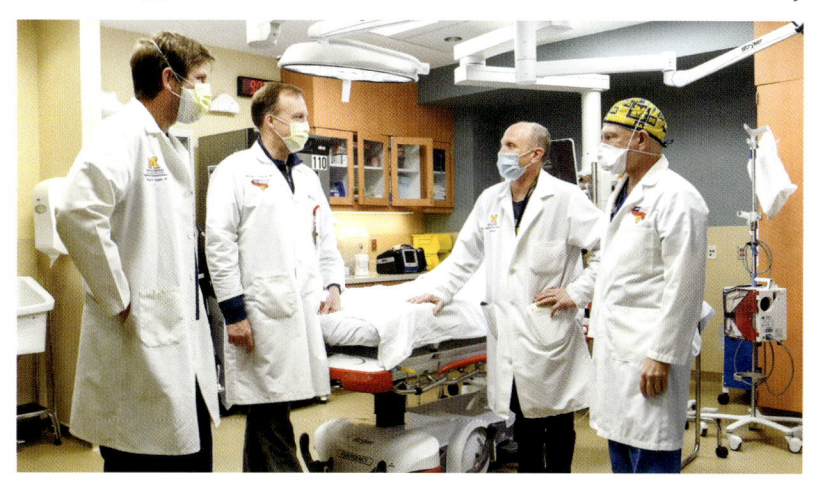

CHAPTER TWO A REGIONAL LEADER IN ADVANCED MEDICAL CARE • 31

> ## Bioethics Committee – Handling the Ethics of Medicine
>
> "I see it as a compelling opportunity to help Hurley patients and their families make challenging and complex end-of-life decisions. Many of these medical problems take a lot of conversation in order to reach a decision to move forward. The Ethics Team may be consulted when families and doctors need to discuss the best course of action for a patient, such as, a family doesn't want their young child to receive lifesaving chemotherapy for leukemia. The ethics board would be consulted to help build consensus between family and the health care team to agree upon the best treatment for the child," said Murray-Wright, who serves on the board of ethics as a community member.

said Michelle Maxson, Trauma program manager. "The 'Golden Hour' is the first hour following an injury, which is the most likely time that a patient can die from their injuries; so, intervening early to stabilize a patient during that 'Golden Hour' gives the best chance of survival."

As a requirement of a Level I Trauma Center, HMC must maintain a registry that catalogues every trauma patient admission in order to accumulate state and national data as to the number, type, and severity of trauma. An injury severity score (ISS) is assigned on all trauma patients and correlates with death, disability, and prolonged hospitalization after trauma. "HMC cares for some of the highest acuity/sickest patients in our state, when compared to other institutions, based upon the data" said John Stewart, RN, BSN, MSA, Service Line administrator.

HMC sought a further designation in support of service-area seniors, and in 2020, it was recognized as a bronze standard—a Level III Geriatric Emergency Department Accreditation (GEDA) Program-accredited Geriatric Emergency Department by the American College of Emergency Physicians, for delivering excellent geriatric patient care in the ED. This furthers Hurley's mission of improving patient outcomes by providing a standardized approach to care that addresses common geriatric issues. It also ensures the optimal transition of care from the ED to inpatient, home, or long-term care. The GEDA program is voluntary and includes three levels, similar to trauma designations. Specific criteria and goals are provided for emergency clinicians and administrators to target, consisting of more than two dozen best practices for geriatric care. A Level III GEDA-accredited Geriatric ED must incorporate many of these best practices, along with providing interdisciplinary geriatric education and have geriatric-appropriate equipment and supplies available.[8]

Breaking the Cycle of Violence

Victim Support

The Trauma Recovery Center (TRC) is a grant-funded program designed to help victims of crime who seek treatment in the ED, such as victims of elder abuse, domestic violence, gunshot wounds, sexual and physical assaults, and human trafficking. Referrals also come from the City of Flint's district attorney, private practice attorneys, and local community agencies. Along with the program coordinator, the TRC has therapists who provide bedside consultations in the hospital and outpatient psychotherapy, and care coordinators who provide emotional support and help

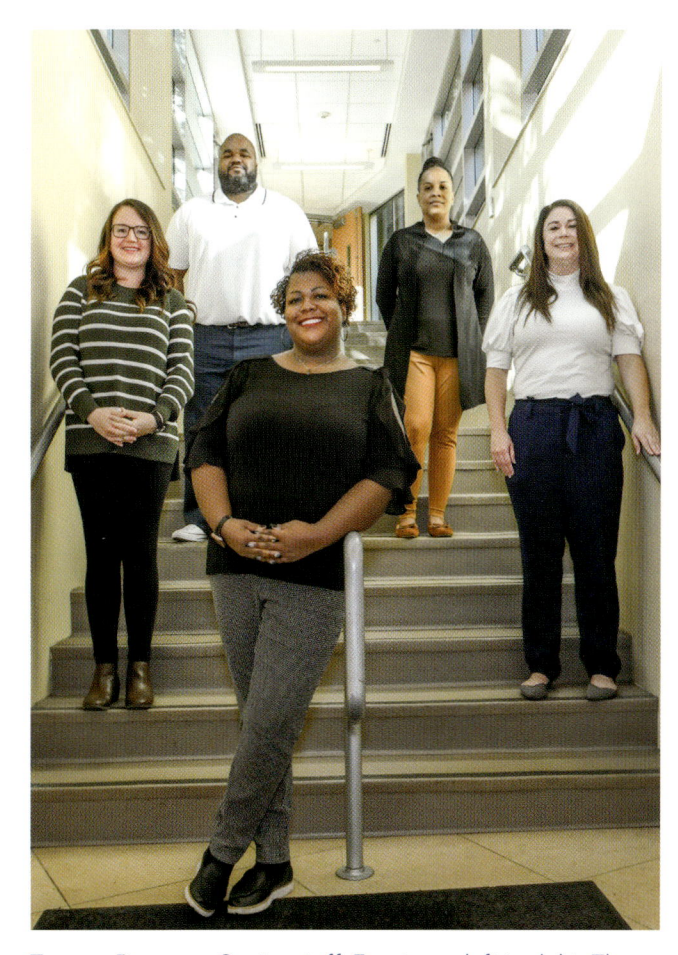

Trauma Recovery Center staff. Front row, left to right: Tianna Stehle, therapist, Tia Coles, coordinator, and Jennifer Thornquist, care coordinator. Back row: Arthur Taylor, care coordinator, and Jamie Holt, care coordinator.

the victims complete compensation applications, attend court hearings, advocate with law enforcement, and complete personal protective orders. They also follow up with loved ones whose emotional and physical health could be affected from hearing or witnessing the pain, injuries, and fear the victim experienced. Emergency shelter, relocation assistance, transportation, and clothing are also provided. Even after a patient is discharged, care coordinators stay in touch until the crisis is alleviated or the victim is stable. "In a city where so many people are hurting, we are grateful to be able to provide support and services to victims that may not have anywhere else to turn to for help," said Tia Coles, TRC coordinator.

HMC and Voices for Children Advocacy Center

Children advocacy centers first began in Huntsville, Alabama, in 1985 as a place where an abused child could go to a single place where law enforcement, medical health, and social services professionals would talk to the child together at one time to determine a case. HMC played a role in developing the Child Abuse and Neglect Protocol in Genesee County in 2000. The program initially started as the Children's Advocacy Center of Genesee County, was later changed to Weiss Child Advocacy Center, and finally, Voices for Children.

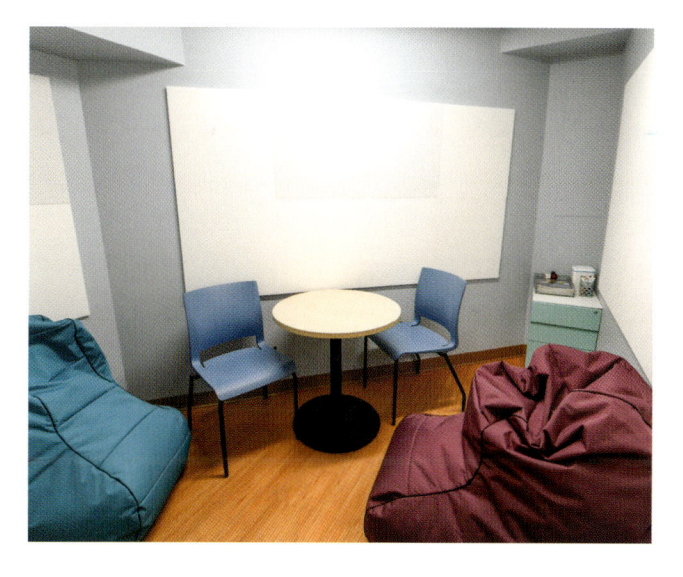

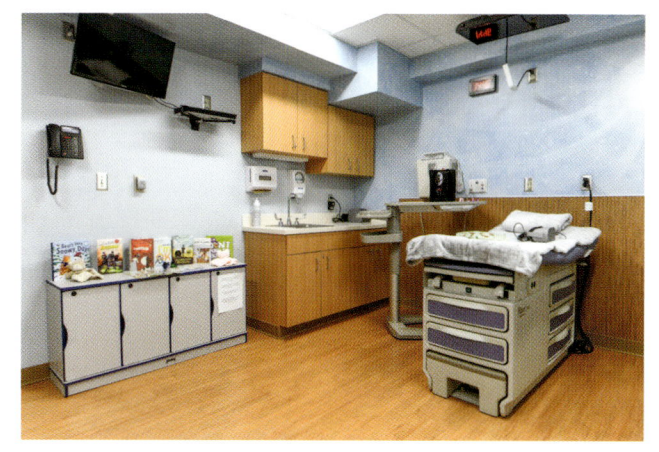

Children's Advocacy Center dedicated interview space and treatment room

CHAPTER TWO A REGIONAL LEADER IN ADVANCED MEDICAL CARE • 33

Patient Advocacy

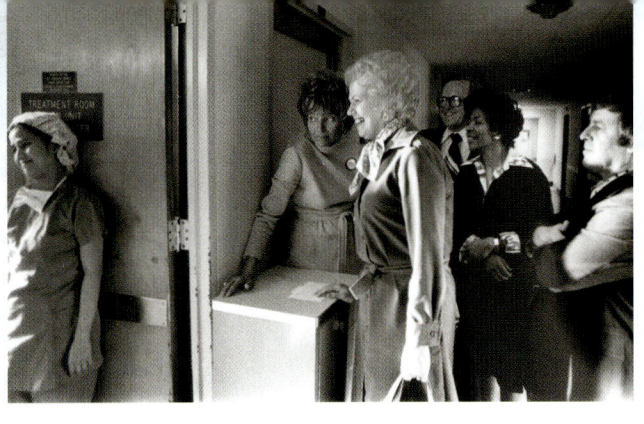

Frankie Perry, RN, LFACHE (second from left), assistant medical center director, started the patient advocacy program in 1977 as part of an administrative effort to make the institution more responsive to the human needs of patients. As the hospital's chief patient advocate, she presented her approach at the American Hospital Association in 1980. Her efforts made a lasting impact not only on HMC but also within the industry as the first female recipient of the American College of Healthcare Executives (ACHE) Lifetime Service Award.

In 2019, HMC built an independent interview space where Voices for Children staff, along with child protective services (CPS) and the police, may hold forensic interviews to obtain vital information while it is still fresh in the child's mind. The surroundings are filled with soft furnishings, child-size tables, chairs, and a chalkboard so that a child can tell their story in the way they are able to communicate. Video recorders and microphones are concealed so that the child is not intimidated.

HMC's Brian Nolan, MD, FAAP, is the region's only board-certified child abuse specialist and one of only eight physicians in Michigan who are board-certified

Family Practice Unit Becomes a Hurley Specialty, 1988

Duane Bailey, MD, chairman of Hurley's Family Practice Department, and Samuel Dismond Jr., MD, led the move to have a medical unit dedicated to the family practice philosophy. "This meant multigenerational care, attention to the individual needs, personal treatment, and family involvement," according to Dr. Dismond. By 1991, about 20 family practice physicians were admitting their adult medical patients to the unit, except when other specialized treatment was warranted. The 20-bed unit, located on the seventh floor in the East Tower, not only provided patient care but also offered teaching service coverage by internal medicine residents. "It has been easy to establish a good working relationship with unit staff," said Dr. Dismond, crediting Nurse Manager Rose Luster for much of the success. "Good communication results in a true interdisciplinary approach."

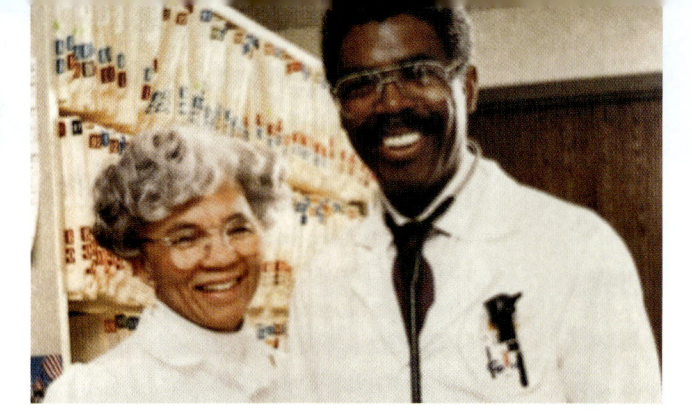

Janice and Samuel Dismond Jr., MD, 1992

in child abuse. He is currently the clinical director of Pediatrics.

"We put the child's care first," said Mattie Pearson, RN, MSN, Service Line administrator for Women and Children Services at HMC. "We are able to provide an independent facility and support for the children and their advocates. Our examination space is located in a separate part of the hospital where it's quiet and kid friendly."

"Hurley is critical to the work that we do, and adds value to us," said Claudnyse D. Holloman, Esq., executive director of Voices for Children Advocacy Center. "Forty-seven percent of our cases start with HMC providing the initial medical care for the child in crisis. This is a positive first step. Many families view

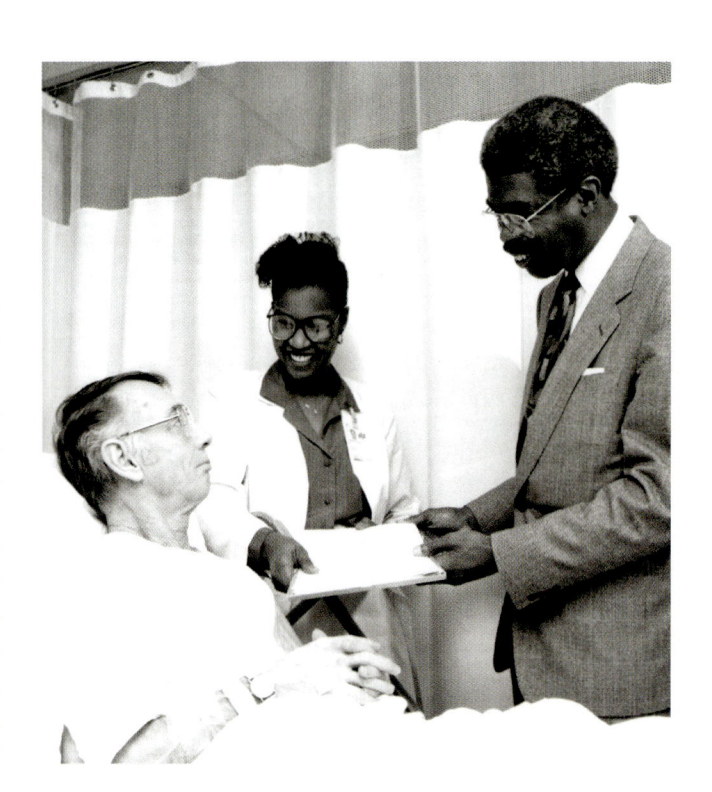

Patients Who Touched Hearts

EMMA HUDSON

Emma Hudson, a lively and vibrant young girl, was diagnosed with acute lymphoblastic leukemia at age 11. She missed two entire school years to undergo 21 months of intensive chemotherapy and radiation. Emma's rare chromosome abnormality made her more likely to relapse. Three weeks after her last chemotherapy treatment tests concluded, she had relapsed. A bone marrow drive was held, resulting in a match and a bone marrow transplant at C. S. Mott Children's Hospital on April 4, 2013. On August 5, 2014, Hudson spoke in front of a crowd of nearly 100 in Hurley's Merliss Brown Auditorium, encouraging everyone to enroll on the bone marrow donor registry. Emma started to introduce who she thought was the next speaker, but what Emma did not know was that she would meet her bone marrow donor, George Schmitz, 26, from Texas. For the first time since April, when she received the information on her donor, she was able to thank him in person.[9] It was an extremely emotional moment for everyone!

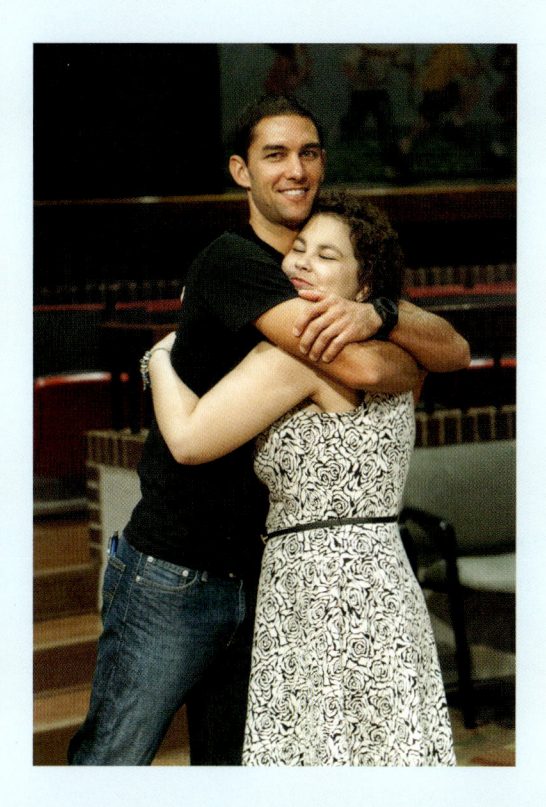

MARK REED

Mark Reed, age 20, had suffered from muscular dystrophy since he was four years old; he had only minor movement in his fingers and face. In May 1980, Mark was rushed to HMC's ER and spent nearly five months in the ICU. He was then transferred to HMC's Transitional Care Unit, where he resided and relied on HMC staff for everything for the next 20 years. Occasionally, staff secured a ventilator to a mobile chair and would take Mark outside to Dort Park. Respiratory therapist Maryanne Strawser, RRT, recalls: "I cared for Mark as a respiratory student and once again after I hired in at HMC. One year for his birthday, he received a stereo with a CD player for his room—which was a new thing at the time. Mark would ask the staff to change the CDs or turn the machine on or off; one day he asked me. I went home and told my husband, 'We need to get one of these!'" The Hurley staff was Mark's family, and he was family to the Hurley staff.

Hurley as a medical place of safety, as many were born there. They trust Hurley to do what is right. And for us, we know that the medical care that they receive will aid the child in hope and healing, which is necessary for them to move forward through the process."

According to Dr. Nolan, "Accidents are common, but we also see children who have been abused. It is important not to accuse parents of abuse when, in fact, the child had an accident and vice versa. We communicate with CPS when we have concerns about possible abuse or neglect."

"Dr. Nolan wears two hats," adds Holloman. "As an expert clinician when the child is brought to the hospital for care, but also to testify on behalf of them in court. All the kids and their parents talk about how great he is because of his expertise. He can find out if a child is not safe and can see through the fear and distrust when they are brought in for treatment."

Traumatic Events with HMC at the Front Line

Bishop International Airport Attack: Terrorism at Home

On June 21, 2017, Lt. Jeff Neville of the airport police was stabbed in the neck at Bishop International Airport. "From our perspective, this was a typical Level I (trauma) activation, but when the patient arrived in the trauma bay, he was accompanied by six to eight law enforcement officers, which is highly unusual," said Leo Mercer, MD, FACS, chief of Trauma Surgery. "Even though there was a high degree of oversight being shown by the officers, we maintained our objectivity and focused on the patient, who was alert and able to talk." After undergoing surgery at HMC, Neville's condition was upgraded from critical to stable and he was discharged June 26, 2017. "I had a truly amazing recovery—[a] life-changing and lifesaving experience at Hurley," said Lt. Neville. "Without Hurley's trauma center, I don't believe I'd be alive today. I feel truly blessed that Hurley Medical Center was here." Airport maintenance worker Richard Krul, a retiree from Hurley's Maintenance Department, attempted to subdue the attacker and was cut on the hand as a result. "Mr. Krul was treated by the ED staff, but his injury did not require trauma services," added Dr. Mercer.

Clara Barton Terrace Convalescent Home Explosion

On the night of November 10, 1999, the boiler supports collapsed in the basement of Clara Barton Terrace Convalescent Home, leading to a gas main rupture that caused a massive explosion and the collapse of the center section of the building. Neighbors and first responders helped to remove people from the building after the 9:00 p.m. blast, but more than 20 injured people were sent to HMC for treatment. According to local news reports, several fire departments responded to the blaze. As county firefighters converged, Battalion Chief Paul Plunkey of the City of Flint Fire Department called for the Urban Search and Rescue Team. In the end, there were 155 survivors and five fatalities.

A Hurley nurse attends to one of the people injured by the Beecher tornado, 1953

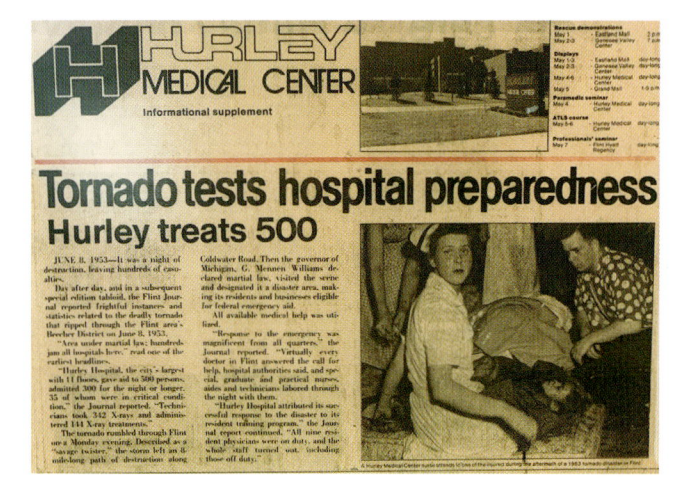

Beecher Tornado Tests Hurley's Emergency Preparedness

On the evening of Monday, June 8, 1953, the deadliest tornado in Michigan's history hit the Flint and Beecher areas. The category F5 tornado touched down in Genesee County and continued on a 27-mile path, causing 126 fatalities, 925 injuries, and an estimated $19 million (1953 US dollars) in damage. Described as a "savage twister," it left an eight-mile-long path of destruction along Coldwater Road northwest of the city of Flint. Only hours later, the community praised Hurley's response. According to the *Flint Journal*, "Hurley Hospital was swamped Monday night and early today [June 9, 1953] as its staff treated more than 300 persons injured in the tornado. Under the circumstances, the hospital staff handled the situation smoothly and efficiently. All three shifts of staff nurses, doctors, volunteer nurses, Red Cross workers and volunteers were busy. They helped ease the pain of patients, assist in emergency room first aid at the rear entrance, comfort anxious relatives, compile a list of the injured and directed traffic. Before the episode was over Hurley Hospital treated 500 people, many who were critically injured."

The community's response to this tragedy was immediate and overwhelming. Unsolicited donations poured in from General Motors, the United Auto Workers, and numerous businesses to a disaster aid fund. Hundreds of local workers gave through payroll deductions; within a few weeks, over $900,000 was collected. In late August 1953, 8,000 volunteers participated in a weekend building spree known as "Operation Tornado." In 90-degree heat, people from all walks of life provided more than 80,000 hours to build 193 houses. For its efforts, Flint was honored as the "All-American City of 1953."[10]

Regional Burn Center – Medical Department of Excellence

Hurley's burn center was founded in 1960 after several surgeons determined that special equipment and specially trained nurses were needed to successfully treat burn victims. The original unit, located in the West Tower, housed five beds and one hydrotherapy tank. After the East Tower opened in 1979, the new

Franklin Wade Burn Unit opening, 1972

CHAPTER TWO A REGIONAL LEADER IN ADVANCED MEDICAL CARE • 37

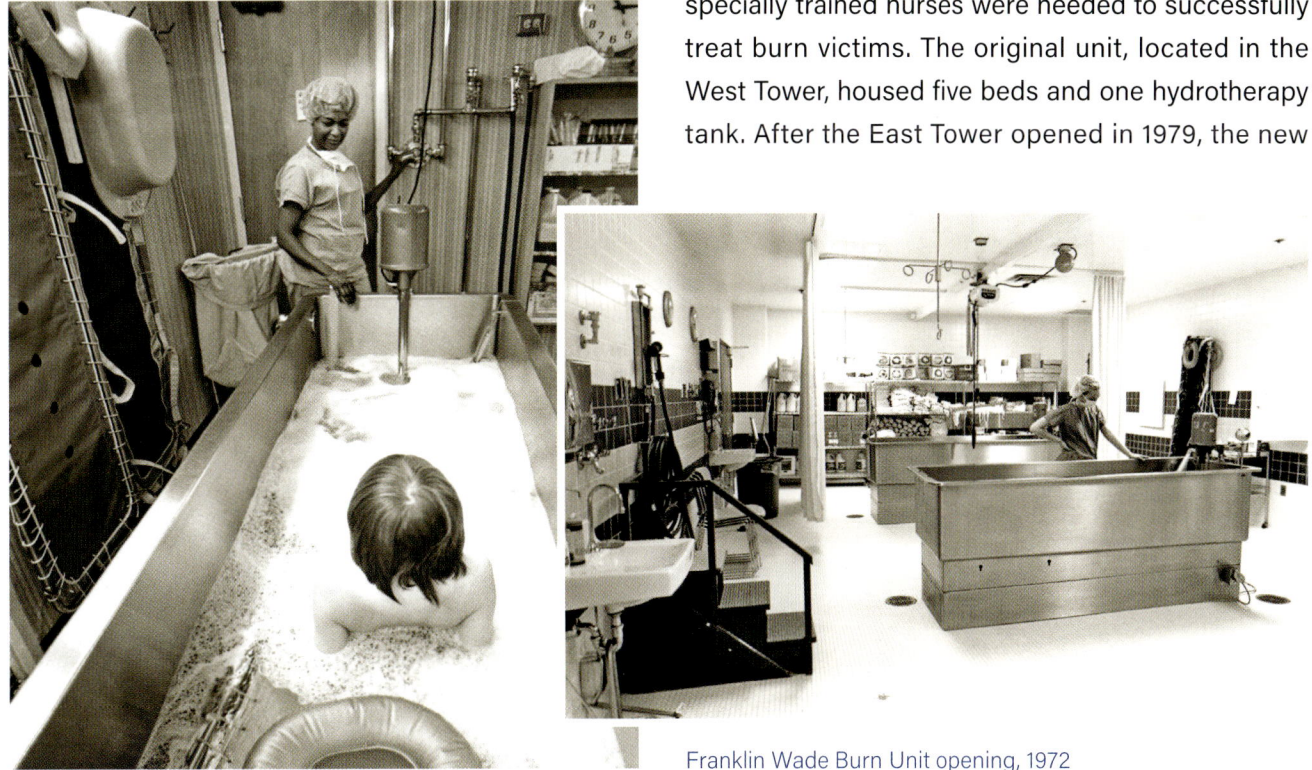

Hurley Cares About Hearts

HMC is one of only 14 Michigan-based hospitals allowed to perform elective coronary angioplasty without open-heart backup, meaning that HMC partners with other institutions for open-heart surgery. Hurley Cardiology Services range from providing outpatient cardiology clinics, which serve as access points for patients to receive medical consultation and referral for testing and intervention, to non-invasive cardiology, which includes echocardiography, stress testing, event monitoring, and other tests to help identify which intervention will be needed to treat the cardiological ailment. HMC performs interventional cardiology and electrophysiology, including diagnostic heart catheters, angioplasty, pacemakers, intra-cardiac defibrillators, right-heart ablations, and electro-physiology studies. The cath lab includes two catheterization suites and twelve pre- and postoperative holding bays to accommodate the annual estimated 2,500 procedures. HMC's cath lab is the only accredited cardiac catheterization laboratory in the Genesee County area, which is staffed by interventional cardiologists, non-invasive cardiologists, registered nurses, and cardiovascular technicians.

In addition to medical and procedural cardiology, patients have access to the cardiac rehabilitation program at HMC, which focuses on the patient's recovery and maintenance of cardiological health after a significant cardiac event. Hurley has invested in improving access and quality for patients suffering from congestive heart failure by developing the congestive heart failure (CHF) Nurse Navigation Program, which assists patients discharged for CHF in improving their lifestyle, complying with physician appointments, and providing education and tools for improved lifestyle choices.

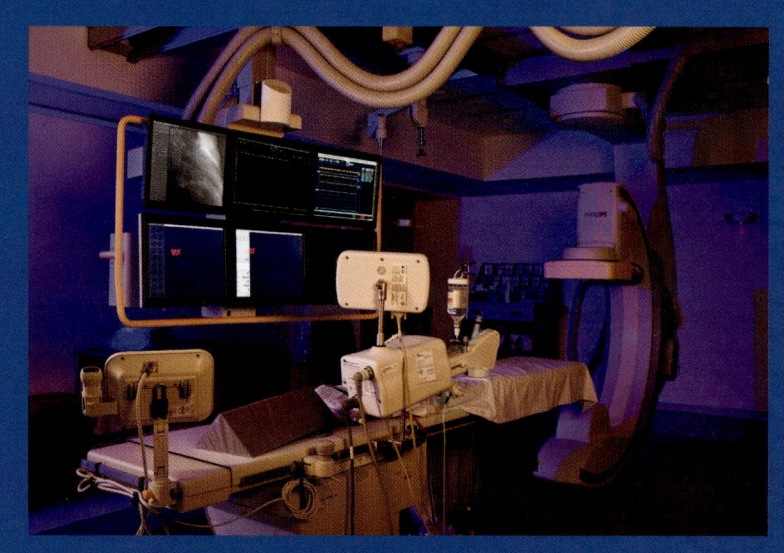

Hurley's cath lab

According to Ron Hubble, MHSA, Service Line administrator for Cardiovascular and Internal Medicine, "Hurley's heart program has been successful by providing access to a comprehensive, high-quality care and affordable program through partnerships with our physician colleagues and other respected institutions. These partnerships allow us to bring multiple levels of expertise to continually improve quality and provide a safe environment for our communities' heart-care needs."

HMC invested in improving access and quality by establishing the Heart Failure Navigator Program, aimed at helping patients with heart failure stay home for care, rather than repeatedly coming to the hospital unnecessarily. The program is accredited by Corazon Inc., which is authorized by the state to regulate the quality of the procedures, ensuring that the heart program stands up to rigorous evaluations and exceeds standards of care.

fifth-floor Burn Unit featured 13 beds, an operating room, a large tank room with four hydrotherapy tanks for immersion therapy, and a physical medicine area for early rehabilitation, plus an outpatient burn clinic.

Sherry Palmer and Mel Nowland marry in Hurley's Burn Unit in September 1976. Sherry Palmer was burned on over 70 percent of her body in an explosion from a propane-tank truck that rolled off of an overpass at I-75 and I-69; she had been a patient in the Burn Unit for 40 days. The couple moved up the wedding after Palmer's accident made them evaluate their time together. Left to right: Helen Palmer, Mel Nowland, Sherry Palmer, and Rev. Edward Azzam.

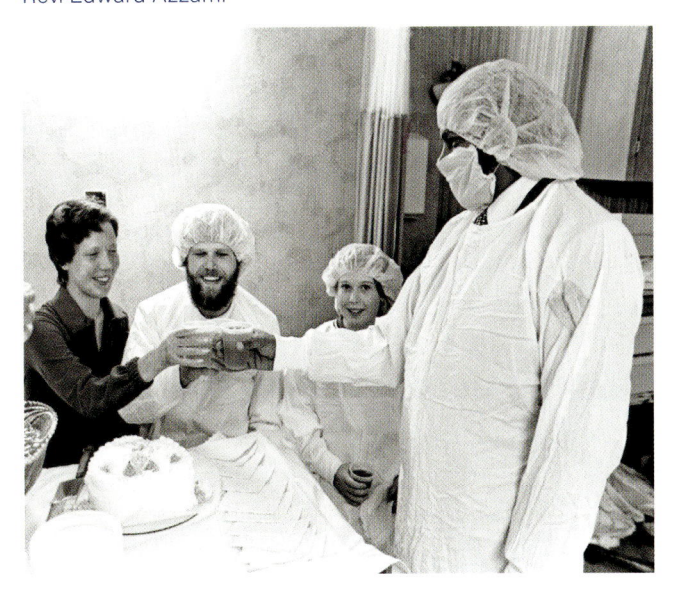

"Statistics have shown that increased survival and improved outcome are much greater in a designated burn center," said Judy Mikhail, critical care clinical nurse specialist in 1990. "The first 72 hours of intensive care are crucial for patients with major burns. Even in the best medical care facilities, healing a burn patient's physical appearance and self-image are forever altered, especially if the injury is severe." HMC's specially trained nurses provide all levels of burn care. Surgeons manage the burns medically and surgically, as complex burns require multiple surgeries, burn debridement, and, eventually, skin grafting.

According to Musa Haffejee, MD, director of the Burn Unit in 1996, "Ninety percent of the surgeries performed are to regain function of injured limbs, and 10 percent are to reconstruct burn scar deformities."

"It's not uncommon for patients to spend two to three months in care and recovery within the burn center. Patients receive intense physical and occupational therapy, along with psychological support. We care for both adult and pediatric burn cases," said Michelle Maxson.

HMC admits about 175 to 200 severely injured burn victims annually, while also caring for hundreds more through the burn clinic, which is an outpatient service. "This allows patients to go home while our team still manages their ongoing care," adds Maxson.

The high quality of care given by the staff at the burn center is best reflected by several former patients turned ambassadors, who have spoken about their positive experience with the trauma burn team. "We even have a former burn patient who volunteers a couple of times a week in order to give back," said Maxson.

Pharmacological Medicine

Hurley Hospital's first pharmacy was established in 1922 and was only 1,232 square feet of space. In June 1981, the pharmacy was upgraded to an advanced dispensing system, which included an expansion to 4,852 square feet of space, with medication and supply refrigerators capable of opening on both sides, a drug information library, and a pharmaceutical purchasing area. Also housed in the new pharmacy was the Poison Control Center, the most comprehensive in the state at the time. There was also a secured patient reception and billing area. HMC was the only Flint-area hospital to use pharmacokinetics to determine the proper dosage levels individualized for each patient, based upon lab results. Pharmacists calculate the precise dosage to achieve optimal therapeutic effectiveness, while reducing the risk of side effects and unnecessary exposure to the drug.

This modern-era pharmacy used a new concept in "unit dose" dispensing to improve economy, accuracy, and speed. Medication was wrapped and packaged in individual doses and stored alphabetically in wall-mounted racks above the work area, where six to eight pharmacy technicians stationed along the "assembly-line style" track would deposit ordered medications into a patient-specific bin that slid past them until the order was complete. A registered pharmacist validated the order for accuracy. A 24-hour medication supply was delivered daily to nursing stations, where they were dispensed as prescribed by physicians.

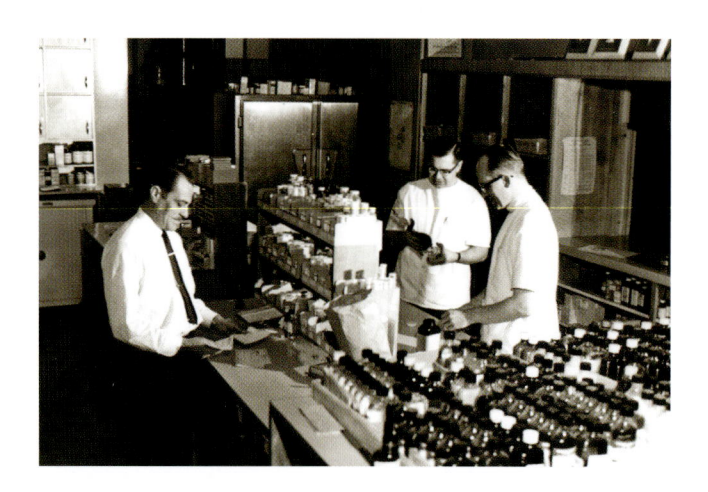

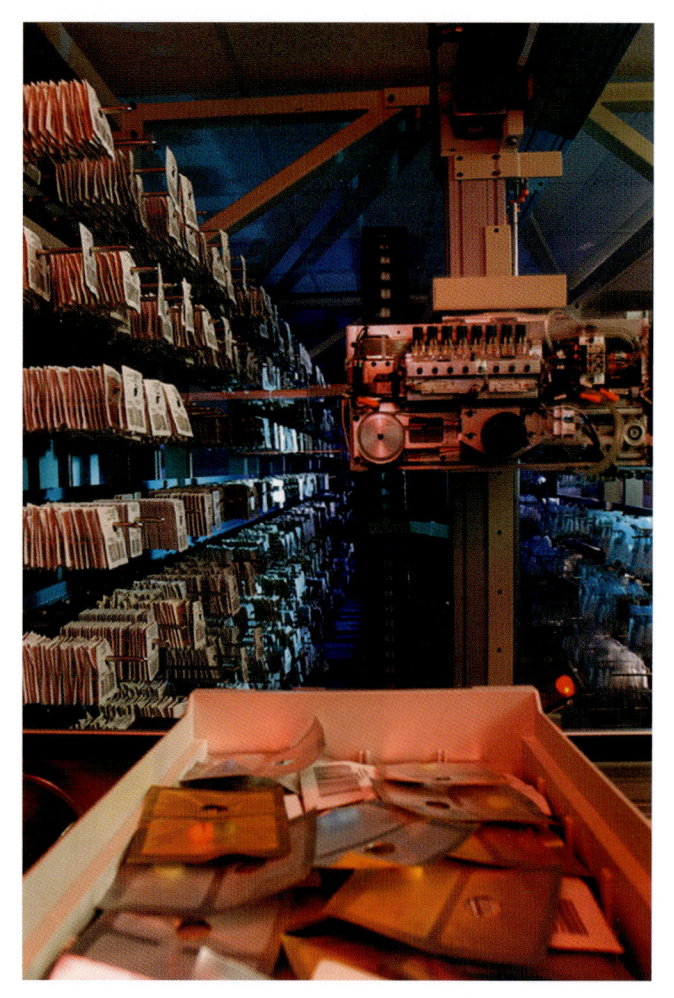

Pharmacy, yesterday and today

In 1990, HMC's Zolton K. Papp Pharmacy (named for Zolton Papp, who served on the Hurley Board of Managers for 41 years) moved to the ground floor of the West Tower, again doubling in size. It included a sterile production room for intravenous (IV) preparations, such as chemotherapy, parenteral fluids, and other IV medications. The new space included a unit-dose production room, a clinical pharmacy area, administrative and purchasing offices, secured space for the storage of controlled substances, and a spacious warehouse for the storage of inventory. The pharmacy dispenses more than 2.5 million doses of medication annually, an average of 18 per patient.

Today, technology plays a huge role in pharmacy services. Medication dispensing is performed with the use of a centralized robotic drug distribution system and automated dispensing cabinets that use barcode technology. These advancements have allowed the pharmacy department to expand their clinical role in ensuring safe and effective medication use in all patient care settings.

Embracing Information Technology and Epic

"The beginning of the Information Technology (IT) Department started prior to the personal computer era in the early 1980s," according to Sherry Ross, business analyst. "Initially, IT was called 'Data Management,' which simply meant that information was manually input onto punch cards by operators. A data processing company transferred this data onto large IBM tapes. An example would be employee timecards; after the timecards were punched by the data entry clerks, the information was sent out to the data processing company, and three days later, we would have all of the reports. In 1986, the management services, finance, and other administrative areas began using personal computers (PCs) in their departments, however none of these were networked together, so information was passed via large floppy disks. In 1989, the first hospital mainframe was installed, primarily for Finance Department processing. The department PCs were connected onto the mainframe; this connection was hardwired, as Wi-Fi did not exist at that time."

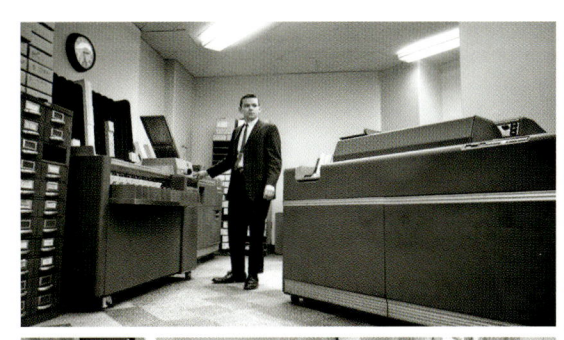

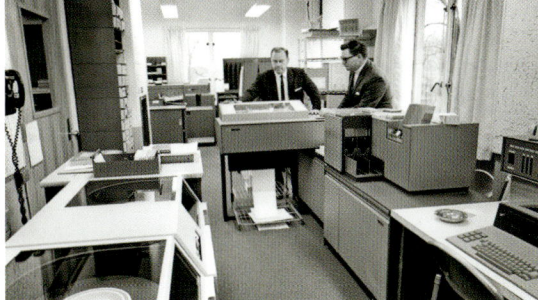

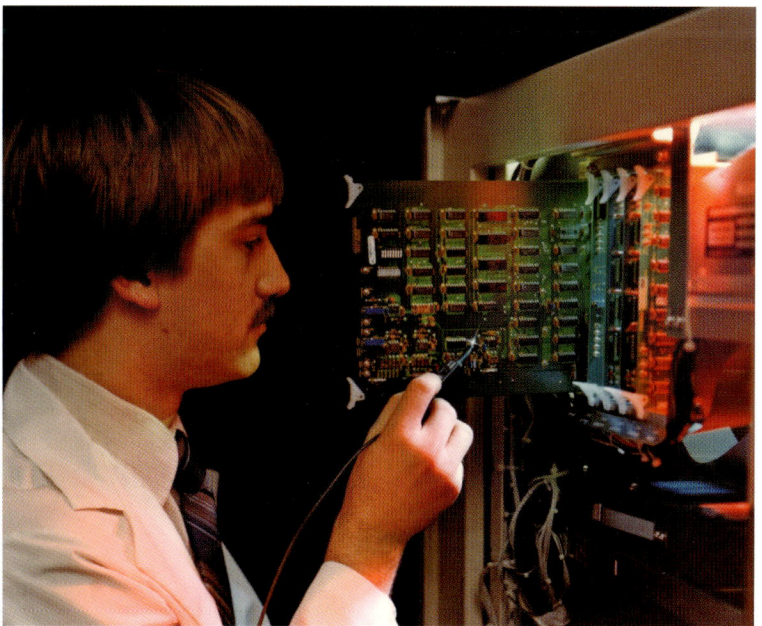

Technology, yesterday and today

CHAPTER TWO A REGIONAL LEADER IN ADVANCED MEDICAL CARE • 41

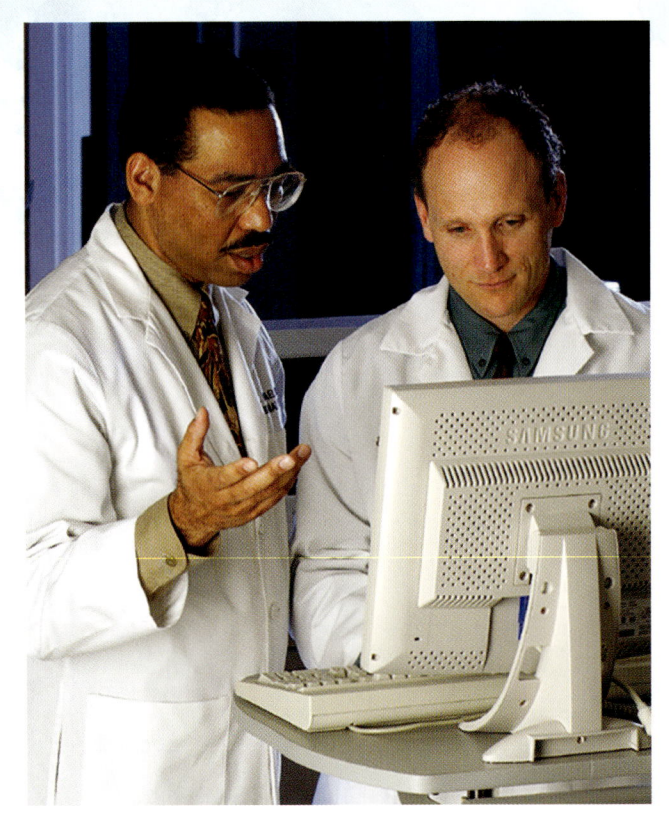

Michael Boucree, MD (2001 Pinnacle Award recipient), and F. Michael Jaggi, DO (2002 Pinnacle Award recipient), review patient records on the first clinical information system (CISCO) used in the 1990s.

"In the early 1990s, the department was renamed Information Services," said Annette Jones, director of Applications Support. "In 1991, we installed the first clinical information system. This was the first time computer technology was used for direct patient care. Hurley was the first hospital in the area to bring technology to the patient bedside. The system was called something technical, so we held a contest among staff members to come up with a more usable name. The winning name was CISCO." According to Michael Roebuck, MD, chief medical information officer, "By today's standards, this was very rudimentary technology, but it was the first step towards the modern Information Technology [Department] in the hospital."

"The 1991 CISCO system allowed providers to enter orders electronically. This was an improvement from the prior process, where physicians wrote patient orders by hand," said Dr. Roebuck. "Handwritten orders required an additional staff member to transcribe the doctor's handwriting, which often required a clarification phone call. The staff member would then enter the patient orders into the computerized order system. This could be a very time-intensive process and also had a potential for error because of the need to interpret physicians' handwriting."

"As part of the national push towards increasing patient safety, in the early 2000s, HMC brought IT to selected clinical areas by installing PCs at nurses' stations and doctors' lounges, allowing physicians direct access and order-entry capabilities at computer stations on every patient floor," said Dr. Roebuck. The system also provided a patient's known allergies, prescribed medicines, and other basic patient information, such as height and weight. This early computerized care system allowed

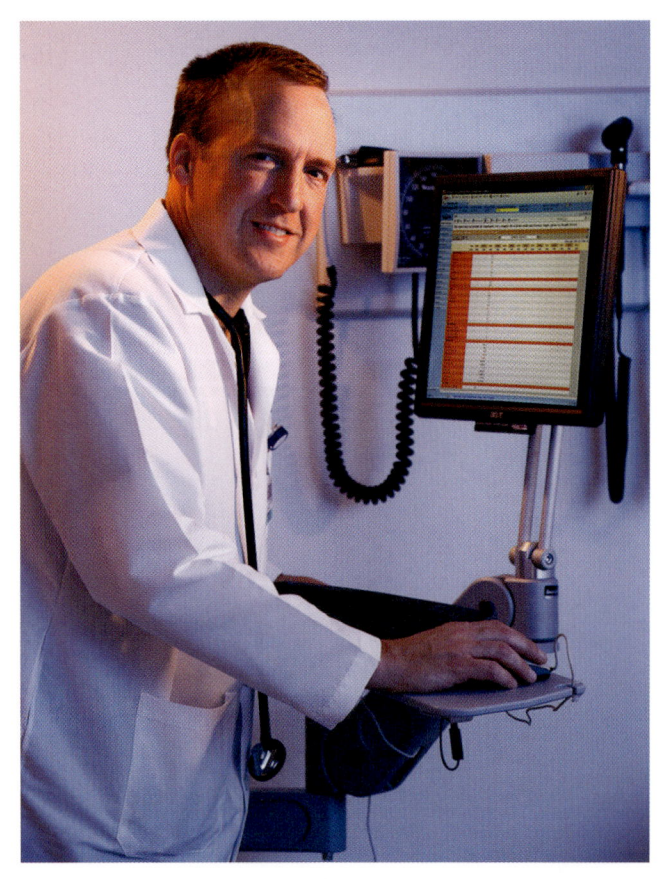

Michael Roebuck, MD, during the installation of the Epic electronic medical record system, 2012

42 • HURLEY MEDICAL CENTER

DID YOU KNOW

... HMC is only one of 10 hospitals in the state of Michigan to receive advance warning of a political dignitary. US Secret Service staff are typically deployed several days in advance to complete an environmental assessment, including aspects such as specific routes to the hospital and internal travel routes to the ED, operating room (OR), and ICU. Security debriefings are conducted with the administrative team, public safety leadership, and various members of the ED in an effort to develop dedicated communication systems and to further identify specific security observation points.

providers to view simple results, such as lab and radiology. "There is no translation required, no handwriting errors, no second steps, no calls for clarification, which resulted in safer, more efficient care," said Dr. Roebuck.

HMC's commitment to excellence in patient care has embraced the rapid innovation in advanced technology. In the fall of 2001, HMC introduced a multimillion-dollar, state-of-the-art picture archiving and communications system (PACS) in radiology. The system distributed and stored images digitally. Instead of examining images on sheets of film held up to a light box, clinicians retrieved and examined images on computer terminals. "This system allowed us to view, manipulate, and compare current studies with past studies," said Dr. Roebuck. "At the time, this was an incredible advancement in technology that greatly enhanced the quality of our radiology studies. As with electronic order entry, Hurley was one of the first in the area to implement such a system."

Beginning in 2009, HMC began preparation for the greatest technology leap ever taken in the clinical areas: implementing the new electronic health system, called Epic. "Providers now enter their orders directly from their phone, tablets, or laptops. Along with the expansion of Wi-Fi in 2008–2009, these two technical advances have really changed how we deliver medical information for patient treatment," said Dr. Roebuck.

"From a technology standpoint, electronic patient care generates billions of data points. It's really gotten quite complicated with the addition of computers into the patient care model," adds Roebuck. "We now work to simplify the data and present it to users in a meaningful way. Although very complicated, this new complexity has come with significant safety advances. Medication administration, for example, now utilizes barcode technology on both the medication and the patient. Each dose of

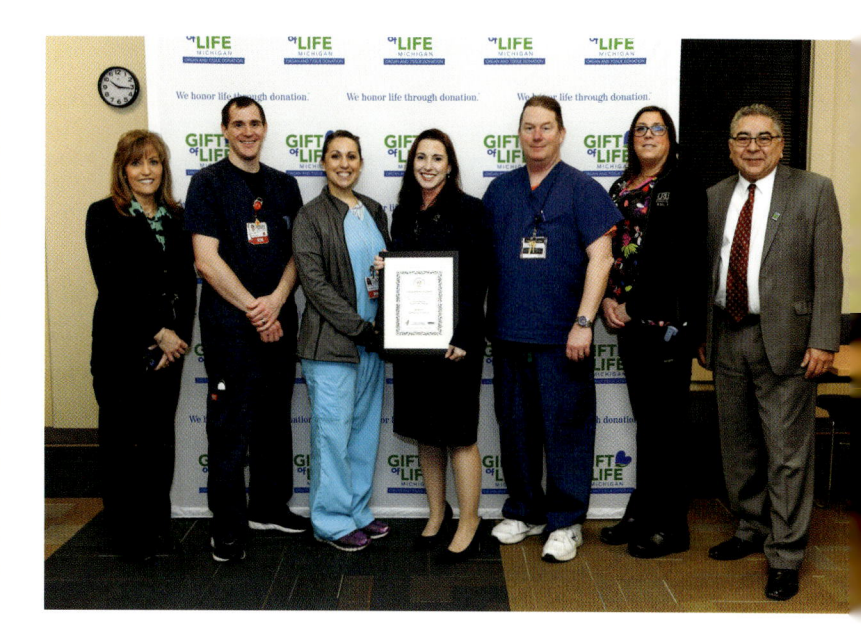

HMC Receives HRSA Gold Award from Gift of Life Michigan
Gift of Life Michigan is the state agency that coordinates lifesaving organ donation. Public awareness, education, and additions to the donor registry increase the number of organs and tissues available for transplant. Valerie Canary and colleagues presented educational sessions and held donor registration drives in the community, which led to an increased number of registered organ and tissue donors. These efforts mean that fewer individuals and their families have to wait for a lifesaving and life-improving organ transplant. Gift of Life Michigan presented HMC with an HRSA Gold Award from the Health Resources and Service Administration in 2020 as a result of 300 new people being added to the Michigan Donor Registry. Left to right: Melany Gavulic, Seth Duquette, Maureen Larson, Valerie Canary, William Thompson, Kim Lipka, and Chris Flores.

CHAPTER TWO A REGIONAL LEADER IN ADVANCED MEDICAL CARE • 43

The Development of Cancer Treatment

As early as 1953, Hurley Hospital was named among the 232 "four-star" United States hospitals that housed a new specialty cancer clinic. Since 1956, Hurley's cancer program has received continuous approval from the ACS Commission on Cancer, meeting the qualifications for a Community Hospital Comprehensive Cancer Program, with a dedicated team of trained oncology specialists involved in every aspect of screening, diagnosis, treatment, recovery, and rehabilitation. Board-certified physicians and nurses develop individual, comprehensive patient- and family-centered treatment plans for each patient.

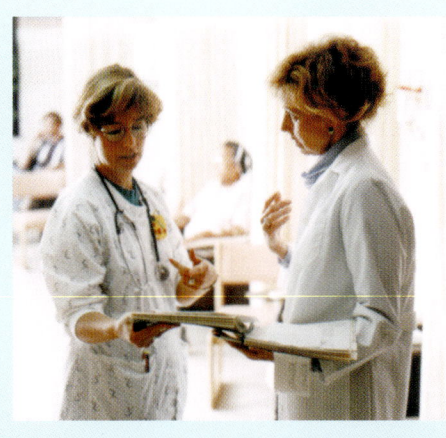

Well-known research nurse Deborah Frick, RN (left), played a pivotal role in the development of the Genesys Hurley Cancer Institute. Frick was in charge of managing a myriad of patient cancer protocols for years. Frick is pictured with Dr. Sharon Dowd, an oncologist.

Hurley established its outpatient chemotherapy clinic in 1977 and served about 650 patients in the first five years; the name was changed to Hurley's Hematology-Oncology Clinic to better reflect the fuller range of services. According to cancer specialist Sharon Dowd, MD, "Death rates for various cancers had been declining since 1960. The survival rates for about a dozen cancers, including Hodgkin's disease and childhood leukemia, have been dramatic." She attributed the progress to the steady advancements in the three traditional methods of treating cancer—surgery, radiation, and chemotherapy—along with new ways to use these techniques to increase the chances of a cure. "Promising new treatments, such as immunotherapy, are being developed and refined to provide even more hope," she added.

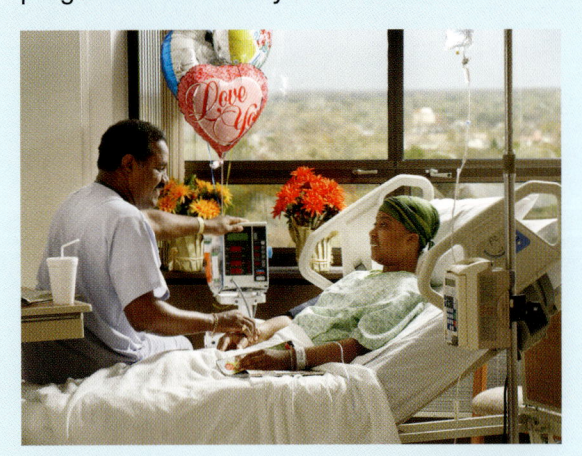

Terry Thomas, RN, sits with a cancer patient, 2008

For many years, Hurley doctors and researchers contributed to the development of cancer treatments over a broad range. In 2001, the new Genesys Hurley Cancer Institute was established as a partnership to broaden cancer treatment in the area.

medication is scanned to be sure the medication to be given is the correct dose, at the correct time, and to the correct patient. This is a huge step forward for patient safety."

"HMC is different than other medical centers in that the IT function and development is handled in-house. We pitch in together to get the job done while wearing several hats," said Mike Joseph, senior director of IT. "System security has come to the forefront of priorities. Over the past five years, the IT team has been working on best practices to protect infrastructure stability," said Joseph. Fast-forward to 2020, and technical capability is of utmost importance.

Technology is also being used at HMC to conduct virtual office visits between physicians and patients. According to Teresa Bourque, RN, BSN, chief nurse, "Maternal fetal medicine started using telemedicine in or about 2013, but outpatient and specialty clinics ramped up their usage in March 2020" in response to the coronavirus pandemic, which limited the physical access of patients to their physicians. The telemedicine program establishes a one-to-one link between patient and doctor. The IT staff helped physicians with the platform and, in turn, help patients use the technology. Telemedicine is different than telehealth, which is a service that provides health-related answers and information. "I think telemedicine will continue to expand into the future," adds Bourque. "Some patients really like the convenience of the service, but others find the technology challenging."

"Hurley has a history of being the leader in this community for utilizing technology in patient care areas, beginning with CISCO many years ago and continuing today with Epic," said Dr. Roebuck. "This commitment was evident when we were validated as a Healthcare Information and Management Systems Society (HIMSS) Stage 7 hospital. HIMSS performs a full-day, on-site survey to validate HMC's electronic patient care capabilities. To be Stage 7, you must maximize your electronic tools and have proven outcomes related to the technology. At the time of our validation, HMC was one of only three health systems in the state to be validated as meeting all Stage 7 requirements. This is an incredible accomplishment for a hospital of our size with our limited resources."

Robotic Surgery

The ability to mimic the surgeon's hand movements with enhanced dexterity is why HMC welcomes surgeons who have expert training in minimally invasive surgery, such as robotics, for a wide range of surgical procedures. Robotics provides an advanced level of technology that takes surgery beyond the limits of the human hand and

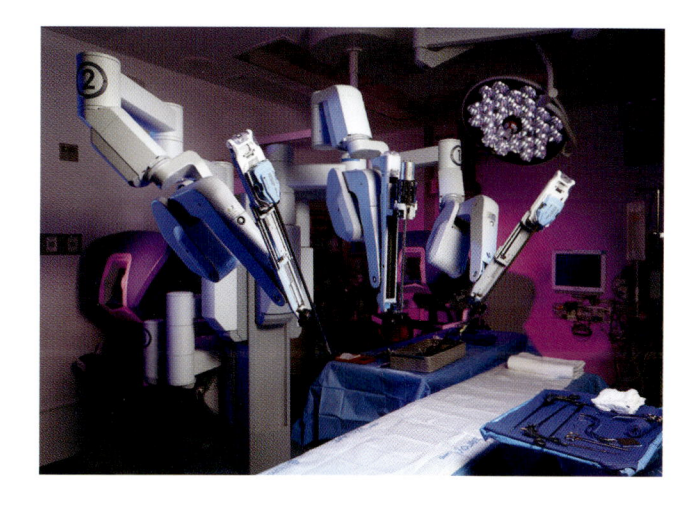

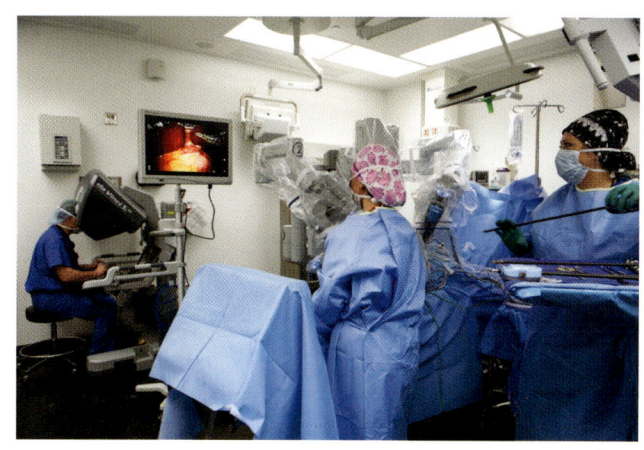

DaVinci robotic surgery system

CHAPTER TWO A REGIONAL LEADER IN ADVANCED MEDICAL CARE • 45

complements the goal of extending minimally invasive surgery to the broadest base of patients. Surgeries such as gallbladder removal, hysterectomies, hernia repairs, myomectomies, removal of adrenal glands, gastroesophageal reflux disease (GERD)-related diagnoses, and esophageal stricture are currently being done with robotics. Some known benefits of robotic surgery are faster healing, lower complications, generally smaller incisions, and higher patient satisfaction.

Laboratory Services

HMC's laboratory is a technologically advanced, full-service clinical laboratory that performs nearly 3.3 million tests per year. The laboratory services team consists of nearly 100 experienced employees, including four board-certified pathologists. Since it was built in 1976, the laboratory has occupied most of the first floor of the North Tower.

Pathologists provide higher-level, complex diagnostic services in clinical and anatomic pathology, and they work closely with physicians from all departments at HMC. Clinical biochemist Harland Verrill, PhD, whose skills added a crucial resource for consultation, test utilization, and interpretation, was part of a research team that investigated muscular dystrophy in the late 1970s. He worked in conjunction with two out-of-state researchers to develop a new test that identified carriers of muscular dystrophy and was considered to be a significant breakthrough at the time in understanding the muscular dystrophy diseases.[11] Today, HMC staff collaborate on unique consultations with faculty from the University of Michigan.

In 2005, construction began on a new, state-of-the-art facility of one of the nation's largest laboratory automation systems. The 63-foot-long Siemens automation track accommodates a total of nine analyzers, two centrifuges, and two sample managers. Tests performed by analyzers on the automation track account for 85 percent of all of the laboratory testing, in the specialties of chemistry, immunochemistry, hematology, coagulation, and urinalysis. HMC provides the largest menu of testing services, in scope and in volume, available in the service area. HMC continued to adapt and evolve the clinical laboratory through the use of advanced technology in 2010, developing the lab's molecular diagnostics capabilities as the wave of the future.

"We have to be able to adjust to all changes and the equipment that we have will keep up with future needs. That, along with close interaction and a high level of staff tenure, efficient and accurate analysis, and a

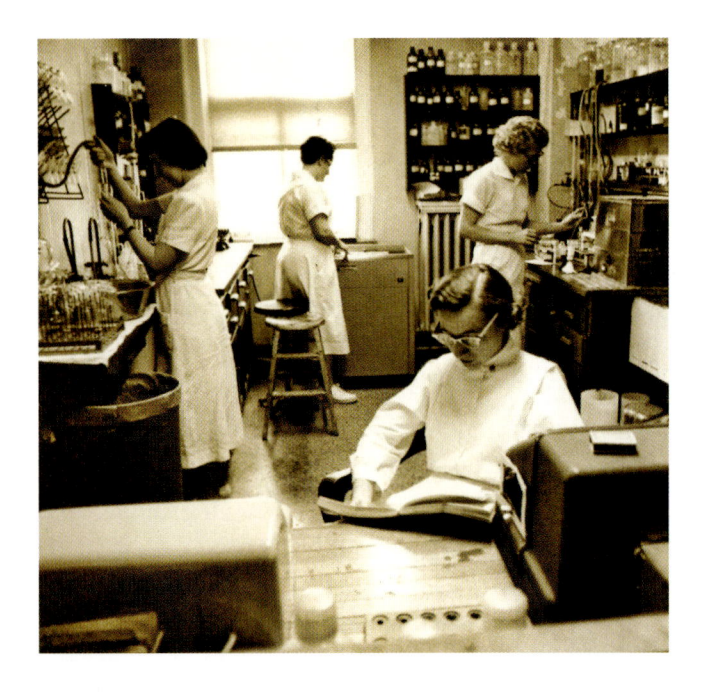

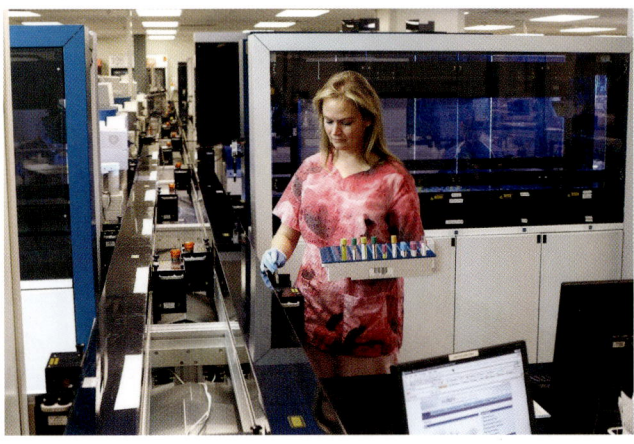

Laboratory, yesterday and today

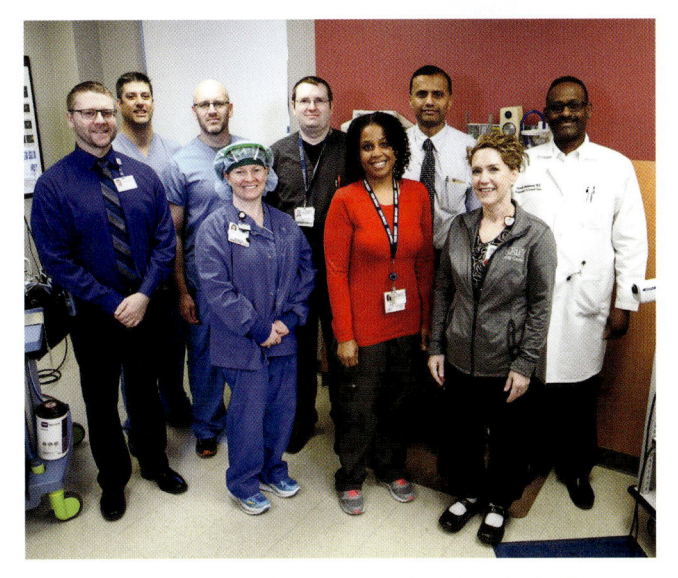

Hurley Lung Center celebrates its 100th patient in the first year, March 2017. Left to right: Rick Barker, RRT, BS; Kevin Reynolds, RRT; Shawn Watts, RRT; Margaret Kohler, RN; Ryan Cohee, RRT; Krysten Chambers, cytology tech; Piyush Patel, MD; Ronise Waite, RN; and Elfateh Seedahmed, MD.

significantly low error rate, enables us to provide precise and quick test results to physicians and their patients more quickly," said V. Mitra Tewari, MBA, MLS (ASCP) SM, administrative director of Clinical Laboratory, who was hired as a staff microbiologist in December 2008.

In December 2019, HMC implemented a rapid diagnostic test (RDT) into the standard microbiology workflow for positive blood cultures. RDTs for bloodstream infections are automatically performed 24/7, in addition to all current lab processes. This diagnostic testing can identify pathogens about 24 hours earlier than the previous method of culture-only. The notable advancement and efficiency of Hurley's laboratory was a major benefit as HMC battled COVID-19 and the extreme demand for testing.

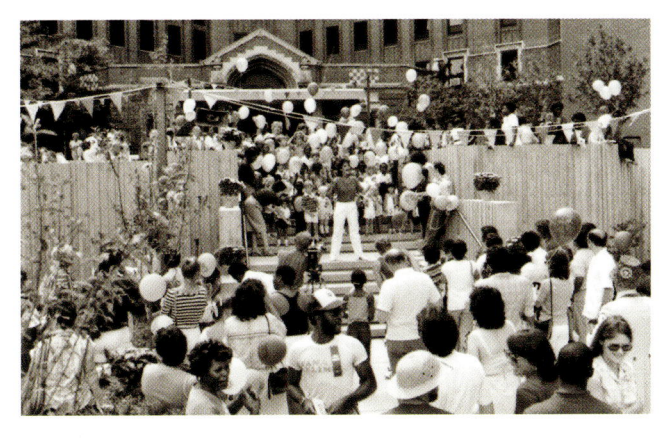

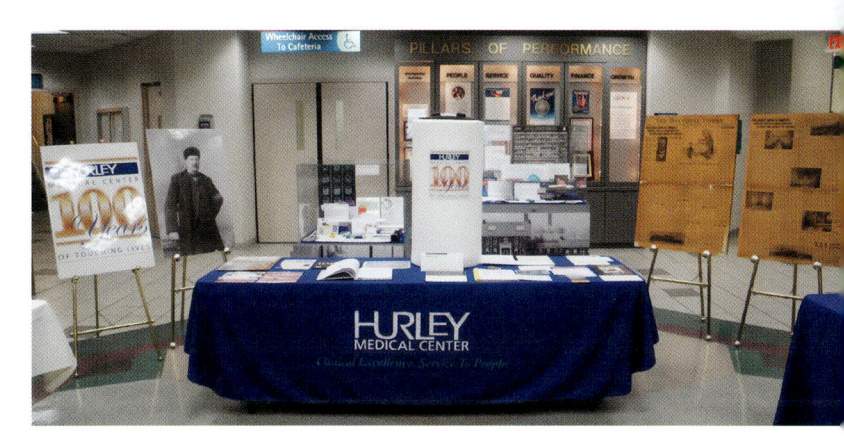

HMC 75th Anniversary, 1983

The three-day celebration took place from Friday, July 29, to Sunday, July 31, featuring a continuing medical education seminar on sports medicine and a pre-race clinic on Friday. The Tuuri 10,000 race was held on Saturday with 1,000 runners, followed by a dinner-dance with Hurley employees, medical staff, alumni, and friends at the Flint Hyatt Regency. On Sunday, a free, public ice cream social was held at Dort Park, adjacent to Hurley's West Lobby. Shown here are children born at Hurley singing "Happy Birthday, Hurley" for those who attended the ice cream social.

HMC 100th Anniversary, 2008

On January 15, 2008, the Historical Society of Michigan unveiled a plaque honoring Hurley's 100 consecutive years in one location. The event was commemorated with numerous elected officials, community members, physicians, and staff, along with a special anniversary cake and photograph displays with artifacts from the past. The Hurley Heritage Festival, a public celebration, was held on August 2 and featured Hurley baby and American Idol singer Lakisha Jones, who performed to a crowd of 3,000 at the "old-fashioned block party." At year's end, each department selected an item that represented the way they serve their patients, along with a message board of staff members' personal messages to their future counterparts, which was placed in a time capsule to be opened in 2108. The message to those who open the capsule in 2108: "To James J. Hurley's turn of the twentieth century dream . . . We begin our next century with a new cardiac center, a completely upgraded state-of-the-art radiology department providing the highest degree of diagnostics, and a focus on patient-centered care. We continue to embrace our role as a model public hospital as we move ahead into our next century of 'Touching Lives Through Better Medicine.'"[12]

CHAPTER TWO A REGIONAL LEADER IN ADVANCED MEDICAL CARE • 47

HMC Distinguished Programs as of 2020

- Level I Trauma Center (highest level)
- Level III Neonatal Intensive Care Unit (highest level)
- Level III GEDA-accredited Geriatric Emergency Department
- Hurley Children's Hospital
- Blue Cross Blue Shield Center of Michigan Designated Blue Distinction Center COE Hip and Knee Replacements
- The ACS Commission on Cancer for the Community Hospital Comprehensive Cancer Program
- Kidney Transplantation Partnership with Henry Ford Health System
- Hurley Diabetes Center
- Hurley Bariatric Center of Excellence
- Project JOINTS exemplar hospital
- The Joint Commission Advanced Primary Stroke Center

CENTER FOR JOINT REPLACEMENT

Among the leading programs in the region and recognized by Blue Cross Blue Shield (BCBS) for expertise and efficiency in delivering knee and hip replacement care, Hurley's Center for Joint Replacement opened in 2007. The center is part of a national initiative to implement proven methods for preventing surgical site infection, high patient satisfaction ratings, and an emphasis on promoting wellness and recovery care tailored to individual needs. Part of an extensive continuum of care that includes an educational preoperative evaluation and postoperative rehabilitation, the surgeons routinely perform shoulder, hip, knee, ankle, elbow, wrist, and finger joint replacement surgeries. HMC is one of only two Project JOINTS exemplar hospitals in the state of Michigan.

KIDNEY TRANSPLANTATION

In September 1966, a six-member committee of physicians gathered to discuss starting an artificial kidney treatment at Hurley Hospital to help relieve the plight of the mounting numbers of desperate patients. They treated patients on the machine in emergency situations and also assessed the patient's chance of benefiting from long-term machine treatment or kidney transplant operations. The program initially accepted four patients with incurable kidney disease. According to a committee spokesman, "The lucky four now are being kept alive in a hospital close to home—so they can lead near-normal lives and make themselves useful in the community, and so doctors can determine whether medically they can be candidates for kidney transplants." At the time, transplantation was still in the experimental stage. The rigid screening process had a patient age limitation of 40 years or younger. "It's all so experimental," continued the spokesperson. "All [kidney] facilities are overloaded. The pressure is tremendous. One doesn't realize how difficult it is to make each selection. When a committee has to make a choice, it's close to playing God." Stanley Biddis was the first Flint-area resident to receive treatment for complete kidney failure at Hurley Hospital on an artificial kidney machine.

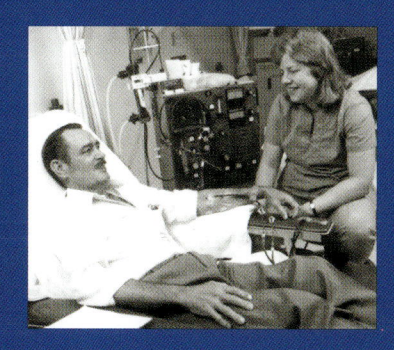

The Flint Journal, February 19, 1967, "Flint Kidney Victims Live with Hope"

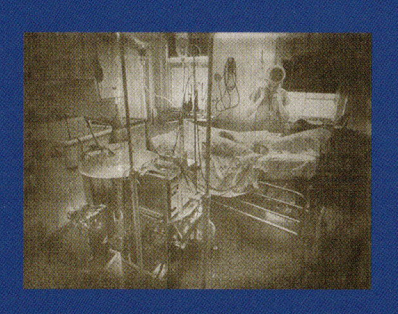

Theda Wright from Clio was the first female and the second of the four chosen to receive treatment on an artificial kidney machine at Hurley Hospital. Ernest "Ernie" Wright inherited kidney disease from his mother, Theda Wright. Ernie's kidneys failed at age 36. When he first started his hemodialysis treatments at Hurley's Renal Center in 1975, the procedure (in which three times each week, blood is pumped out of his body and through a machine, cleansed, and returned to his body) took four to five hours. After many years and with medical advancements, his treatments were completed after only three hours. Ernie did not let his reliance on the kidney machine stop him from living a full life. Starting in 1987 and after his Friday treatments, Ernie drove to ballroom dancing classes and regularly participated in dance competitions; at age 57, he won first place in the waltz! "You can live a full life as long as you have the right attitude. But I don't know what I would have done if Hurley hadn't been there for me," said Wright.

Today, the kidney transplant program at HMC holds an outstanding partnership with Henry Ford Transplant Institute (HFTI). Performing transplants since 1968, the HFTI has built one of the nation's most successful programs, performing more than 100 kidney transplants each year. As one of the multiple-organ transplant centers in Michigan, they also transplant bone marrow and all other primary organs.

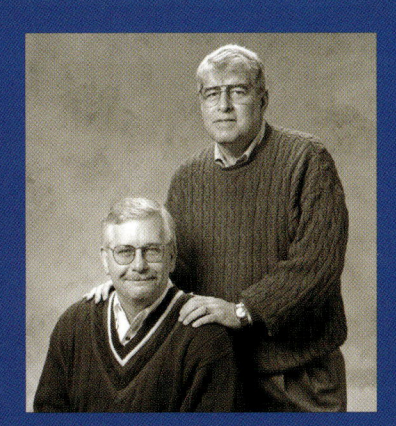

Hurley's first living, unrelated kidney transplant took place in 1996 between Ron Colavincenzo (right) and donor Mike Charlier. Ron had a family history of kidney disease and was diagnosed in 1975; his condition was managed with medication until 1994. He went on the kidney transplant waiting list, but his close friend and Bible study member, Mike, offered to donate his kidney.

CHAPTER TWO A REGIONAL LEADER IN ADVANCED MEDICAL CARE • 49

HURLEY DIABETES CENTER

A comprehensive diabetes program offering inpatient and outpatient services opened in 2000 at the Hurley Eastside Campus. The diabetes education program is the largest program in Genesee County, offering an adult diabetes education program, diabetes-during-pregnancy education, and pediatric diabetes education. This program is recognized by the American Diabetes Association and certified by the Michigan Department of Community Health as a quality, self-management, diabetes education program.

HURLEY BARIATRIC CENTER OF EXCELLENCE

Hurley Bariatric Comprehensive Surgery Center with BCBS Blue distinction opened in 1999. Highly skilled, board-certified surgeons specialize in bariatric surgery and are credentialed in critical care at a Level I Trauma Center. More than 5,000 procedures, such as the Roux-en-Y gastric bypass, sleeve gastrectomy, and adjustable gastric band, have been performed. In 2006, Hurley Bariatric Center was designated a "Center of Excellence" by the ACS. Hurley was the first bariatric center in Michigan to be given this designation, and one of only five in the nation with this accreditation.

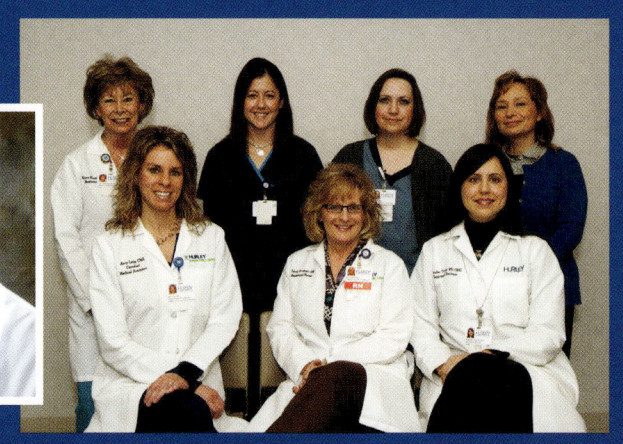

The bariatric team (back, left to right): Kaye Kaufherr RN, BSN; Jennifer McCracken, insurance specialist; Triena Rudder, program assistant; Dee Cassels, insurance specialist; (front) Amy Benner, MA; Linda Krueger RN, bariatric clinical coordinator; and Jennifer Traub, RD.

Left: Jamal Farhan, MD, FACS, bariatric surgeon

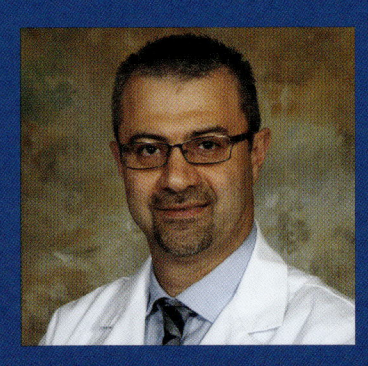

ADVANCED PRIMARY STROKE CENTER

HMC is designated as a Primary Stroke Center by the Joint Commission for providing patients with the highest-quality stroke care based on scientific research and improvements in treatment. Providing exceptional stroke care while educating communities, HMC received the Get with the Guidelines – Stroke Gold Elite Plus Quality Achievement Award from the American Heart Association and the American Stroke Association for consistently giving the most-appropriate treatment according to nationally established, research-based guidelines.

Mohammed Al-Qasmi, MD, Director, HMC Stroke Program

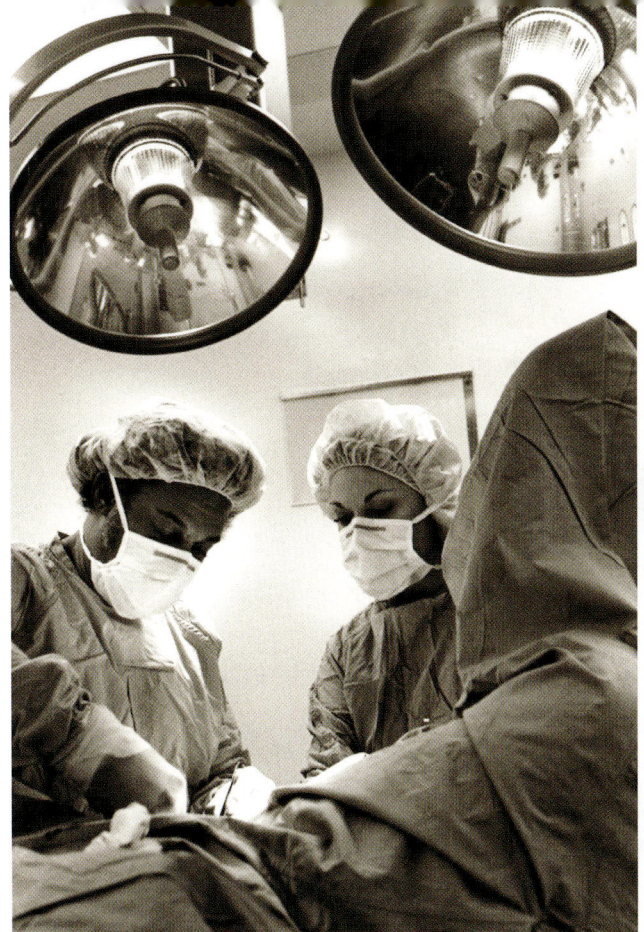

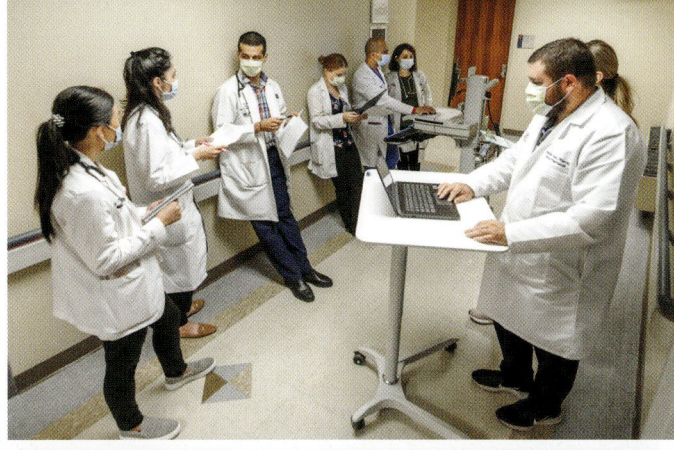

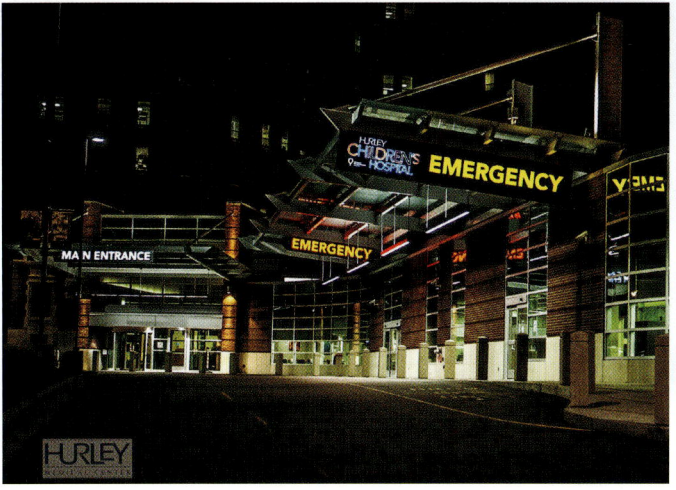

Top right: Clockwise from the left: Kathleen Dinh, medical student; Hina Amin, MD, resident physician; Adiraj Singh, MD, attending physician; Sara Clements, RN, nurse case manager; Pujan Kandel, MD, resident physician; Ann Sedeeq, MD, resident physician; and Brandon Flues, PharmD, clinical pharmacist.

Much of the information in this chapter about early Hurley Hospital history is from the 80th anniversary publication of Inside Report *in 1988, published by the Hurley Foundation in Flint, Michigan.*

NOTES

1. https://journals.lww.com/em-news/Pages/emhistory.aspx.
2. http://www.connectionnewspapers.com/news/2006/may/31/the-alexandria-plan-a-national-model/.
3. Hurley Foundation, *Inside Report* (Summer 1990), p. 6.
4. Ibid., p. 6.
5. https://journalofethics.ama-assn.org/article/social-justice-egalitarianism-and-history-emergency-medicine/2010-06.
6. Hurley Foundation, *Inside Report* (March 1980), p. 4.
7. Hurley Foundation, *Inside Report* (Number Two, 1991), p. 34.
8. Hurley Foundation, *News You Can Use* (*NYCU*) Vol. 17, Issue 3 (March 2020), p. 2.
9. Sara Schuch, MLive.com, August 5, 2014, https://www.mlive.com/news/flint/2014/08/im_a_survivor_teen_cancer_surv.html.
10. Sloan Museum and Longway Planetarium: https://sloanlongway.org/beecher-tornado-of-1953/.
11. Hurley Medical Center Annual Report, 1978–79, p. 8.
12. Hurley Medical Center, *News You Can Use* (December 2008), p. 1.

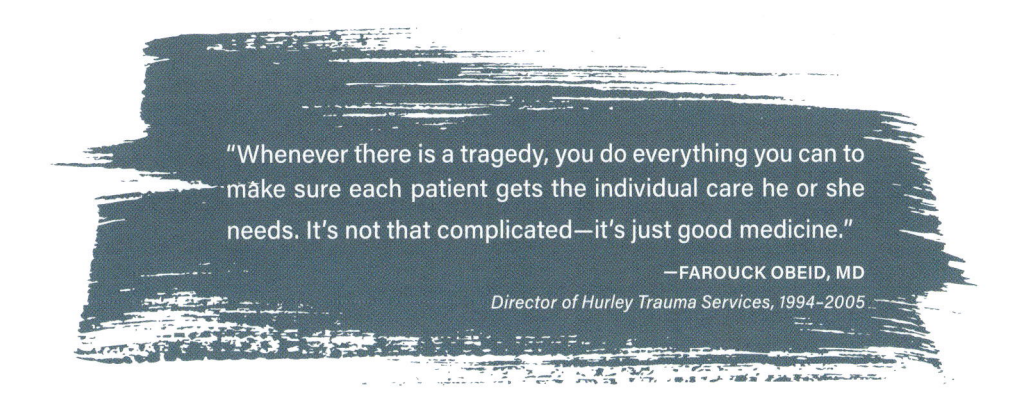

"Whenever there is a tragedy, you do everything you can to make sure each patient gets the individual care he or she needs. It's not that complicated—it's just good medicine."

—FAROUCK OBEID, MD
Director of Hurley Trauma Services, 1994–2005

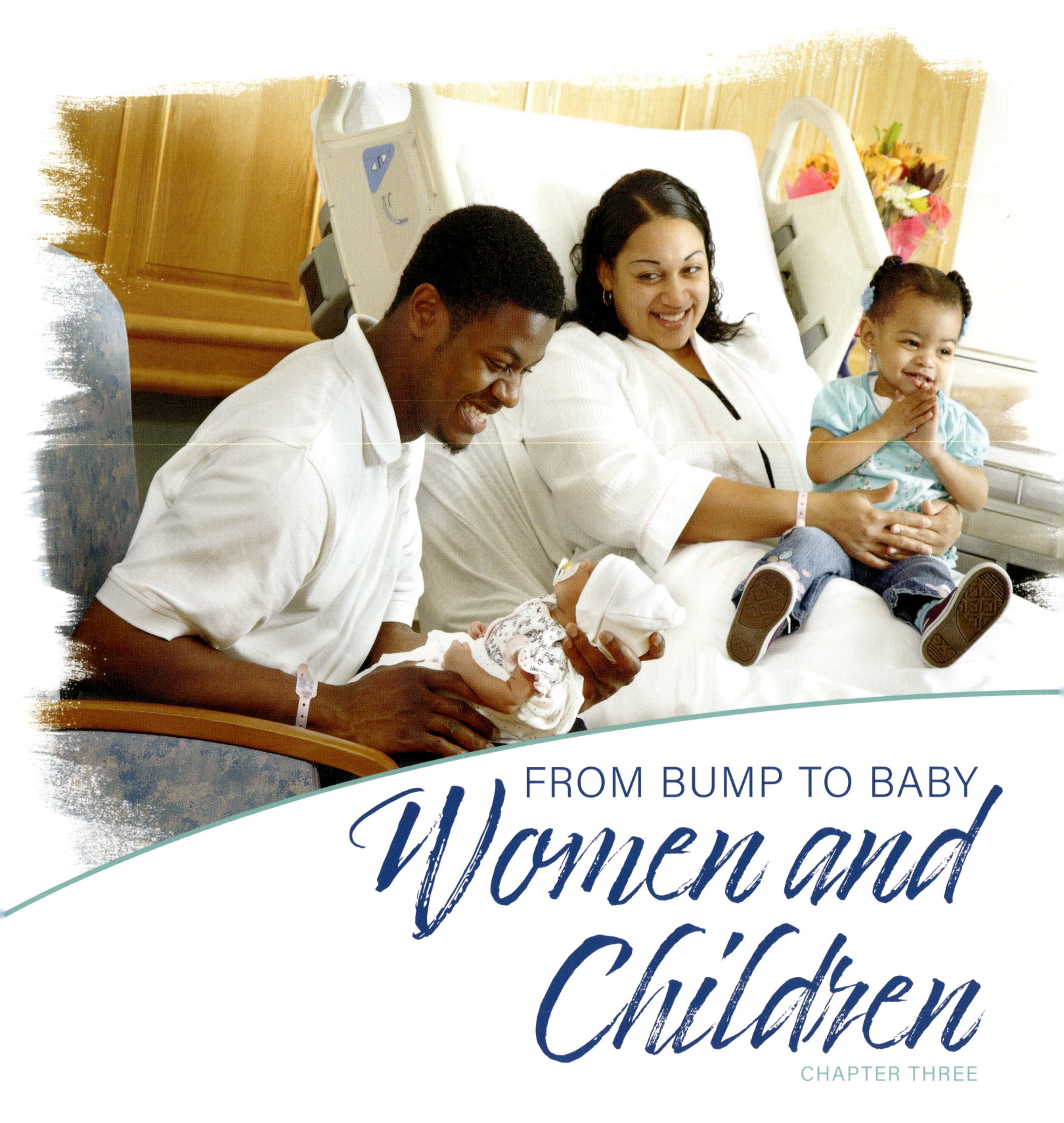

FROM BUMP TO BABY
Women and Children
CHAPTER THREE

Obstetrics and Gynecology

The best services. The best equipment. The best staff. The best variety of choices. Hurley babies have the best.[1] That is the declarative statement from staff and administrators in 1993, and it continues to be true today. Hurley started Flint's first Obstetrical Care

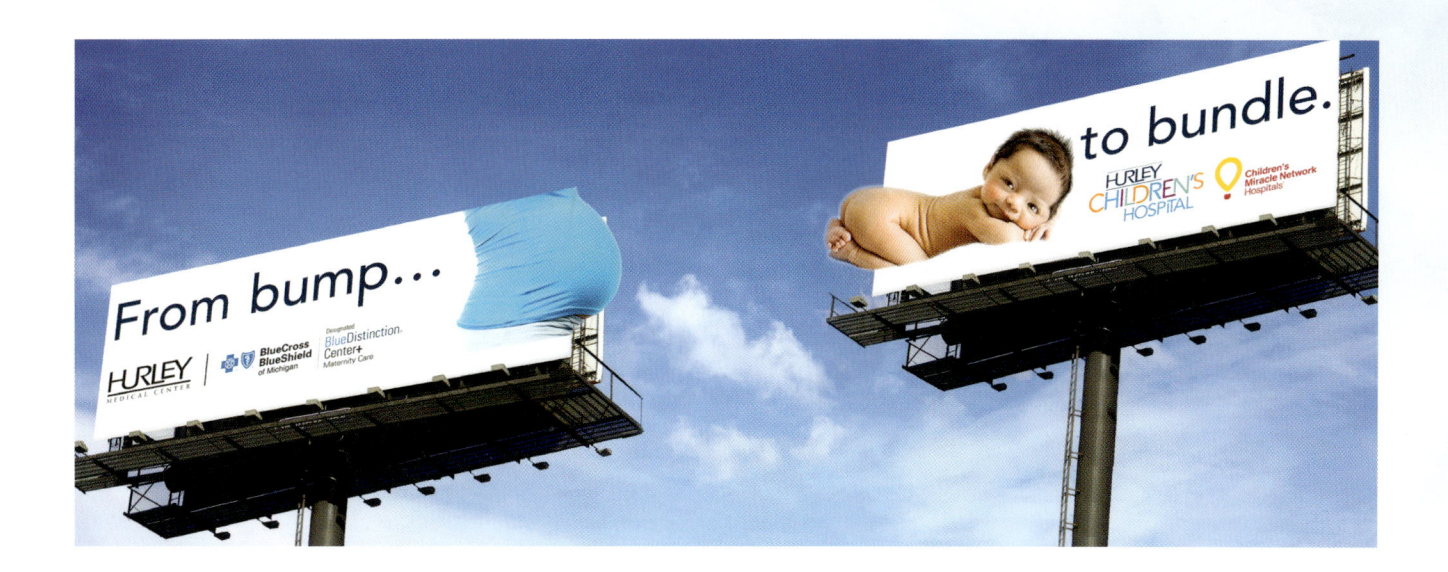

Unit in 1908, with six bassinets. On February 13, 1913, a women's group organized to propose the building of a "Maternity Hospital and Children's Home." The nucleus of this group was from the former Women's Auxiliary Hospital Board, which had disbanded the previous year. The goal was to build close enough in proximity to Hurley Hospital as to be operated by the same management and heated by the same power plant.[2] On March 7, 1913, at a meeting that included Flint's mayor, C. S. Mott, and Hurley Hospital's superintendent, Anna M. Schill, it was decided that the "Women and Children's Hospital" should be built as a unit of Hurley Hospital rather than as an independent hospital. Funds were raised from the Mary Stockdale estate for the $18,386 to be used for the addition, and the ladies group agreed to furnish the equipment. Taxation appropriations of $42,835 were needed for the "great increase in the cost of building materials"

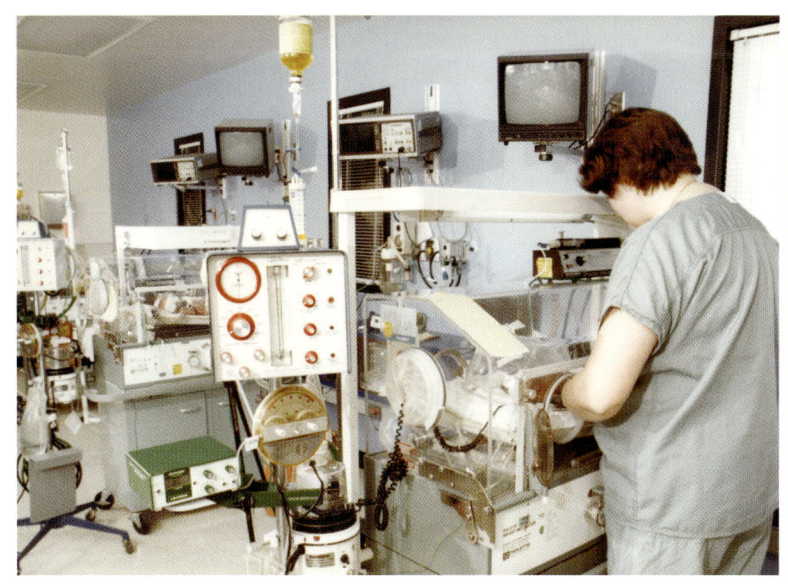

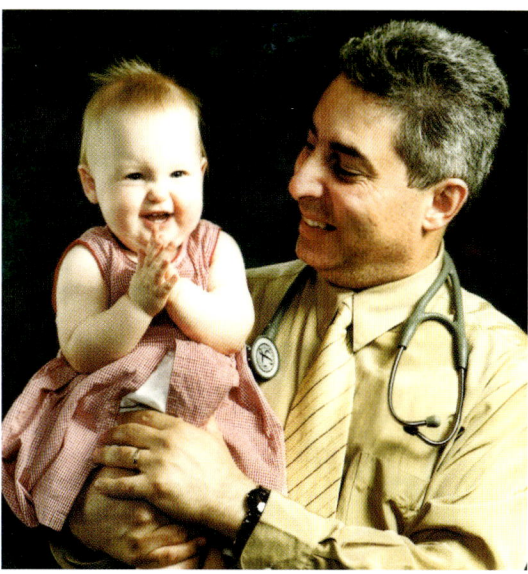

Left: NICU circa the 1990s

Right: Many area couples have been blessed with babies due to the expertise of Mostafa Abuzied, MD, as a pioneer in reproductive and infertility medicine.

CHAPTER THREE FROM BUMP TO BABY – WOMEN AND CHILDREN • 53

to see this project to completion.[3] The Maternity Unit opened in the spring of 1917 and was attached to the nurses' residence. The new building offered 26 beds, 26 bassinets, a delivery room, and other facilities. The building later became a Venereal Disease Center, and then the Psychiatric Unit.[4]

Many levels of expertise are readily available at HMC, from conception to birth. Mostafa Abuzeid, MD, reproductive endocrinology and infertility specialist, was the first in the United States to treat male infertility through intracytoplasmic sperm injection (ICSI) in 1994. ICSI is a procedure in which a single male sperm is injected into the cytoplasm of an egg. He also pioneered microsurgery and laparoscopic techniques to cure infertility in women and resolve gynecological disorders. Generations of Flint residents have begun their lives at Hurley. HMC's reputation has become "the place" for expectant mothers to have their babies, especially if complications arise. In fact, the average number of births per year at HMC ranges around 2,700 annually.

"The obstetric experience for women in the 1970s was a much different experience," said John Hebert III, MD, program director for the Obstetrics and Gynecology (Ob-Gyn) Residency Program, former department chair from 1986 to 2011, and 2001 Hurley Pinnacle Award recipient. "Pregnant women would arrive and be placed in a labor room and then for the actual birth they would be moved to a delivery room. After delivery, they would be taken to a recovery room and, finally, to a postpartum room on another floor. There was a trend across the US back then to change this outdated tradition to a concept that allowed women to labor, deliver, and recover in the same family-centered room. During my tenure as department chair, this concept was adopted and implemented in the 2 North Tower Labor and Delivery Unit and in the 1 East Tower Birthing Center," said Dr. Hebert. In 1991, HMC piloted a labor-delivery-recovery program, and in 1993, construction began within the 1 East Tower wing on single-room maternity suites, for laboring, delivering, and recovery, that offered mother and baby a homelike atmosphere.

Along with a significant number of Ob-Gyn faculty physicians who care for patients on an inpatient and outpatient basis, HMC is happy to welcome the patients of a number of private practice Ob-Gyn physicians for their deliveries and other hospital-based needs. In addition, HMC has offered midwifery services since 2014, which offers an alternate care model for mothers to use for their delivery.

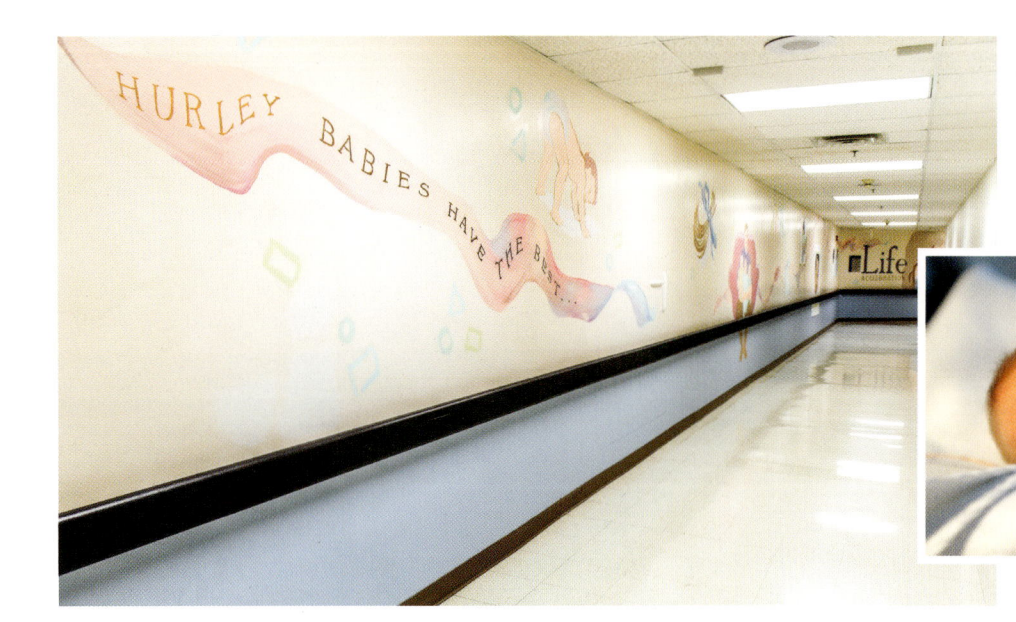

Hurley babies wall

High-Risk Obstetrics

HMC has devoted resources, caring staff, and specialists in high-risk obstetrics, as well as the area's only Level III (highest level) Neonatal Intensive Care Unit (NICU), allowing comprehensive care for high-risk pregnancies and deliveries. Hurley's team of ob-gyns provide expert and compassionate care for routine pregnancies to the most-complex cases. Maternal-Fetal Medicine (MFM) and the Diabetes in Pregnancy Program (DPP) provide specialists with advanced training in medical and surgical complications of pregnancy, as well as prematurity and prenatal diagnosis of genetic and birth defects. Patients from the Perinatal Center are supported by HMC's Neonatal Intensive Care Unit. Hurley perinatal/neonatal services are unique in the region.

Level III Neonatal Intensive Care Unit

Caring for the most-at-risk premature babies was the major goal in establishing the regional Neonatal Intensive Care Unit in 1973. Neonatal care was a relatively new medical subspecialty at the time, and it was under the direction of Raymond Chan, MD, a neonatologist, who had a direct impact on infant mortality in the region. Flint fell from having the highest infant mortality in Michigan to below the state average within four years. By 1977, the NICU renovation had expanded the facility and earned a Level III status (the highest level).

In 1983, HMC was still the only hospital in the region that could perform surgery on premature babies. "In the first few minutes of life for these babies, every second counts," said Dr. Chan, who was a major force in the neonatal complex design. "That's our goal here, to lose as little of that precious time as possible. To make the most of those vital seconds, the delivery room is adjacent to a stabilization room. From there, a child can be whisked away to the 'mission room,'

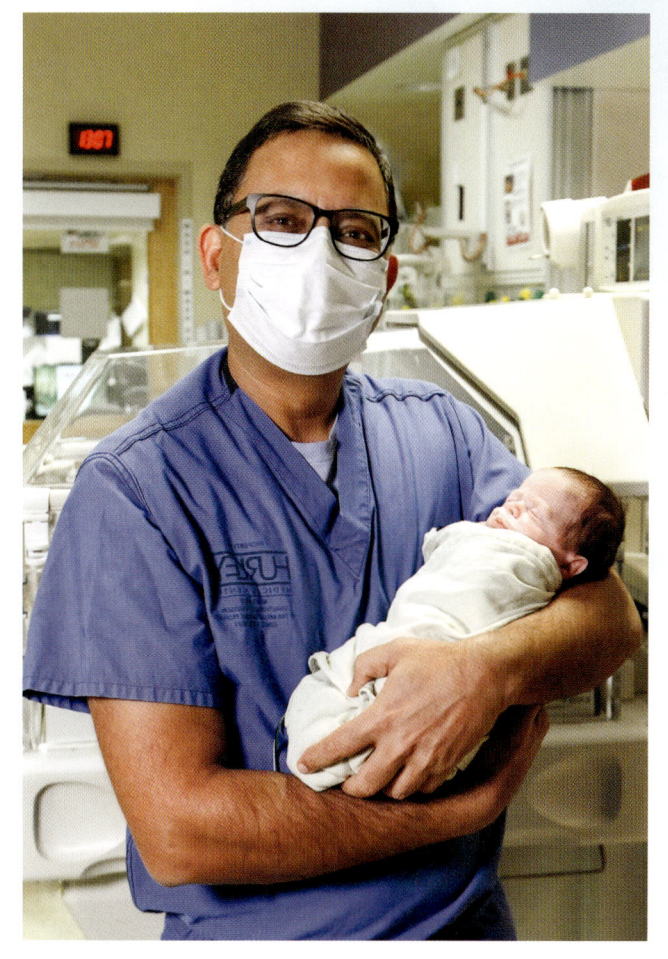

Ranjan Monga, MD, with NICU patient

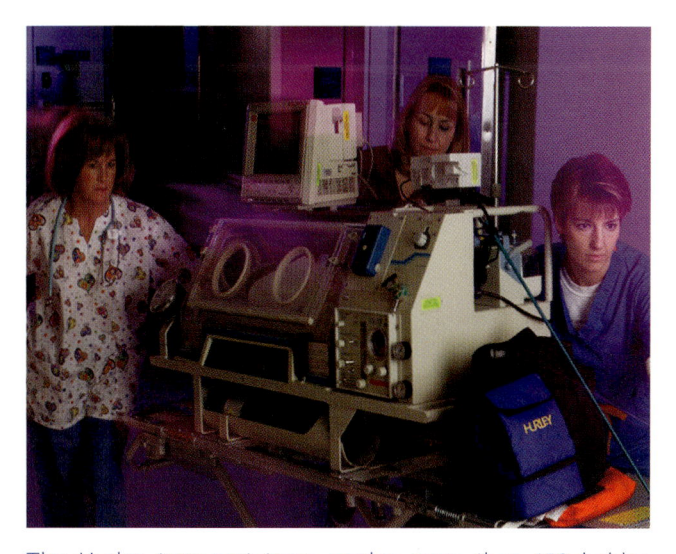

The Hurley transport team carries more than 150 babies annually to the NICU. The team was dispatched to pick up babies throughout the region from the 1980s to the 2000s with a specially equipped transporter to monitor the baby. Left to right: Lynn Neeland, RN, Darcy Coon, RN, and Mary Miller, RRT.

CHAPTER THREE FROM BUMP TO BABY – WOMEN AND CHILDREN • 55

Top left: Nurse with NICU baby

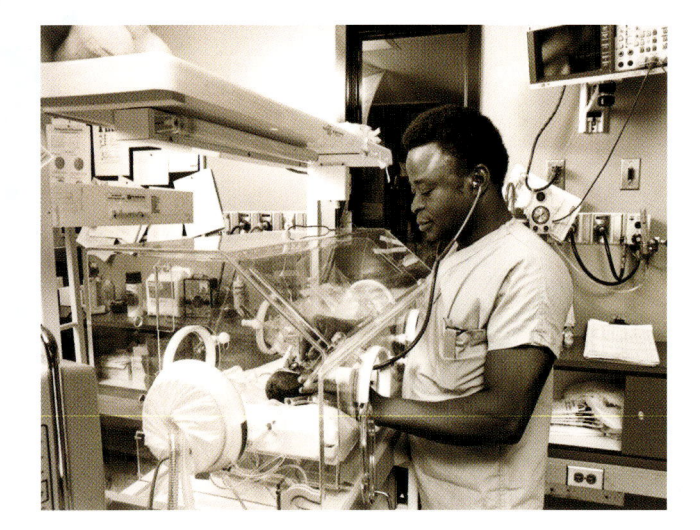

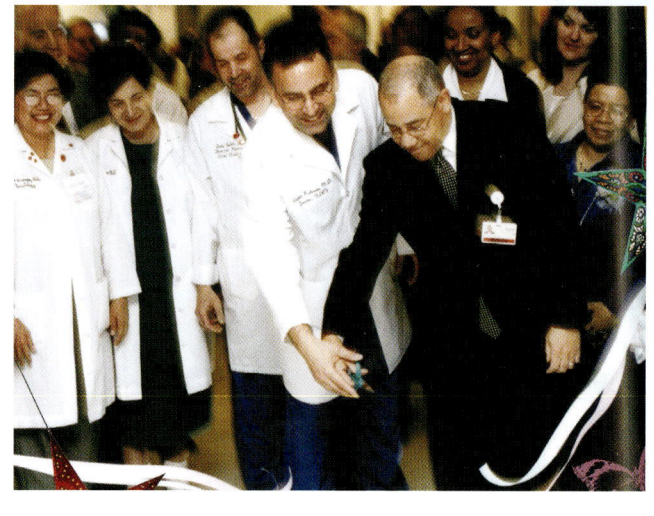

Top right: Julius Spears, Hurley CEO (right), NICU renovation ribbon cutting, 2003

Left: Flint mayor Woodrow Stanley (left) congratulates Raymond Chan, MD, director of Neonatology, at the 20th anniversary of the regional NICU in front of thousands who showed up to celebrate the 15,000 NICU graduates who had received care.

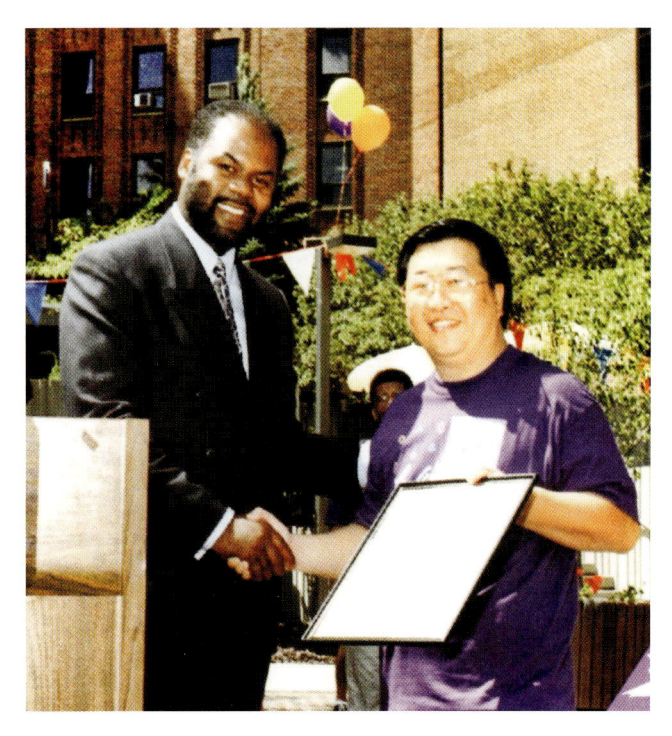

where a respiratory therapist is always on hand to assist the doctor and nurse. An X-ray room and lab are just a few steps away, allowing the physician to have the X-ray and vital information in their hands in 90 seconds," Dr. Chan explained.[5]

At the 20th anniversary in 1993, the NICU had provided care for between 800 and 900 newborns annually, who had needed the unit's highly specialized equipment and uniquely skilled nursing expertise.

In 2000, the Hurley Foundation kicked off a NICU renovation campaign called "Give Our Babies Room to Grow," with a goal of raising $2.5 million. Funds were used to upgrade equipment and lighting, and to create physical space for patient treatment, family interaction, and technological support. The project included expanded space for patients, high-frequency ventilation equipment, and specialized isolettes for premature infants. The new unit opened on March 26, 2003. For the 150 babies who are born at other hospitals each year and need to be transported to Hurley for specialized care, there is a Hurley transport team that picks up the baby in a specially designed Transport Unit that helps the team protect and monitor the baby until they arrive at HMC's NICU.

Today's NICU provides care for close to 800 babies each year[6] and is designed specifically to support dangerously ill newborns, most of which are premature;

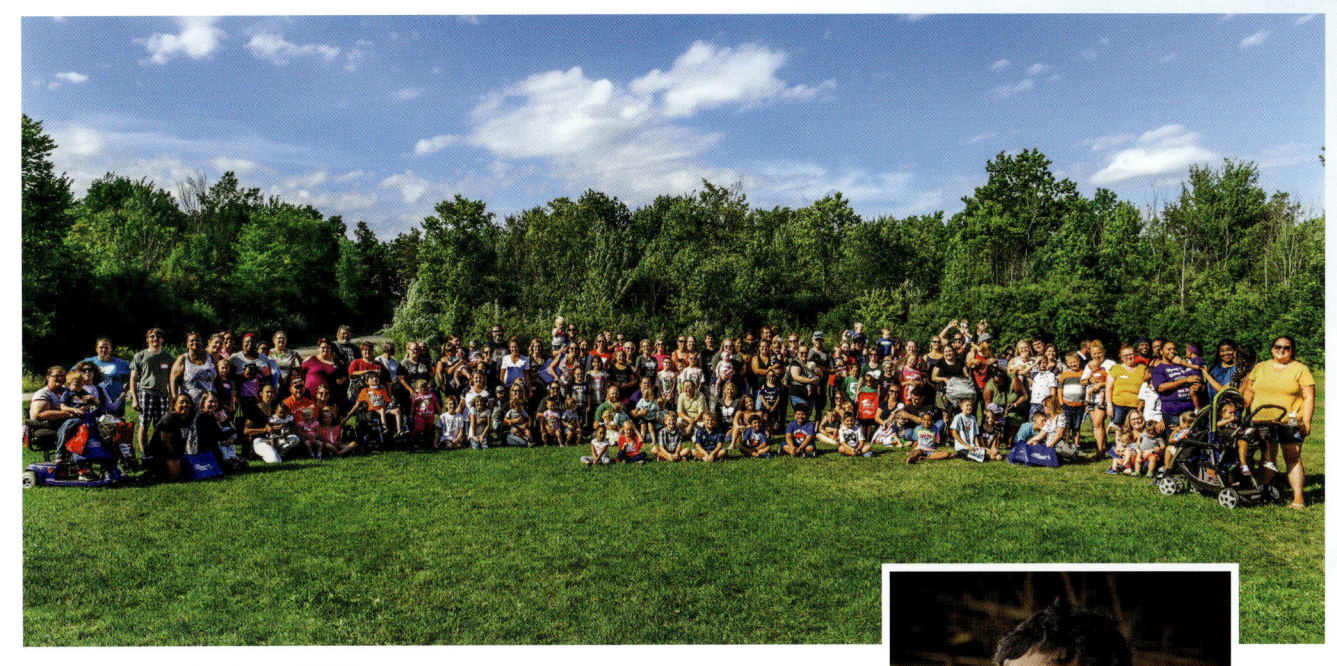

Connected by Miracles – NICU Reunions
In 2019, more than 250 people, including doctors and nurses, joined together at Bicentennial Park in Grand Blanc to celebrate NICU grads, who are lifelong members of the Hurley family. Every five years, Hurley Children's Hospital hosts a special NICU reunion for families of children who began life requiring the specialized care of Hurley's NICU staff.

Right: Cashton Cruz Mingo celebrates life.

babies may also have congenital problems, diseases, or infections. Though these cases are severe, most survive, thanks to the team of skilled experts. Once the patient leaves the hospital, their progress is followed by both Hurley and Mott Children's Health Center staff.

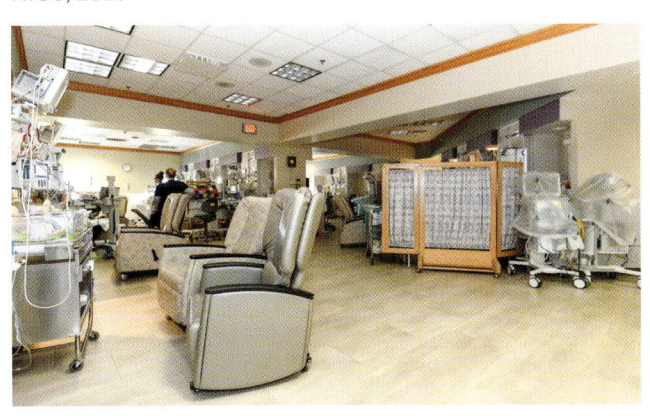

NICU, 2020

The Early Years

On October 2, 1939, a small health clinic that the Mott Foundation funded through the Flint Board of Education moved to Hurley Hospital in a 1,400-square-foot space, and it officially became known as the Mott Children's Health Center (MCHC). According to C. S. Mott, "If anyone is going to do anything on earth to help humanity, doing something for children is a good place to start." At that time, children's health services only amounted to what was provided within school systems, such as immunizations, school and camp physicals, and general health advice. Dr. James Olson, director of Flint's school health program,

CHAPTER THREE FROM BUMP TO BABY – WOMEN AND CHILDREN • 57

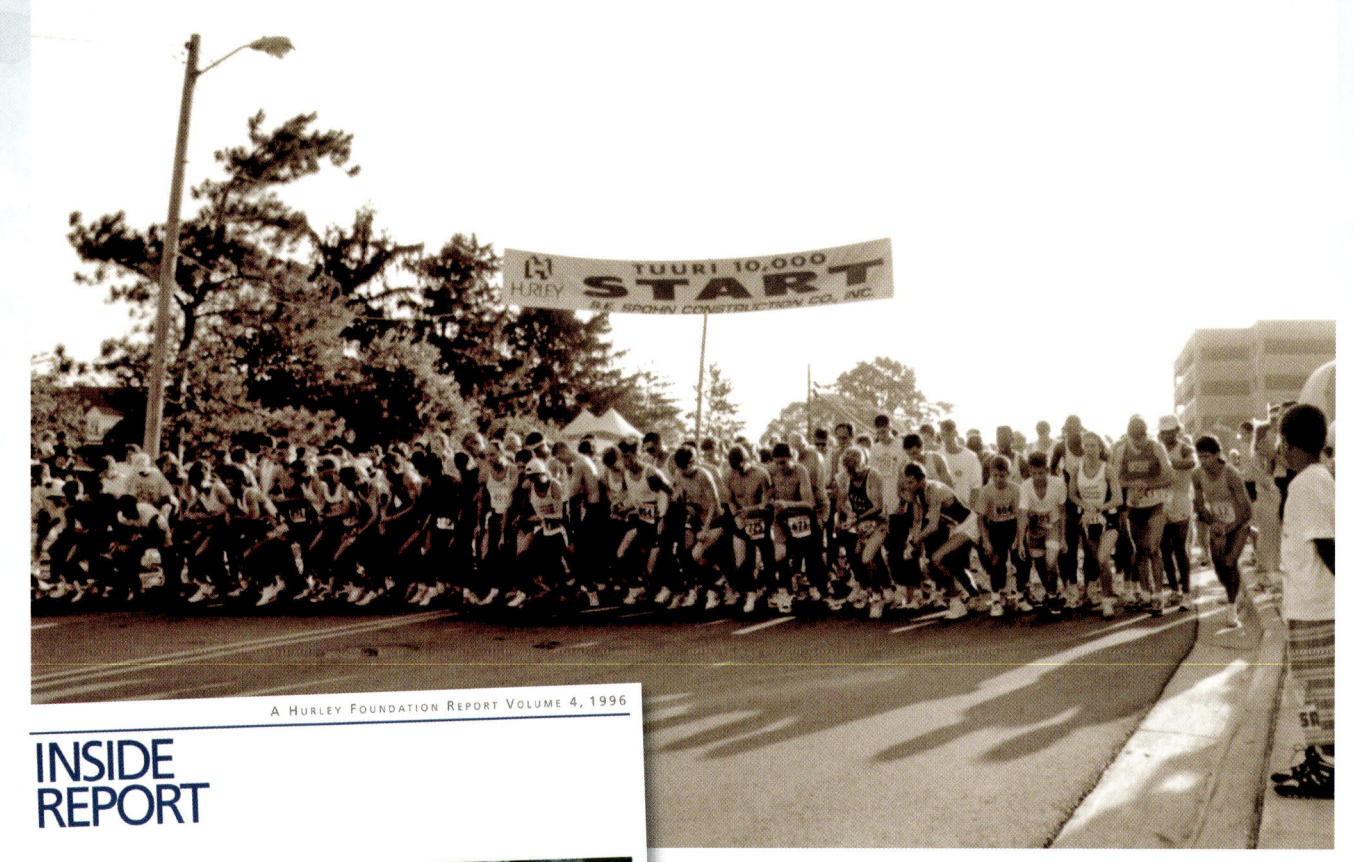

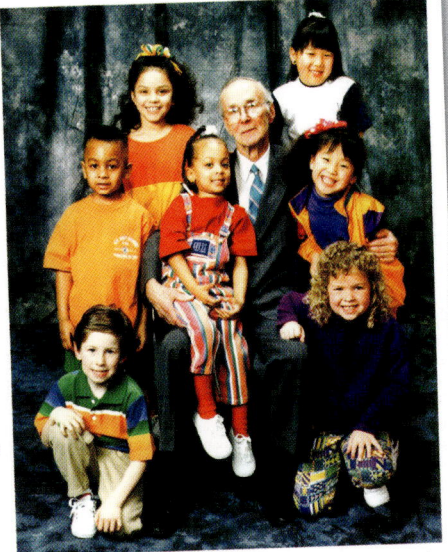

Tuuri Road Race – A 31-Year Fundraising Tradition

Beginning in 1979, runners have lined up outside Hurley every July for the Tuuri 10K (and, since 1984, the 5K) Run for Children's Health, named for Arthur Tuuri, MD, to raise funds for pediatric services at HMC. The race developed into a major fundraiser for the Children's Miracle Network at Hurley. The first race raised $5,185 and attracted nearly 600 runners. The 10K course followed a winding route through tree-lined streets of Flint and ended back at Hurley. The Tuuri 10K was voted "the most challenging urban course" and one of Michigan's top 50 road races by readers of the Michigan Runner. At the 10th anniversary race on July 22, 1989, the event had raised more than $100,000 toward HMC's comprehensive pediatric services and the Children's Wish Fund. The race grew beyond the 5K and 10K races to also include a Children's Challenge and a One Mile Miracle Walk. The final race was held in 2010.

became the first director of MCHC; he was replaced nine years later, when renowned pediatric physician Arthur Tuuri, MD, arrived and transformed children's health services.

"During the early days, the one name that comes to mind is Dr. Arthur L. Tuuri," said Linda Tracy-Stephens, director of the Children's Miracle Network. "He was a pediatrician who was considered a 'world authority' on polio in the 1950s." Dr. Tuuri came to Flint in 1948, intending to stay for only one year, but his passion led him to a lifetime of providing medical care for low-income children in the Flint area, where he also created a pediatric residency program. Dr. Tuuri's "whole child approach" gave way to a new generation of pediatric specialists who helped to meet the needs of increasingly complex cases.

In 1962, MCHC moved to its own 24,000-square-foot building directly across Patrick Street on the western

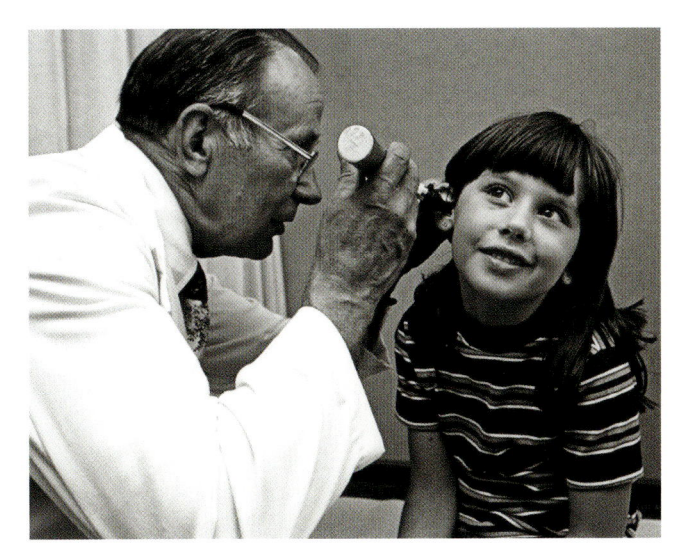

Arthur Tuuri, MD, with a patient

DID YOU KNOW | ... a healthy baby is usually born at 40 to 42 weeks' gestational age and weighs at least 5.5 pounds (2,500 grams). Over 90 percent of Hurley NICU babies weighing between 1.98 and 8.81 pounds (900 to 4,000 grams) survive.

side of the hospital. "Hurley still provided steam to heat the new structure," said Dr. Tuuri. "Those types of things led to a long relationship between Mott and Hurley. I have a very warm place in my heart for Hurley Medical Center because it has done a lot for Mott Children's Health Center, and the children of this community."

Dr. Tuuri served as co-chairman of the East Tower fundraising drive, where the current Pediatric Units are located. On November 4, 1979, the newly renovated second floor of the East Tower was named the "Arthur L. Tuuri Pediatric Center." A few months later, in March 1980, the region's only Pediatric Psychiatry Unit opened on 1 East Tower. The Pediatric Psychiatry Unit offered a 10-bed unit, providing emotional rehabilitation for youngsters ages 10 to 16 years. "More children are treated now for emotional or learning problems stemming from disruption of the family. Economic difficulties caused by termination of employment or one-parent families also create current medical problems," said Dr. Tuuri in 1988.

Hurley's outpatient clinic for children and adolescents moved to larger quarters on the third floor of the West Tower, which allowed for more services and expanded clinic hours. "The laboratory was just down the hall from us, and Hurley did all of the patient's

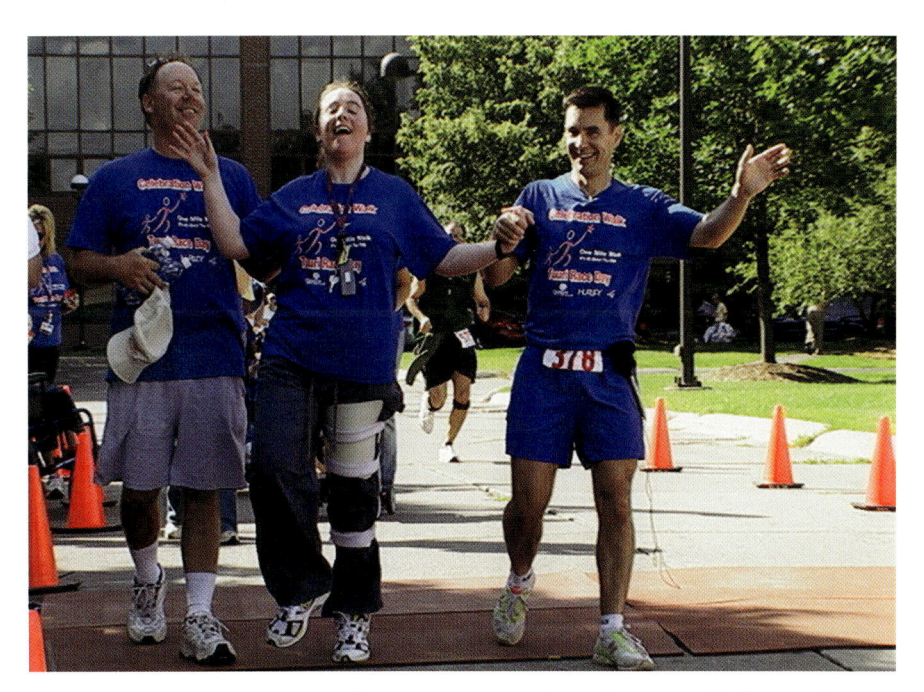

In 2006, the One Mile Miracle Walk was a new race-day option created in honor of Regina Stoolmaker (center). On August 21, 1996, Regina was a passenger in a car accident involving six teenagers; four died, and Regina was one of two survivors, with extensive injuries. At the time, she had earned a college scholarship for soccer but was not expected by doctors to ever walk again. Fast forward to 2006: Regina's brother, Richard (right), who was totally devoted to her recovery, helped her train so that she could participate in the Tuuri Race. Regina displayed extraordinary effort and willpower to cross the finish line: "It looked like she was winning the Olympics," according to participants.

CHAPTER THREE FROM BUMP TO BABY – WOMEN AND CHILDREN • 59

lab work," said Dr. Tuuri. "There was no such thing as Aid to Families with Dependent Children or Medicaid at that time, and most patients didn't have any insurance. Being a municipal hospital, Hurley never turned down any of our patients."

In 1985, Dr. Tuuri became the president emeritus of MCHC and was succeeded by Roy Peterson, who would serve as president of MCHC until 1999.

In 1989, Dr. Tuuri suffered a severe heart attack, but he continued to work from offices in MCHC until his death in January 1996. At the time of his passing, Chief of Staff Samuel Dismond Jr., MD, said, "He was the human link between the clinical practice of pediatrics—and much of the medical center—and the driving force to expand our services to the community. He was a powerful advocate for making changes and increasing our coverage to children who needed help. He was a relentless fundraiser . . . when he asked you to do something or to help, you always knew that it was because he was doing it as well, that he had already given his all. So, you could never refuse him."[7]

Pediatric Hematology and Oncology

An important subspecialty that made HMC a regional referral center for pediatric care is pediatric hematology and oncology. In 1986, Ralph Gordon, MD, pediatric residency program director, and Sharon Dowd, MD, medical oncologist, asked Susumu Inoue, MD, FAAP, to join Hurley to start a pediatric hematology/oncology department. "This was after 20-plus years at the Children's Hospital of Michigan in Detroit, where I started in 1966 with my pediatric residency and fellowship in pediatrics, hematology, and oncology," said Dr. Inoue.

In January 1987, Dr. Inoue arrived as HMC's director of Pediatric Hematology and Oncology. "When I first arrived here, we had to work hard to be an independent, recognized, regional pediatric oncology center. In the beginning, we were only a satellite institution of the Detroit Children's Hospital. It was a huge project, and the transition from the satellite to independent pediatric oncology center took about three years."

"Dr. Roderic Abbott would send us the children, but physicians would bypass HMC after we made a diagnosis, and transfer patients to U of M and Detroit

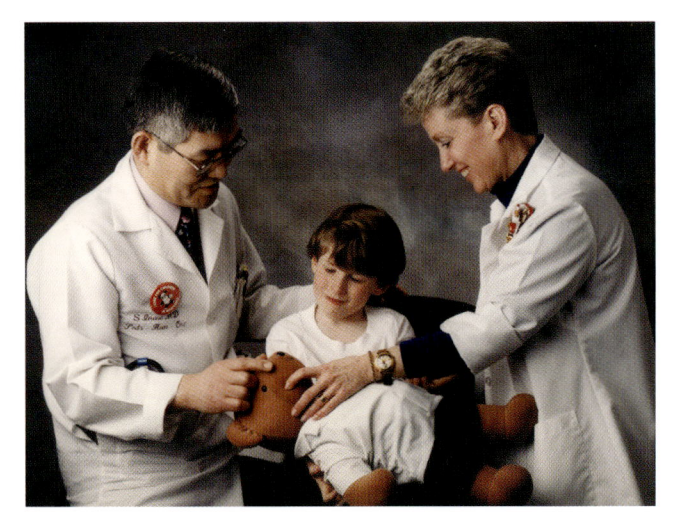

Susumu Inoue, MD, FAAP (left), and Mary Mitchell-Beren, RN, with a patient

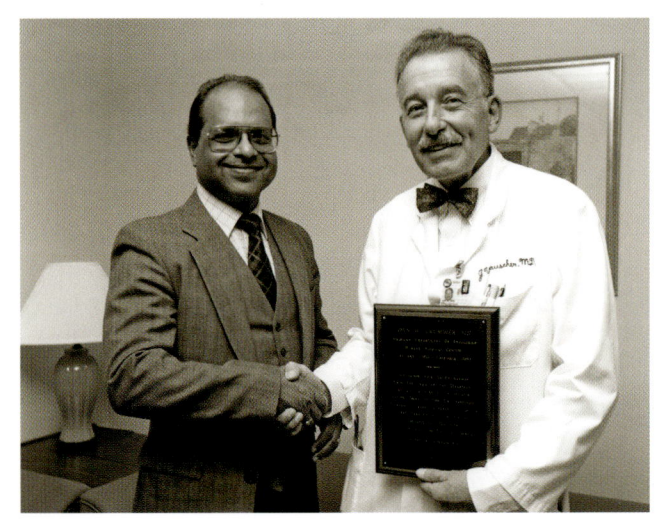

Amitabha Banerjee, MD, congratulates John Tauscher, MD, on his retirement and being chairman of the Department of Pediatrics from January 1980 through December 1989.

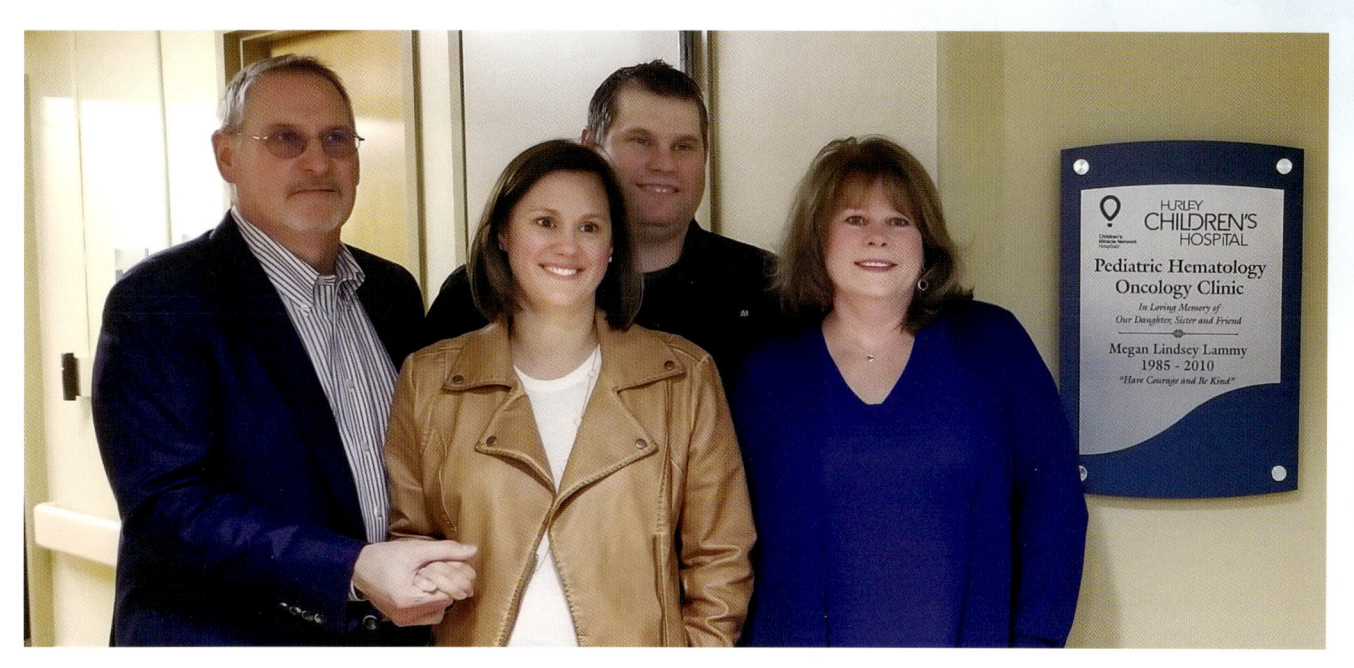

The Art of Caring – Megan's Legacy

Megan Lammy of Flushing was diagnosed with leukemia in 1990 at five years old. Her team, led by Susumu Inoue, MD, FAAP, took care of the many complexities of her disease over an eight-year period. The Hurley family became a second home to Megan, as she gave up her formative years going through treatment, rather than at school with friends. Her family reflected on why they think she did so well with her treatment, and it came down to three things: her positive attitude, her unending sense of humor, and quality care from both her family and the team at Hurley Medical Center. Although she lost her battle to secondary cancer at age 25, her legacy of strength lives on through family and friends. Her family honored their daughter by supporting the remodeling of the new pediatric hematology/oncology clinic on the 11th floor of the West Tower, as well as wall-mounted Touch2Play entertainment units for the clinic's treatment rooms. "This is exactly what Megan would have wanted to see this space become, a place of healing and courage," says Ronald Lammy II, Megan's father. "Our hope is that each patient and family member who walks this clinic floor for years to come is provided with the same care and support that our family received."

Children's, even if it meant greater difficulty for patients and their families getting to those bigger institutions," said Mary Mitchell-Beren, RN, pediatric hematology/oncology nurse. The benefits of a pediatric hematology and oncology center at HMC was immediate. Inoue's prior clinical experience with hundreds of patients with a variety of disorders allowed families with leukemia and cancer the option for treatment closer to home.

HMC became an official member of the Pediatric Oncology Group (POG), a multi-institutional research organization with officially approved therapeutic protocols; it is funded by the National Cancer Institute (NCI). Because of this affiliation, Dr. Inoue was able to expand the scope of the experimental studies and gain immediate information. "Many of these therapeutic protocols are experimental and free for the children. This offered HMC prestige in that we knew our patients would receive the same therapies given at the larger children's hospitals," said Dr. Inoue.

Dr. Inoue noted that "interacting with the kids every day—even though they are sick—is the most rewarding part of my work. Most of the time, kids get sick quickly, but then they get better quickly too. That's a good thing. We meet parents, grandparents, aunts, and uncles, and we keep in touch with them by attending graduations and weddings; it's a lot of fun. Fortunately, their babies are regular, healthy kids, even if their parents received chemotherapy as kids."

Hurley Children's Hospital – A Children's Miracle Network Hospital

In 1990, Hurley's extensive pediatric services and demonstrated expertise were recognized by an invitation to join a group of special hospitals, the Children's Miracle Network (CMN) Hospitals, because "HMC provides the most outstanding, kid-centered care in our region to every child who needs it, regardless of the family's ability to pay," said Tracy-Stephens. "At that time, CMN was composed of 160 of the most prestigious hospitals across the United States and Canada, dedicated to providing the very best care for sick and injured children. As a CMN Hospital, we help kids with cancer, birth defects, diabetes, asthma, accidents, trauma, and almost any other health issue you can imagine. CMN Hospitals have changed the face of care and given all children, facing all illnesses, a better hope for the future." Today's network of 170 hospitals serves 10 million children and their families every year—more than any other children's cause.

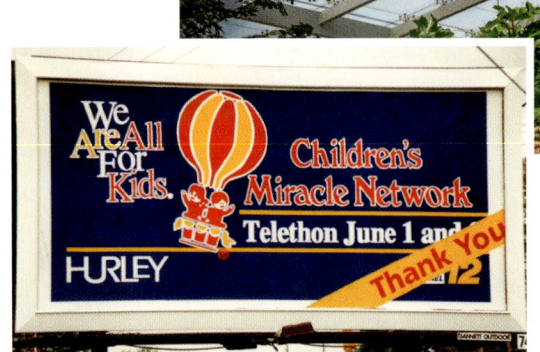

Hurley CMN Children's Hospital sign and billboard sign

Upon joining CMN, Hurley's pediatric service-area territory grew to 15 counties, extending as far north as Alpena, Mount Pleasant to the west, and a

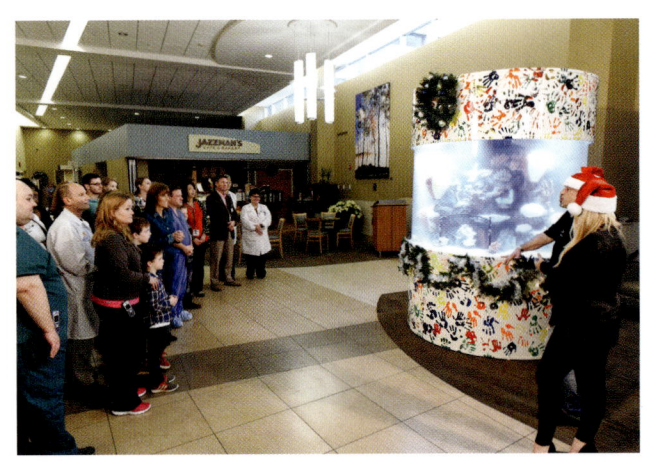

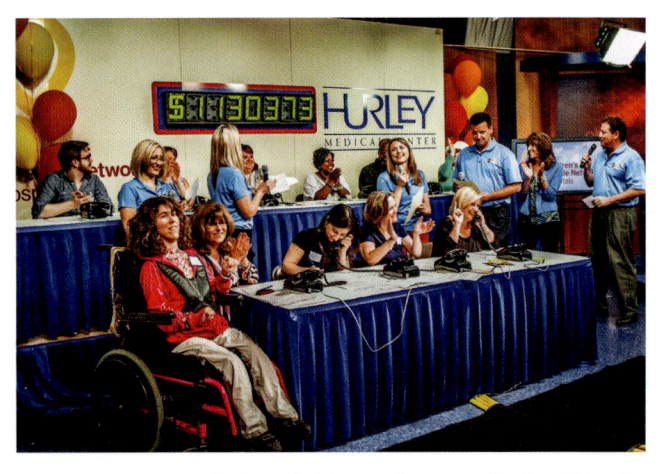

Left: In 2016, the CMN Children's Hospital lobby aquarium was donated by Animal Planet's hit TV show *Tanked*. Within the 850-gallon, four-ton glass enclosure are CMN balloons, Flint Vehicle City arches, an image of Longway Planetarium, and a guitar representing 2016 CMN Teen Ambassador Ali Simpson's music. Hurley's Pediatric Art Program is called out by artist palettes.

Right: Annual Fundraiser for Miracle Children – CMN Telethon, 2014
The telethon was an annual live-TV broadcast that spotlighted local and national partners for CMN fundraising efforts. Hurley's Miracle Kids were celebrated, and Hurley Children's Hospital medical staff, employees, and volunteers were highlighted. The final telethon aired on June 5, 2016.

Hurley Celebrate Six Sets of Healthy Quadruplets

The first quadruplets were delivered on June 7, 1990, by Hurley's "quad squad" (led by Clinton Dowd, MD, Hurley's Ob-Gyn residency program director), who were ready to assist mom Deborah Rowden from Davison. The first one born was Stephanie, followed by David, Tyler, and William. All four were featured in the CMN Telethon. The second set of quadruplets came in a leap year, on February 29, 1992. Renee and Carl Diener selected Hurley to deliver their four babies: Nicholas, Rachel, Katherine, and Robert, who arrived 12 weeks early. Twenty-five years later, all four were photographed for a Hurley publication. The third set of quadruplets, born ten weeks early on June 1, 1997, were the Bannister quadruplets: William, James, Raydean, and Randi-Leigh. All of them made their appearance simultaneously while the CMN Telethon was airing. The fourth set of quadruplets, born on October 26, 1999, were the Nelson quadruplets: Kylie, Karly, Kayla, and Alan, all weighing less than two pounds and three months premature. The fifth set—all boys—were born on January 8, 1999, to Kim and Darrin Wade: Aaron, Nigel, Nicholas, and Zacary. Hurley's sixth set of four, the Harden quadruplets (Evelyn, Jeffrey, Bethany, and JoAnna), were born on July 11, 2006. They were born two months early, but all were healthy, except for premature lungs.

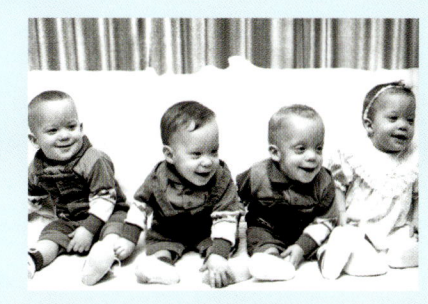

The Flint area's first set of quadruplets, born on June 7, 1990, at nine months old (left to right): Tyler, David, William, and Stephanie Rowden.

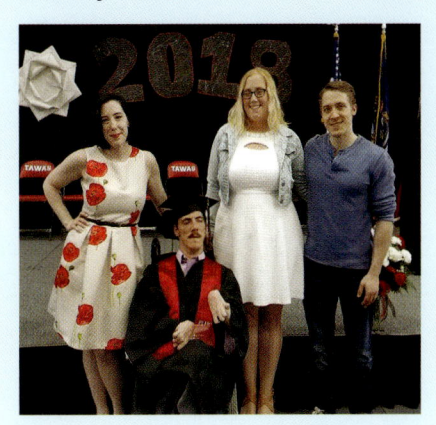

The Diener quadruplets at 25 years old are all happy and lead busy lives.

portion of the Thumb, as well as all of Genesee and Shiawassee Counties. Today, 17 counties are now in the service territory.

According to Tracy-Stephens, "Operating under the umbrella of the Hurley Foundation, the primary focus of CMN is to raise funds for a variety of pediatric services at the hospital, to initiate or expand special programs, or to purchase major pieces of equipment. Of primary concern is raising funds for capital expenditures to replace old equipment to keep pace with the advances in medical technology; the cost for specialized equipment is high, but so is the need. Additionally, CMN donations help provide special inpatient programs like art and music, and comfort items like stuffed animals, books, and toys. Twenty-five percent of funds raised go into a pediatric endowment fund to benefit children for years to come." CMN is best known for their $1 paper-balloon fundraisers; when a donation is given through a CMN-sponsored activity, it stays in that community, helping local kids. The annual CMN Telethon offered an opportunity for many from the Hurley family to staff phone banks and share their own thoughts about the care they provided to Hurley pediatric patients. Aftab Aftab, MD, longtime chair of Pediatrics at HMC, brought a group of pediatricians and pediatric specialists together to staff the phone bank for an hour during each telethon. This offered many people an opportunity to see their doctors on TV and to see yet another example of the commitment to the care they all rendered.

On November 15, 2011, HMC announced the creation of Hurley Children's Hospital—a hospital within a hospital. This new designation recognized the wide range of specialty physicians and services, skilled nurses, and advanced treatment options offered. Ahmad Kadurrah, MD, FAAP, pediatric neurologist, and Hurley Pinnacle Award recipient, shared, "Adding the title of Hurley Children's Hospital allows families who would otherwise have traveled south of us to realize they have the pediatric specialty experts right in their own region." In addition to individual donors, service clubs, schools, and other local fundraising activities, Hurley Children's Hospital benefits from the ongoing financial support of many national and local CMN partners, which include (in alphabetical order) Ace Hardware, CO-OP Financial Services, Credit Unions for Kids, Dairy Queen, various "Greek" partners like Phi Mu and Phi Delta Epsilon, Kiwanis International, Panda Express, RE/MAX, Rite Aid, Sam's Club, Speedway, and Walmart, among others. "National contests have also provided much-needed funding and serve as a platform for energizing awareness and support of the importance of being a CMN Hospital," said Tracy-Stephens.

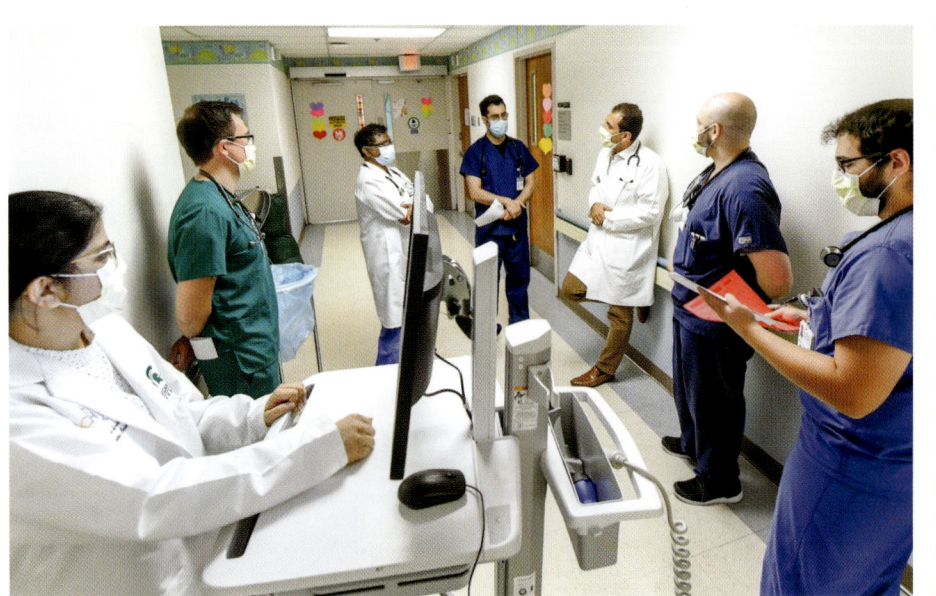

> In keeping with Flint's "Vehicle City" moniker, a 1993 baby-information packet described the outstanding design features of Hurley babies as follows: two-lung power, free squealing, continuous bawl bearing, economical feed, automatic exhaust, changeable seat covers, and jet propelled; along with a "handle with care" label.

Pediatric clinical rounds, 2020. Left to right: Tazeen Qureshi, MD, pediatric resident; Albert Tamayo, MD, visiting resident; Chandrasekhar Kothuru, MD, med/peds resident; Shahin Shafiei, MD, visiting resident; Yaseen Rafee, MD, attending physician; Antonio DiCarlo, DO, visiting resident; and Ryan Avery, MD, pediatric resident.

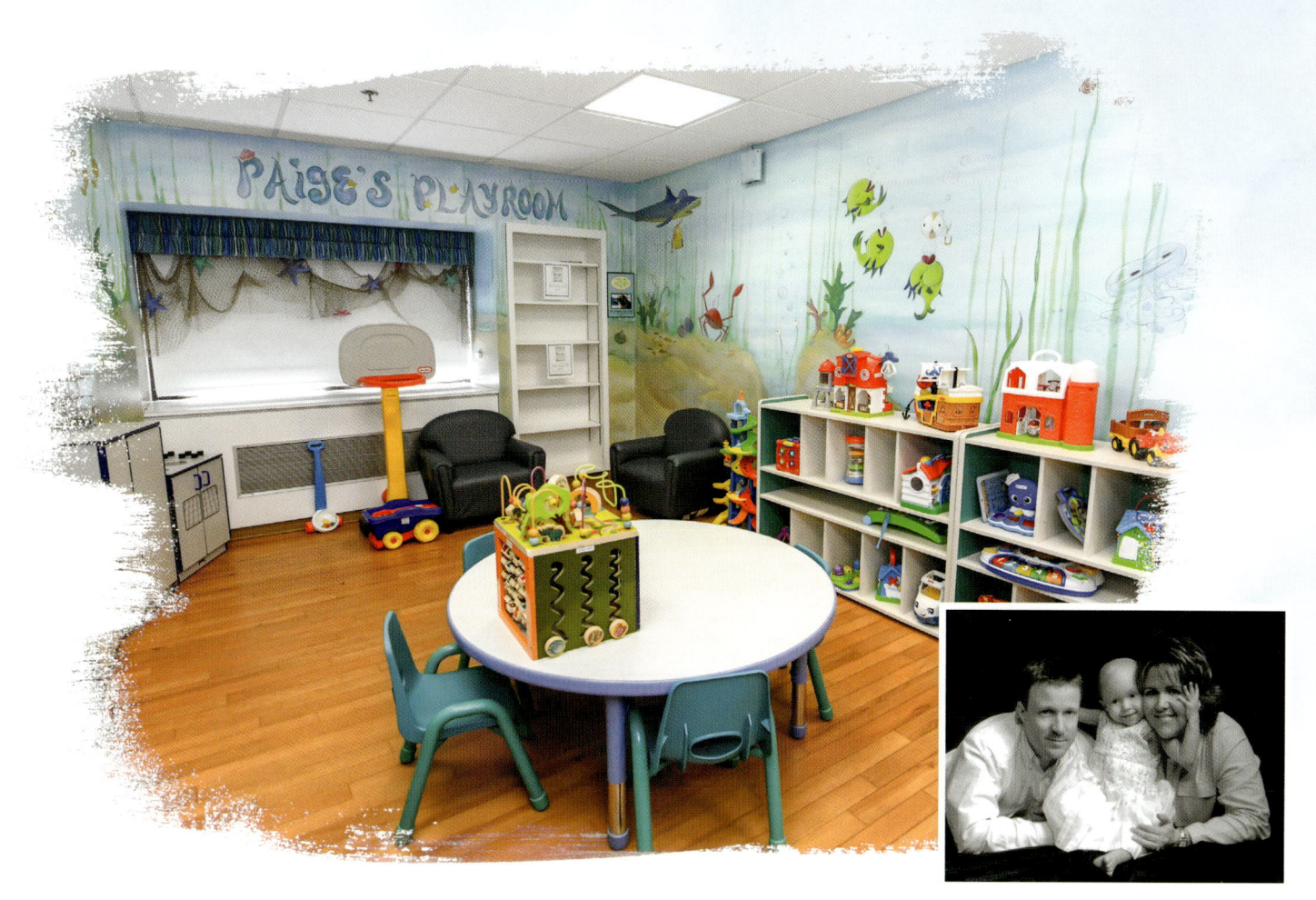

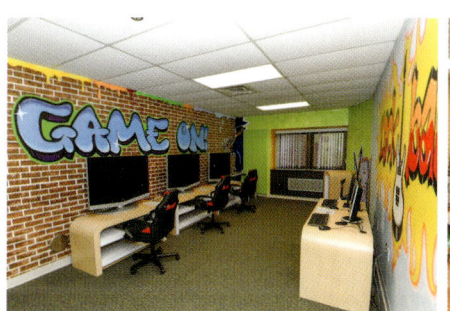

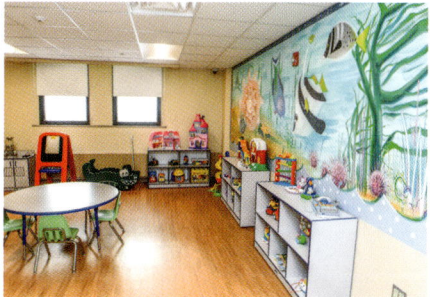

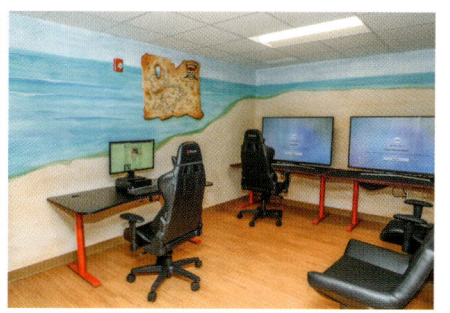

Top: Paige's Playroom, on the pediatric floor, was dedicated on September 19, 2006, in memory of three-year-old Paige Rutter, who lost her battle with neuroblastoma. Paige's parents both work at HMC: Andy, trauma PA-C, and Sandra, RN, in the Neuro-Trauma Unit.

Above left: **The Xbox Game Room Makeover – Miracles Do Happen!**
In 2009, Microsoft offered to donate an Xbox Game Room Makeover to three CMN Hospitals in an online contest, and Hurley rose to the challenge. Participants could vote online up to 10 times a day during the six-week challenge. The Hurley spirit was ignited, and the effort went viral as HMC employees, friends, and family maximized their votes. Against all odds, HMC (as a small regional hospital) came in first place with 2,156,400 votes! "This was truly a David versus Goliath story, as Hurley, with 42 pediatric beds, took first place, while the second-place finisher had 190 beds and third place had 250 beds," said Linda Tracy-Stephens. She continued, "In addition to the $10,000 donated by Microsoft for the Xbox game room, another $10,000 was given by the Sheppy Dog Fund, Alan Klein, DDS, advisor. The Xbox room, constructed within the Pediatric Unit, allows Hurley pediatric patients, ages 10 and older, an escape from tests and procedures. In this magical room, they can have fun and just be kids. That in itself is a miracle."

Above middle: The 11th-floor Pediatrics Unit offers private waiting rooms and a new playroom that was funded by the Child Welfare Society.

Above right: The media dimension room (teen game room), designed for pediatric patients 10 years and older, was funded by Josh Stinson and Extra Life Gamers; it opened on February 8, 2018.

CHAPTER THREE FROM BUMP TO BABY – WOMEN AND CHILDREN • 65

"Taking care of children is very different and requires a significant commitment from a specialized hospital, of which Hurley historically has always been," said Dr. Nolan. "Our current CEO, Melany Gavulic, is very committed to pediatrics," adds Nolan. "The development of Hurley Children's Hospital is a visual demonstration of this hospital's concern for our community. The relationship with CMN is very important in helping support our service."

On February 8, 2018, HMC revealed their new patient-family-focused Pediatric Unit on the 11th floor of the West Tower (in addition to the existing Pediatric Unit on the second floor of the East Tower), which included 14 private patient rooms, a meeting space for staff and families, a new children's playroom, a teen game room, and a nutrition center. "In a pediatric environment, it's more than just the pediatric patient in the bed that the care team is servicing; it tends to be family as well. From nurses to physicians and other care providers, and various learners in the environment, there can be a lot of people not just addressing a patient, but an entire family. This just gives us more breathing room for that and for the families to have more privacy. We can't express enough how important our donors are to these projects. We wouldn't have this without their generosity, but it's not just their monetary support that is important; to us, it's a validation from them that they have confidence in the mission we serve and confidence in the care we provide," said Melany Gavulic, RN, MBA, president, CEO.

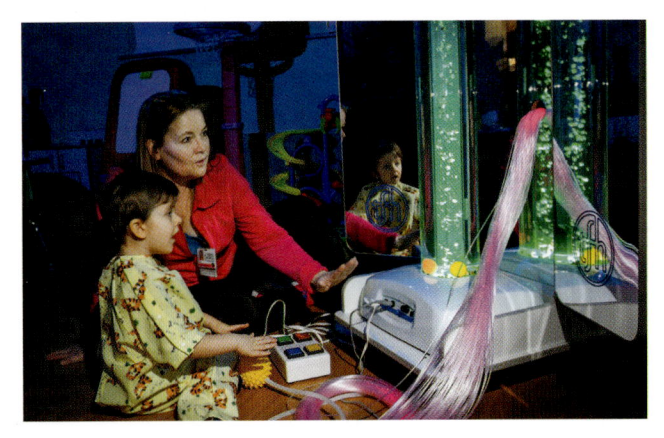

Child Life Services director Laura Parcels with Maxwell Williams in 2019 at the multisensory Vecta machine that was donated by Dairy Queen. Vecta provides a distraction to calm the anxieties of youngsters facing procedures, giving them a sense of control that they otherwise might not have.

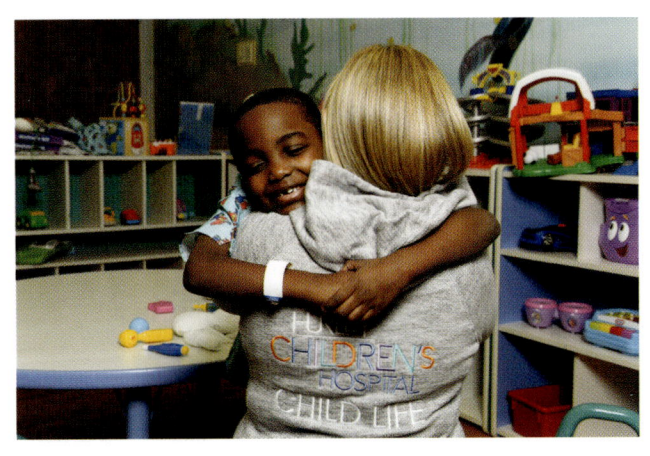

Child Life

Child Life Services

A hospital experience for young patients is made better by the Child Life professionals who help reduce the anxiety that children and their families may feel. These specialists understand that play is an important part of healing and serves a number of purposes when a sick or injured child is trying to cope with pain; therapeutic and recreational play has positive outcomes—play is actually distraction therapy. Child Life specialists provide non-medical preparation and support for kids who will undergo tests, surgeries, and other medical procedures. CMN donations provide valuable support for this program.

Level II Pediatric Trauma Center

Brian Nolan, MD, FAAP, completed HMC's pediatric residency program between 1976 and 1979 and went on to complete a neonatal-perinatal medicine fellowship at Children's Hospital of Michigan from 1986 to 1988; he is board certified in pediatric critical care, general pediatrics, child abuse pediatrics, and neonatal-perinatal medicine. Dr. Nolan was a 2010 Pinnacle Award recipient. He is the clinical director of Pediatrics

CMN Fundraisers

SPEEDWAY MIRACLE TOURNAMENT

Every year, as part of the CMN Hospitals, HMC participates in a national fundraising campaign sponsored by Speedway. The 28th Annual Speedway Miracle Tournament was held in Ohio in 2019, with local child ambassador Edrin Sims accompanied by his mother, Treasa Swinton. Edrin was a brave seven-year-old cancer warrior who participated in all the special events, including a photo shoot with Miss America. As an added bonus, his artwork was used for a special Snapple label, which resulted in increased funding for the Children's Miracle Network Hospitals. In 2018, Speedway raised $9.5 million for kids treated at the 61 participating CMN Hospitals. Edrin, with Mark Matczak of MEM Construction and Edrin's tournament sponsor, shows off his winning Snapple artwork, which says: "Hope, Strength, Faith, Courage."

RADIOTHON – THE POWER OF RADIO HELPS KIDS

The first annual CMN Radiothon was held in 2001 at Courtland Center Mall. In 2006, the event moved to Genesee Valley Center, and beginning in 2009, the CMN Radiothon was presented from Hurley's West Lobby. Over the years, hundreds of miracle families have shared their stories of hope and inspiration, encouraging listeners to phone in and donate. This special event has demonstrated the true power of radio. This fundraiser continues to generate financial support for various pediatric programs at Hurley Children's Hospital.

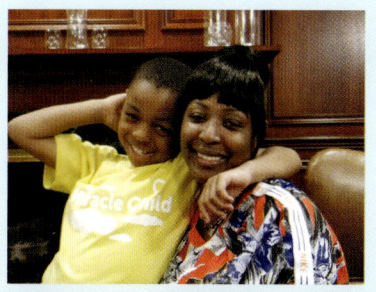

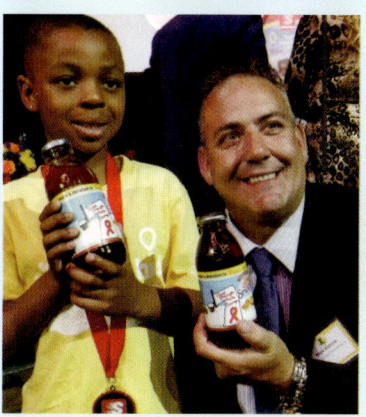

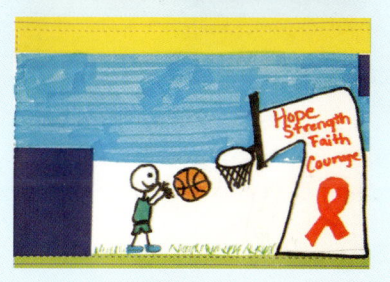

CMN BOWLATHON

In 1990, the Doyle family, owners of Colonial Lanes in Flushing, stepped up to present the first annual CMN Bowlathon for family-friendly fundraising. The 30th anniversary CMN Bowlathon was held in 2020.

and former clinical director of Pediatric Clinical Care, which is a role now held by Mahesh Sharman, MD. HMC opened the region's first Pediatric Intensive Care Unit (PICU) in 1974, with advanced technology designed to treat critically ill and/or injured infants up to age 21. The newly enlarged unit had ten beds, including eight private rooms, and was led by two board-certified intensivists in pediatrics and critical care at that time, which included Dr. Nolan.

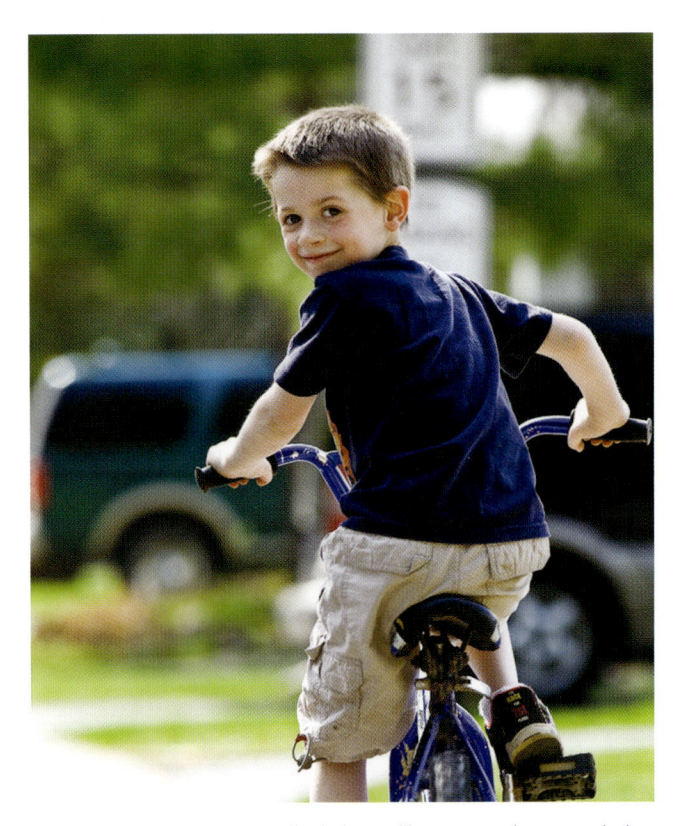

Brian Nolan, MD, FAAP

Archer Granger, like most lively boys, likes to run, jump, and play, but on August 19, 2009, his life changed forever. He was struck by a commercial riding mower near his home and severed 95 percent of his foot, including two tendons and two of three main arteries. He sustained significant bone loss and lost one and a half toes. He was airlifted from Marlette Hospital to Hurley, where Hurley trauma and orthopedic surgical teams successfully repaired the partial amputation of his foot with four surgeries, a skin graft, and pins in both feet to stabilize his broken bones. According to his mom, "Hurley is the place to go for children. I'll never go anywhere else. Archer's recovery is a complete miracle. Hurley saved both of his legs." In March 2010, Archer was named Pediatric Ambassador for the 29th Annual Benefit Ball, which raised $200,000 for the Pediatric Emergency and Trauma Department renovation.

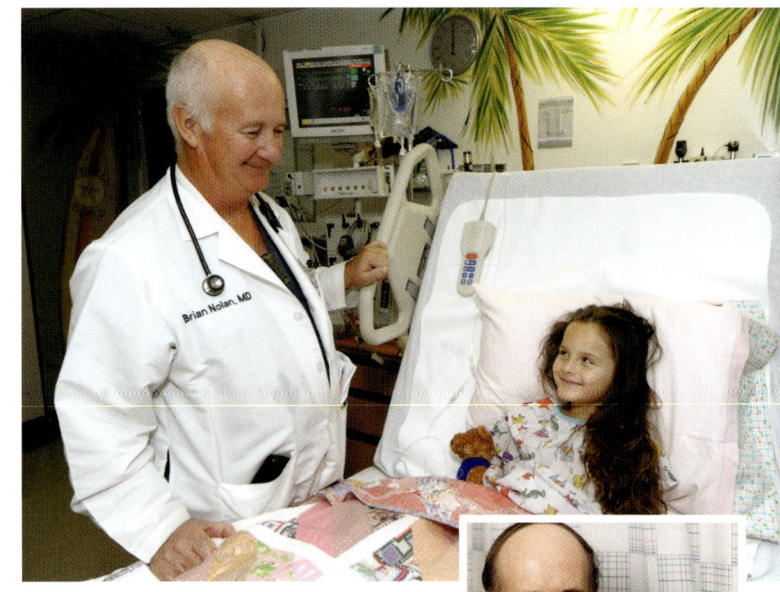

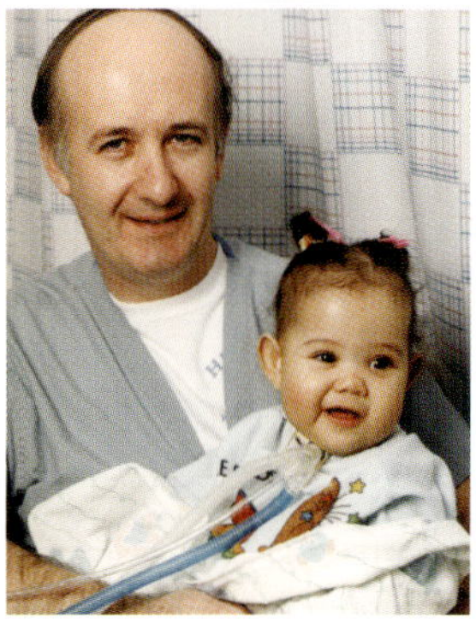

In 1998, with dedicated pediatric-trained staff, HMC opened the service area's only dedicated Pediatric Emergency Department (Peds ED), providing pediatric service 24 hours a day and located adjacent to the adult ED. Over the years, Dr. Nolan has seen many specialists come to Hurley. "Forty years ago, we had very few pediatric specialists, but we now have multiple specialists based at Hurley and others who come from the U of M, Children's Hospital of Michigan, and MSU." Some of these specialties include pediatric cardiology, surgery, nephrology, and psychiatry. In addition, there are Hurley-based pediatric specialists for neurology, neonatology, critical care, infectious diseases, gastrointestinal, hematology, psychology, endocrinology, and adolescent medicine. Dr. Nolan added, "What we try to do is assess what the Flint area and mid-Michigan needs are and develop a strategy to meet those needs so that children don't have to travel long distances for care."

"We get many applications from other states and abroad from doctors who want to come to work with us," said Dr. Nolan. "When they get situated, they tend to stay here.

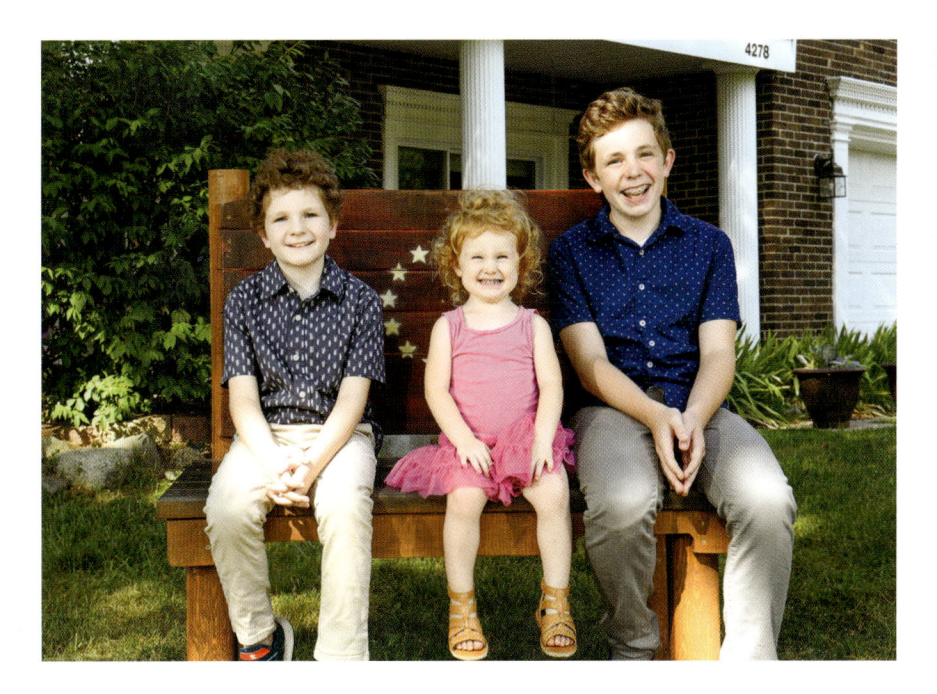

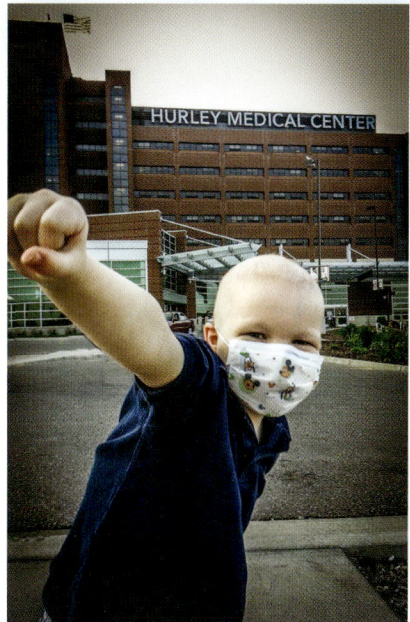

Above: Rowan and Winnie Neumann
Ben and Emily Neumann from Clio had two wonderful sons, Tristan and Rowan, when their daughter, Guinevere (Winnie) Neumann, was born. She seemed perfectly healthy, but when she became continuously fussy and her tummy seemed distended, her parents took her to Hurley Children's Hospital. After many tests and procedures, three-month-old Winnie was diagnosed with stage 4S neuroblastoma; a malignant tumor on her adrenal gland had metastasized to her liver and bones. This was not the first time Ben and Emily had received such shocking news: their son Rowan had been diagnosed with precursor B-cell acute lymphoblastic leukemia at 22 months old; genetic testing showed no connection. The skilled HMC team saw Winnie through every inpatient round of chemotherapy. As Winnie's cancer journey began, Rowan's was supposed to be ending, but that was not the case—he had relapsed for the third time. Rowan received a bone marrow transplant in November 2017. Rowan and Winnie have the kind of special bond that only comes from sharing a common experience. When Rowan was younger, he thought all kids had cancer and got medical ports—it was the only way of life he had ever known. The entire Neumann family has been on this journey for the past seven years. Through it all, big brother Tristan has been caring, optimistic, and resilient. Today, Winnie is doing well, and her future looks bright. She and Rowan share something else in common: their cancer does not define them. Thanks to their amazing parents and support network of family and friends, the Neumann family is finally becoming that "typical" family they have longed to be.[8]

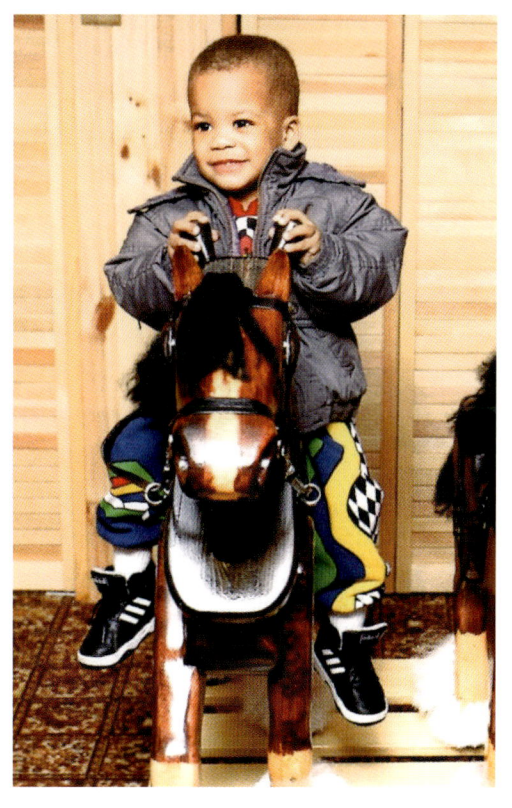

Right: Brok Mabry at 22 months old looks like a typical toddler, but five days after he was born, several heart defects were diagnosed, which doctors hoped he would outgrow. He was placed on medication and scheduled for frequent checkups. Three weeks later, Brok experienced heart failure and was admitted into the Pediatric Intensive Care Unit (PICU) at Hurley, where physicians and nurses worked to keep him alive. After eight weeks, he left Hurley's PICU and received surgery at Children's Hospital of Michigan. He is now a normal, happy baby who visits his pediatric cardiologist annually. His mom credits Hurley's PICU staff for keeping her baby alive: "They cared for him just as I would, and they acted just like he was their baby. They kissed and caressed him . . . there was so much caring there."

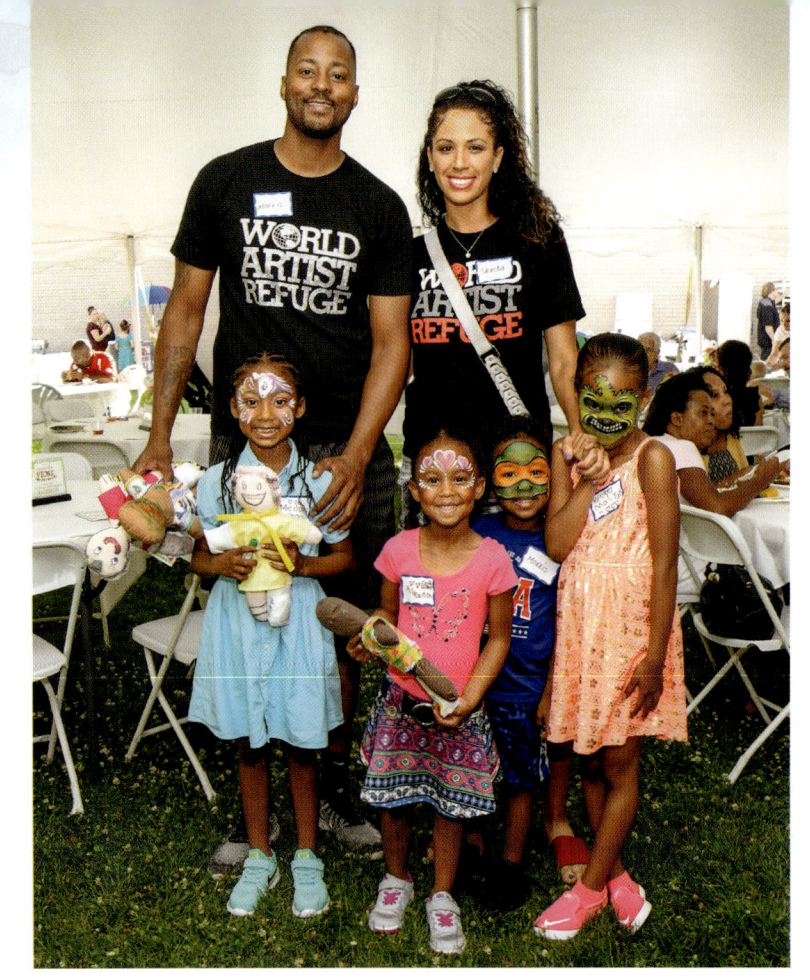

Famous Hurley Babies

Mark Ingram, New Orleans Saints running back and Flint's only Heisman Trophy winner, came back to HMC in 2010 as the headliner for the Men's Fest health fair. NFL player Brandon Carr and NBA player Morris Peterson (owner of local restaurant MoPetes Sports Retreat) visited pediatric patients in 2016. Clarissa Shields (professional boxer and the first American woman to win an Olympic gold medal in boxing), Anthony Dirrell (professional boxer and two-time WBC super-middleweight champion), and Terry Crews (actor, comedian, and former professional football player) were all born at Hurley. Crews paid a "virtual visit" in 2020 to a pediatric sickle cell patient. American Idol singer LaKisha Jones was born at Hurley and performed at HMC's 100th anniversary celebration. Below, NFL player Brandon Carr visits with a pediatric patient in 2016. To the left, former NBA player Morris Peterson and his family attend the Miracle Picnic.

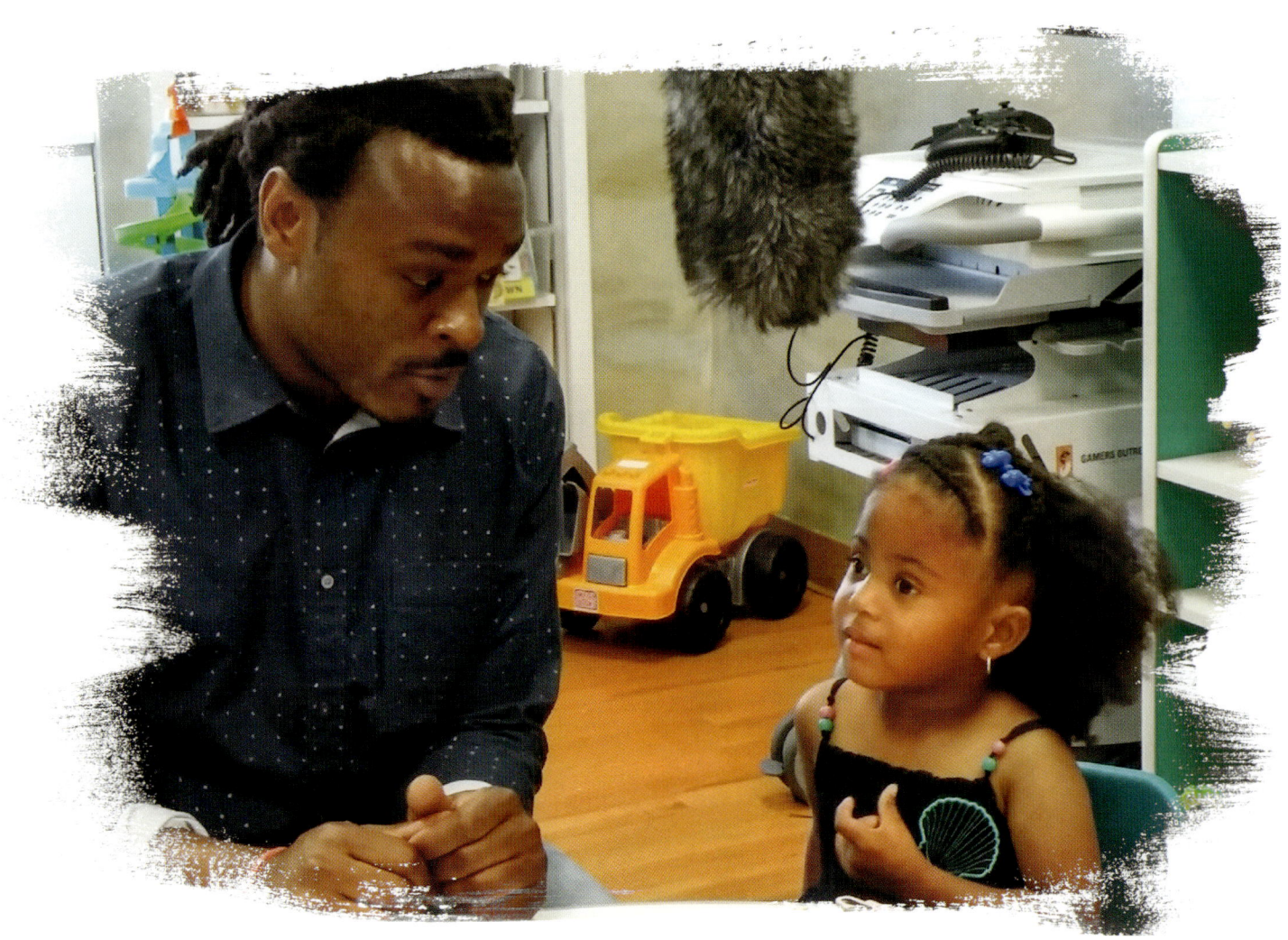

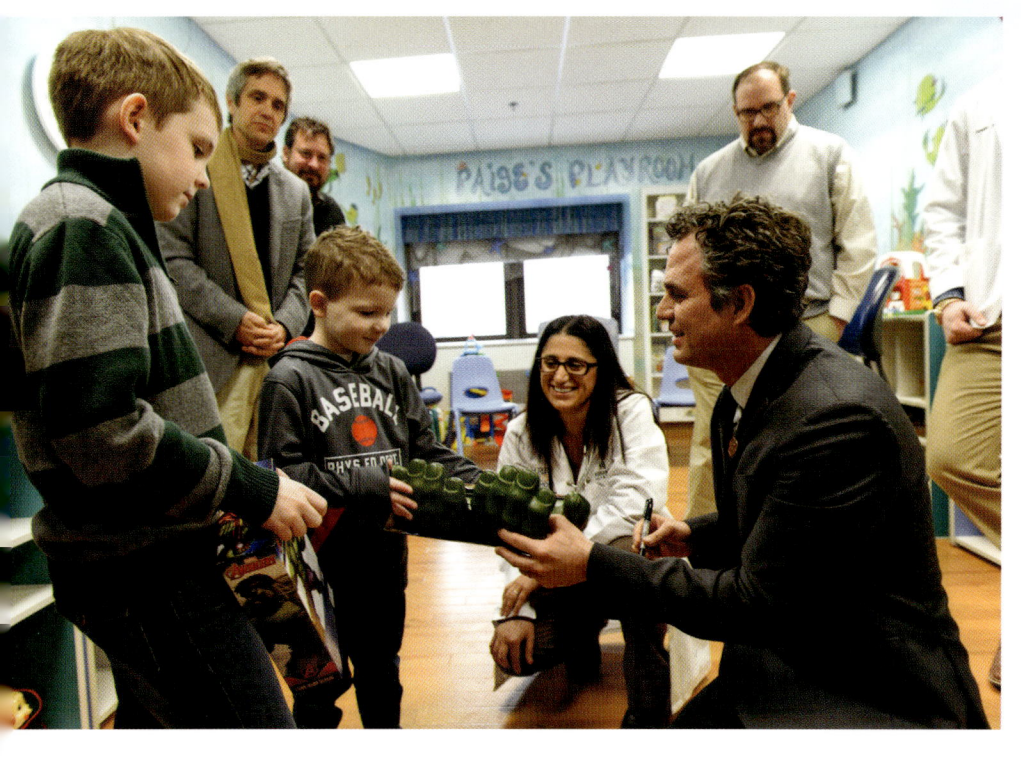

Actor Mark Ruffalo (right) visits Hurley Children's Hospital in 2016 while Mona Hanna-Attisha, MD (center), and Michigan State Senate minority leader Jim Ananich (background right) look on.

Below: Harlem Globetrotter Crissa "Ace" Jackson visited the Pediatric Unit in January 2020.

All of this to say that I am very positive about how HMC is capable of taking care of the kids in the community. We have a Level II pediatric trauma service as designated by the ACS, which means that HMC treats a greater volume of pediatric patients than most, while maintaining high-quality measures with specialized staffing."

The construction of the Paul F. Reinhart Emergency Trauma Center included a Pediatric Emergency Department, which opened on March 4, 2012. The Peds ED, with a separate entrance and a separate waiting area from the adult ED, offers a kid-friendly environment with a sea-life theme, wall murals, and electronic games designed to keep young children engaged while doctors use specially sized medical equipment for diagnosis and treatment to meet the needs of young patients and reduce their anxiety during treatment.

In 2015, the ACS awarded HMC a Level II pediatric trauma designation. "We see more than 25,000 kids in the Pediatric ED every year," said Stewart. "We admit around 300 severely injured into the hospital, though a majority of them heal and return to the activities of daily living."

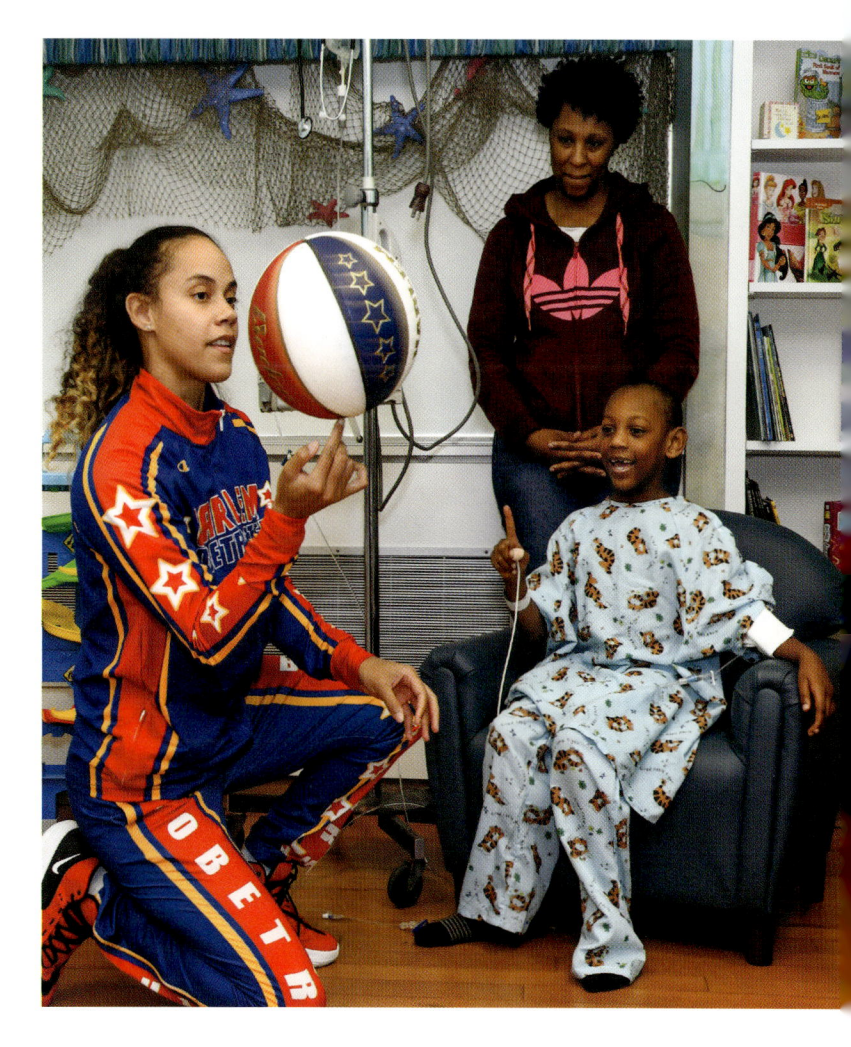

CHAPTER THREE FROM BUMP TO BABY – WOMEN AND CHILDREN

Like Father, Like Son – Larry Young, MD, and Omari Young, MD

Omari Young, MD, was born at Hurley. He completed his obstetrics and gynecology (Ob-Gyn) residency training in 2017. That same year, he moved back to Flint and joined the faculty of the Ob-Gyn residency training program at Hurley and is a clinical assistant professor at MSU CHM.

Dr. O. Young recalls what it was like to grow up in a family in which his dad was a doctor. "The positives definitely outweigh the negatives. My fondest memory as a child is that most every time we were out in public, he would see a patient or colleague and they would be so appreciative of his care. On the flipside, Dad always had a busy schedule, and there were times that he couldn't attend family events."

Dr. O. Young considers his father, Dr. Larry Young, to be one of his best friends and his biggest role model, crediting his dad for influencing his desire to pursue a career in medicine. "Being a Hurley baby, I didn't want to pass up the opportunity to serve my community," said Dr. O. Young. "Furthermore, as a black physician, diversity was important to me. It has been a privilege to call my dad a colleague, along with other black physicians I admired growing up, such as our [residency] program director, Dr. John Hebert, and many others."

Larry Young, MD, completed his Ob-Gyn residency at Hurley in 1987, and he has served in private practice in Flint ever since. He has held multiple leadership roles at HMC, including a term as department chair. He was the 2013 Hurley Pinnacle Award recipient. He has also been recognized for his contributions to the increasing delivery and surgical volume at Hurley.

Both doctors endorse the stellar reputation that HMC holds for women, maternal/fetal, and neonatal health in the Flint area. "Hurley earned this due to the vast experiences of the Ob-Gyn Department staff," said Dr. O. Young. He continues, "A diverse group of faculty physicians, residents, private physicians, MFM [maternal-fetal medicine] and other subspecialists, CNMs [certified nurse midwives], mid-level providers, and nursing staff. We are also privileged to have a strong Pediatric and NICU Department, which allows us to offer comprehensive care for high-risk pregnancies."

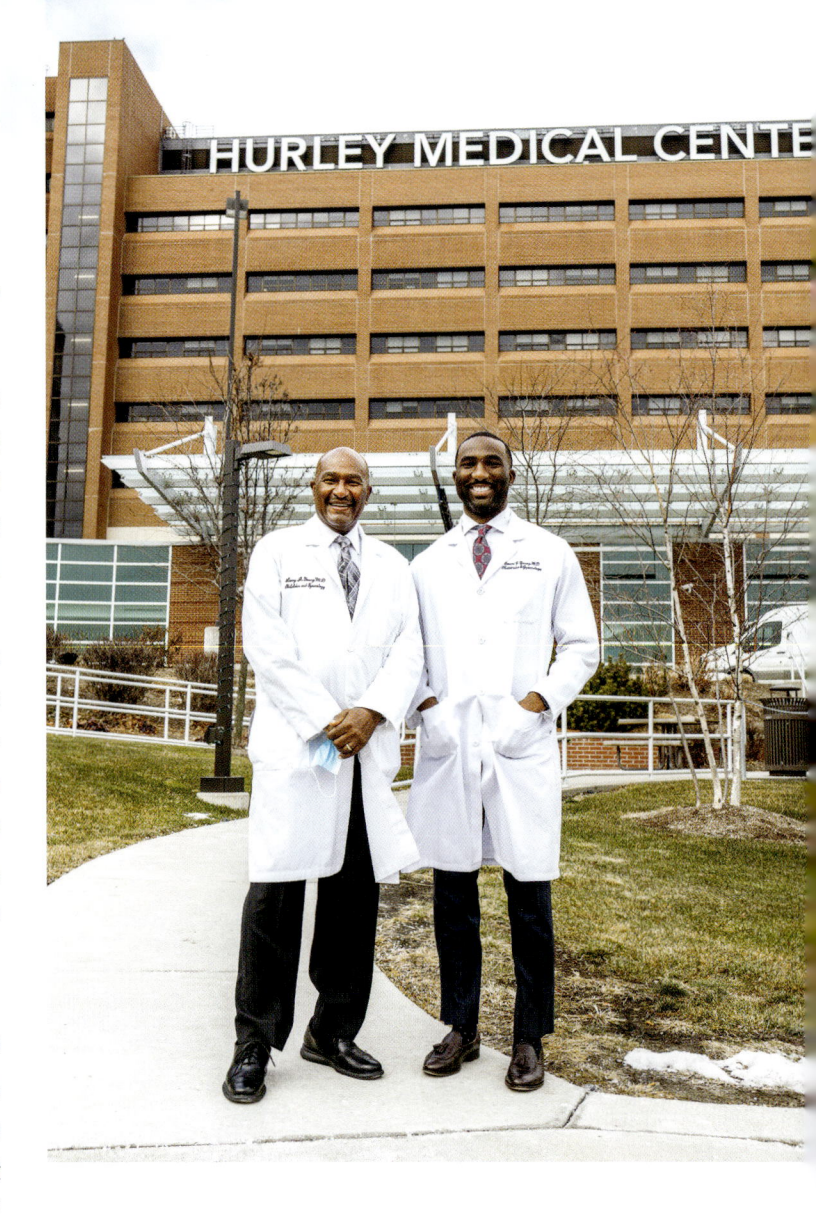

Dr. O. Young recalls an early experience when working alongside his father: "Monday mornings are protected time for resident education/didactics, which are usually covered by our CNM colleagues and faculty physicians. I'll never forget when I had the opportunity to be first assist on a cesarean section with my dad. It was a surreal moment that the entire operating room team took in and enjoyed."

When asked about his goals, Dr. O. Young replies, "I always have two goals in mind. First and foremost, is to always think of ways to improve the experience and patient safety for the women we serve; and second, to improve the educational experience of our resident physicians and medical students." Dr. O. Young is following in his father's steps in leadership positions, such as serving as co-chair of the 39th Annual Hurley Benefit Ball Committee in 2020, with proceeds benefiting the Ob-Gyn Department.

Pediatric Public Health Initiative

In January 2016, Hurley Children's Hospital and MSU formed the Pediatric Public Health Initiative (PPHI), based at Michigan State University College of Human Medicine (MSU CHM) Downtown Flint Campus, across from the Hurley Children's Clinic at the Farmer's Market, to address the Flint community's population-wide water crisis and to help all Flint children grow up healthy and strong. PPHI was divided into five work teams: Child and Health Development, Nutrition, Exposure Assessment, Health Informatics, and Child Health Policy & Advocacy. These teams work closely with the PPHI Parent Partner Group and the PPHI Flint Kids Advisory Group. PPHI works with many partners, as a center of excellence, to mitigate the impact of the Flint water crisis and to serve as a national resource for best practices.

"The creation of this PPHI will give Flint children a better chance at future success. This initiative will bring in a team of experts to build a model pediatric public health program, which will continue to assess, monitor, and intervene to optimize children's outcomes," said Mona Hanna-Attisha, MD, director, MSU-Hurley Children's Hospital PPHI, and former HMC pediatric residency program director.

According to its website, "The foundation for this new initiative is based on MSU CHM's 48-year medical education collaboration with HMC. It leverages MSU's 2014 Flint expansion of its Division of Public Health, which was supported by the Charles Stewart Mott Foundation, bringing new public health researchers to Flint to study the community's most pressing public health needs, with 'boots on the ground' in Downtown Flint."[9]

Since its inception, the PPHI has worked to develop robust evaluation and to lay the groundwork needed for a Flint water-crisis registry. In early 2017, the

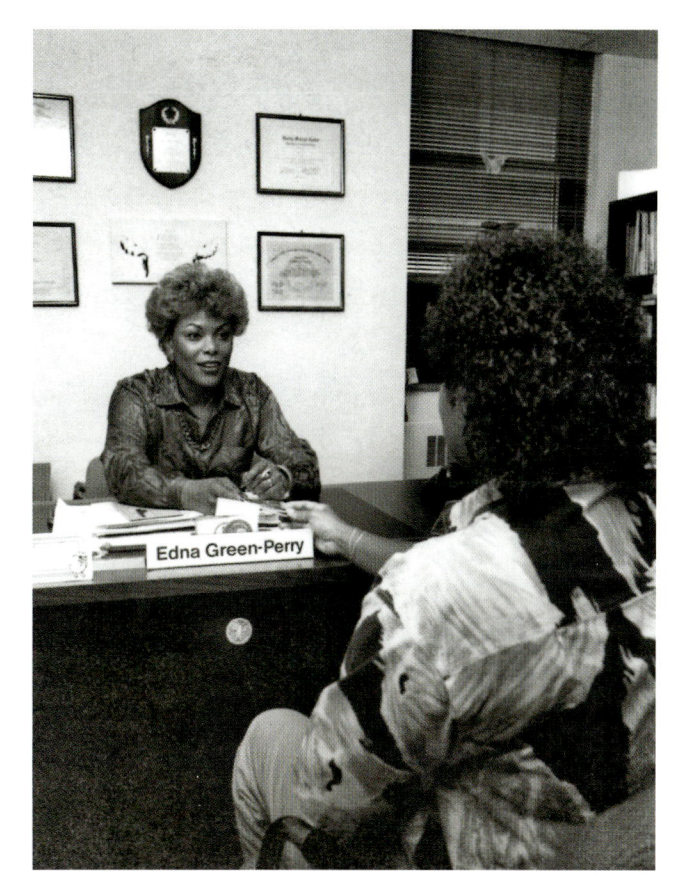

Edna Green-Perry, RN (shown here in 1989), contributed much towards women's health with a community support group, Women Reaching Women, that she started in 1980. The free substance abuse recovery program not only aided in their addictions but also addressed the underlying problems that aggravated recovery. Green-Perry served for many years on Hurley's board after her retirement from HMC in 1995.

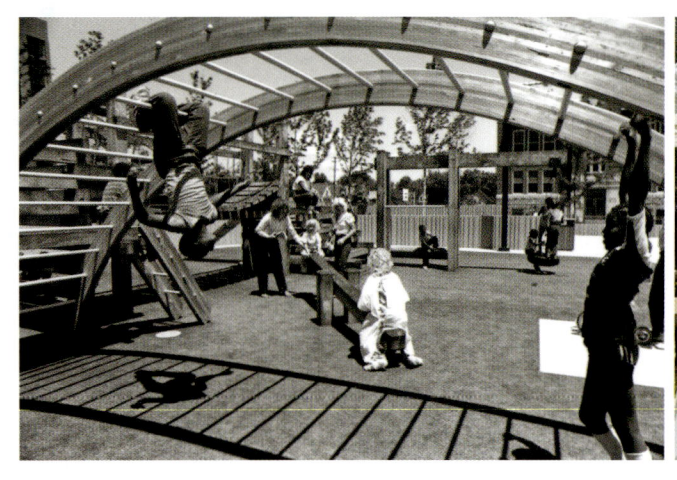

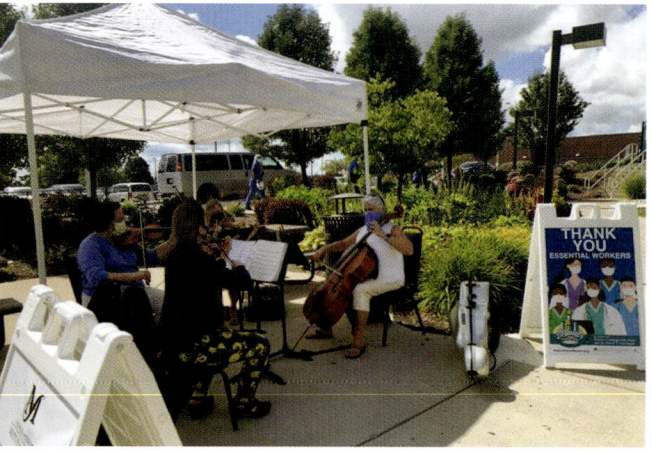

Dort Park, Then and Now
Mr. and Mrs. David T. Dort established the Marcia W. and J. Dallas Dort Park on the Hurley campus in memory of David's parents. His father, J. Dallas Dort, served on the first Hurley Board of Managers in 1905 and helped raise funds to build the hospital. Dort Park offered a place for therapeutic activities to enhance wellness, an aesthetic spot for family and friends to visit, a relaxing place for employees and volunteers, a playground for children, and an appealing neighborhood attraction. The park was dedicated in 1981. In 2012, part of the park's grounds was used to make way for the new emergency room lobby. Walkways, picnic tables, and flowers are still part of the old Dort Park. In 2020, musicians from the Flint Symphony Orchestra played there in an open-air concert series.

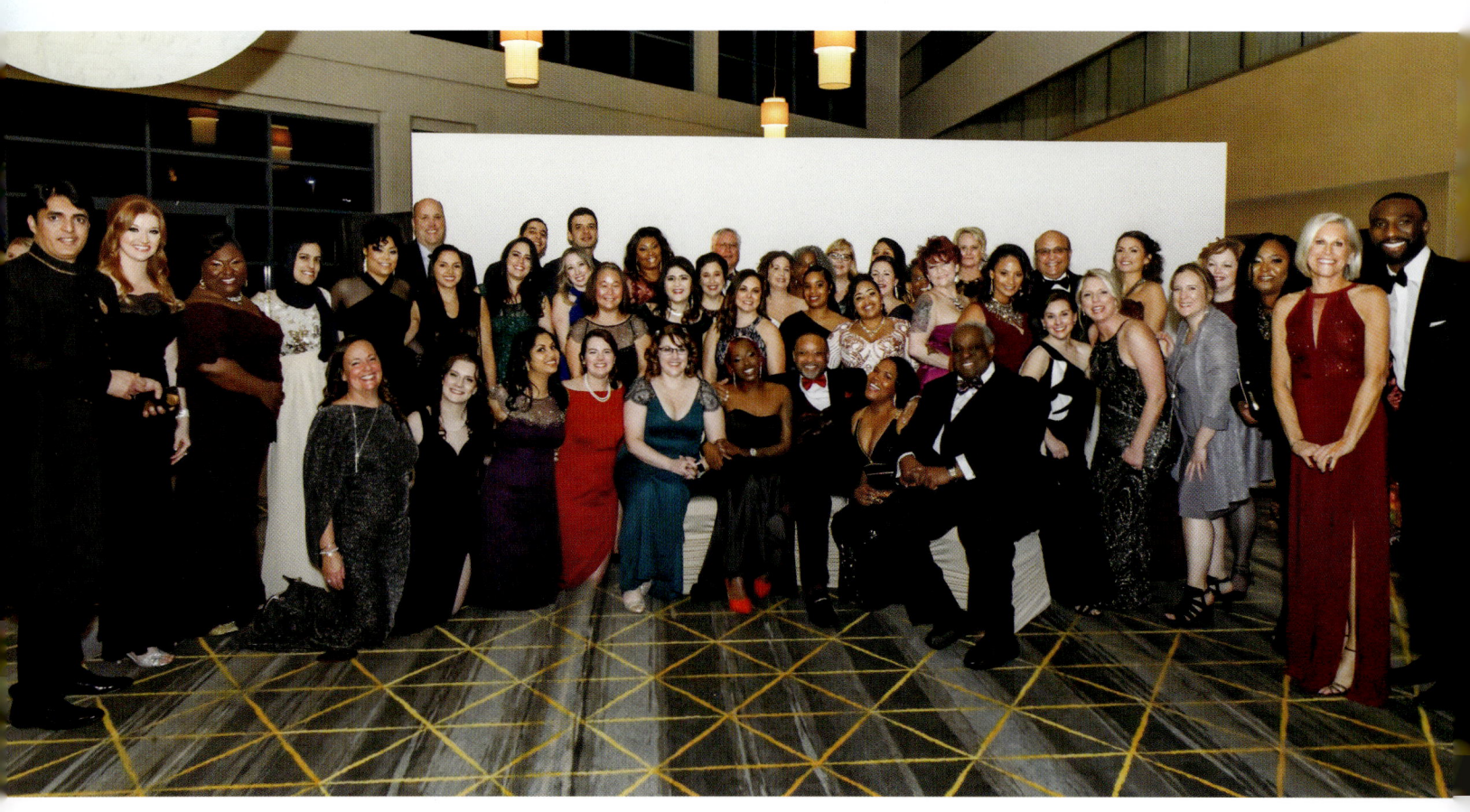

Many of the members of the Ob/Gyn Department turned out for the 2020 Benefit Ball. These individuals, many of whom have known each other for years, work together every day in caring for Hurley moms and babies. It was an enjoyable evening for them to dine, dance, and mingle while raising money to benefit the obstetrical service.

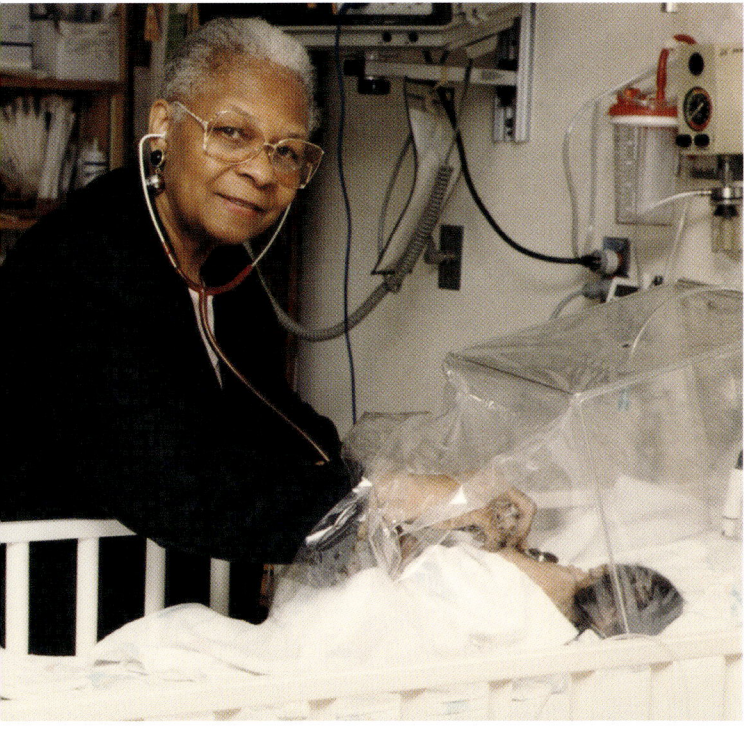

Vivian Lewis, MD

Crystal Cederna-Meko, PsyD, pediatric psychologist, with a patient

Michigan Department of Health and Human Services announced that it awarded a one-year, $500,000 grant to the PPHI for the planning of a registry of Flint residents.[10]

"Much of our work in Flint is just beginning, including efforts to mobilize long-term sustainability of interventions and assessments," said Dr. Hanna-Attisha. "However, we are hopeful and optimistic that the future for our Flint children will be as bright as ever!"

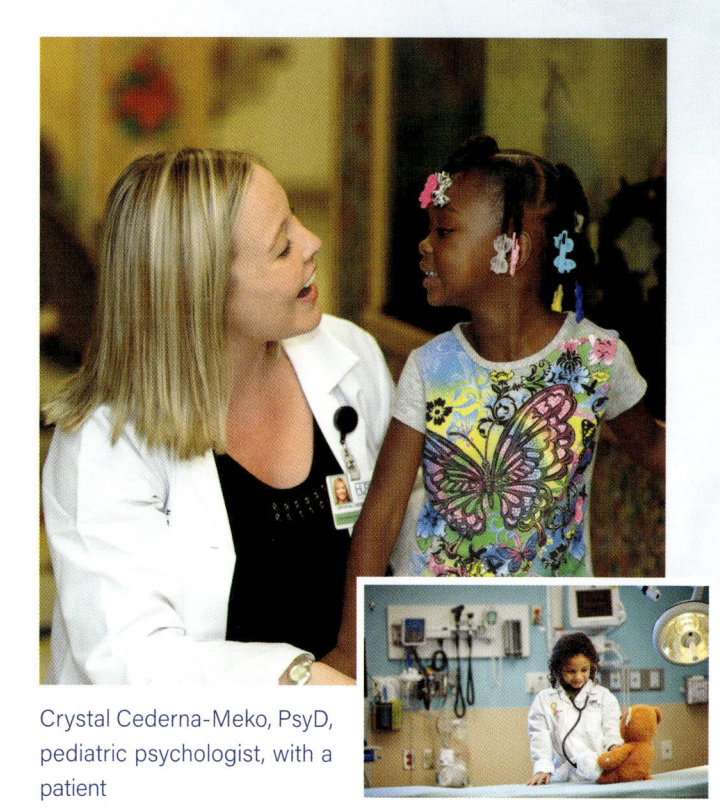

NOTES

1. Hurley Foundation, *Inside Report* (Winter 1993), p. 4.
2. Edwin Wood, *History of Genesee County, Michigan: Her People, Industries and Institutions* (Indianapolis: Federal Publishing Company, 1916), p. 806.
3. Ibid., p. 808.
4. The New Face of Hurley development campaign, 1977.
5. Elizabeth Shaw, "Birth Mark," *The Flint Journal*, September 8, 1988, p. C1.
6. Hurley Foundation, *Inside Report*, 2018–2019, p. 36.
7. Hurley Foundation, *Inside Report*, Volume 4 (1996), pp. 6–7.
8. Hurley Foundation, *Inside Report*, 2018–2019.
9. https://msuhurleypphi.org/about/overview.html.
10. Ibid.

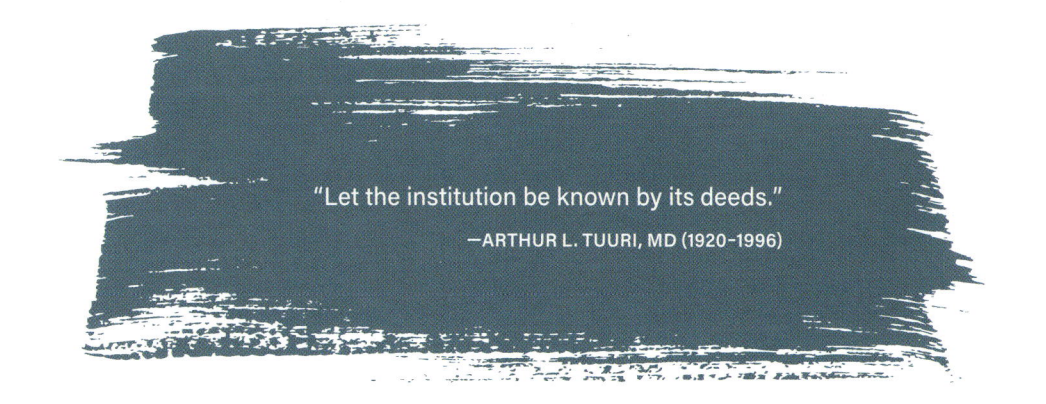

> "Let the institution be known by its deeds."
> —ARTHUR L. TUURI, MD (1920-1996)

AN EDUCATION Leader

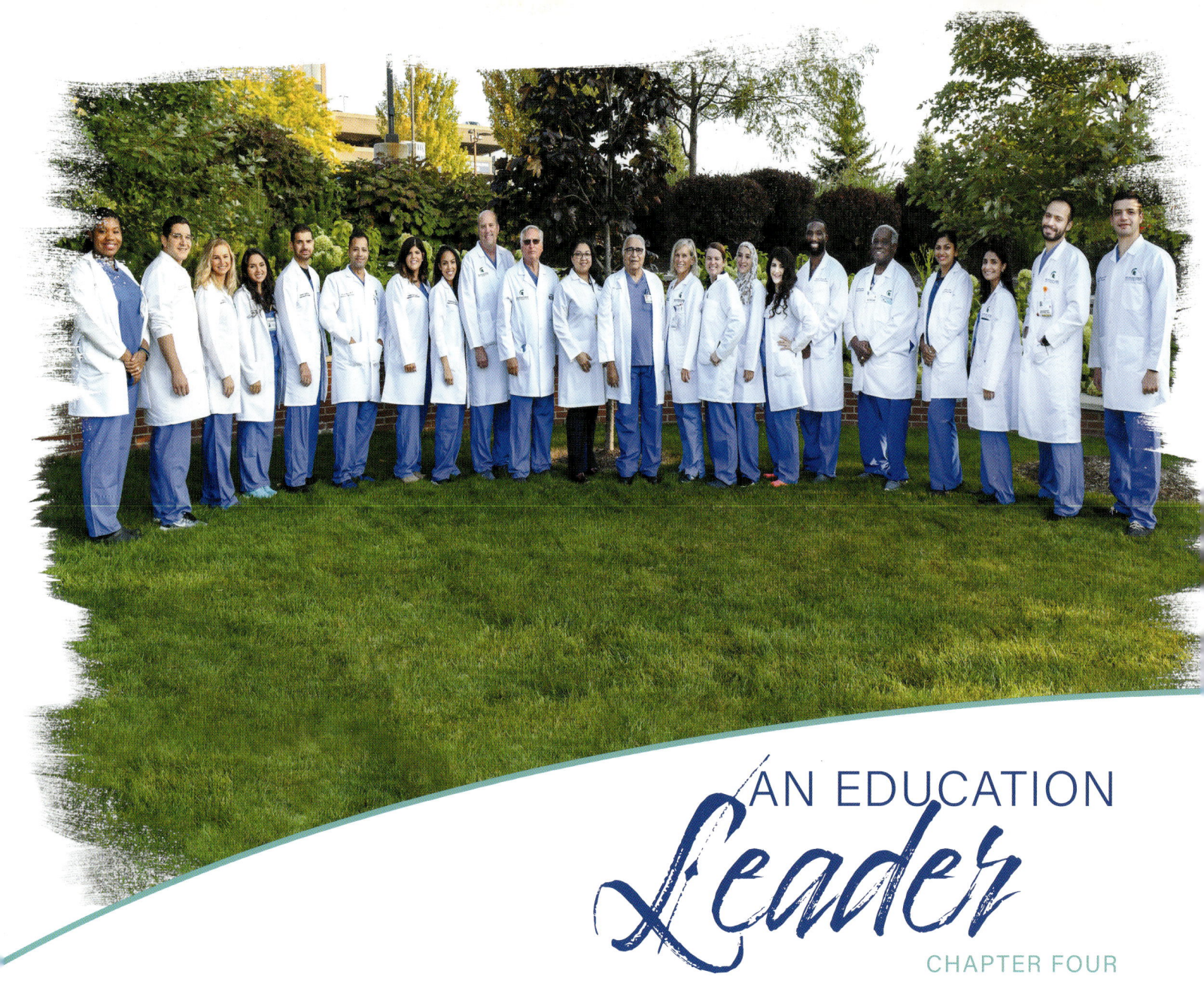

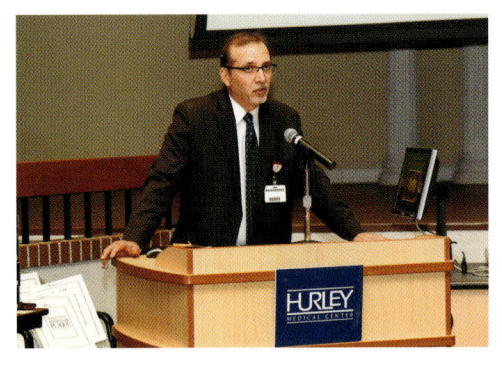

CHAPTER FOUR

Jim Buterakos talking to residents

Top: HMC residents with faculty. Top: Obstetrics and Gynecology,

As a premier public teaching hospital, Hurley provides a range of clinical experiences simply unavailable anywhere else in the region. Hurley's stellar reputation is due in part to the excellence of its educational programs and teaching, continuing medical education, and research opportunities. HMC is considered to be an exceptional place to learn from top professionals in their fields, while also gaining experience working with one of Michigan's largest and most diverse patient populations.

Leading the residency training programs is Jim Buterakos, chief academic officer and designated institutional officer (DIO), who has worked in the Hurley system for nearly 38 years. "GME [graduate medical education] works closely with all Hurley's residency training program directors to ensure their programs meet accreditation

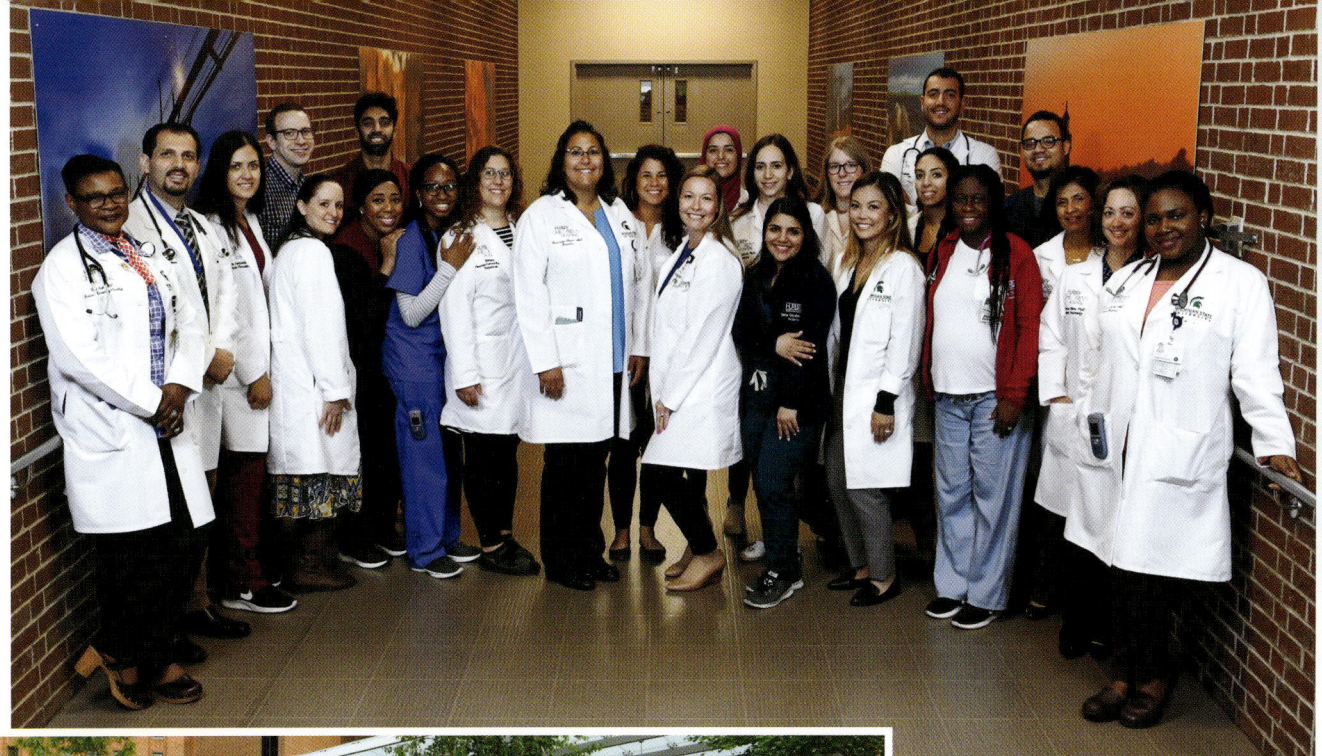

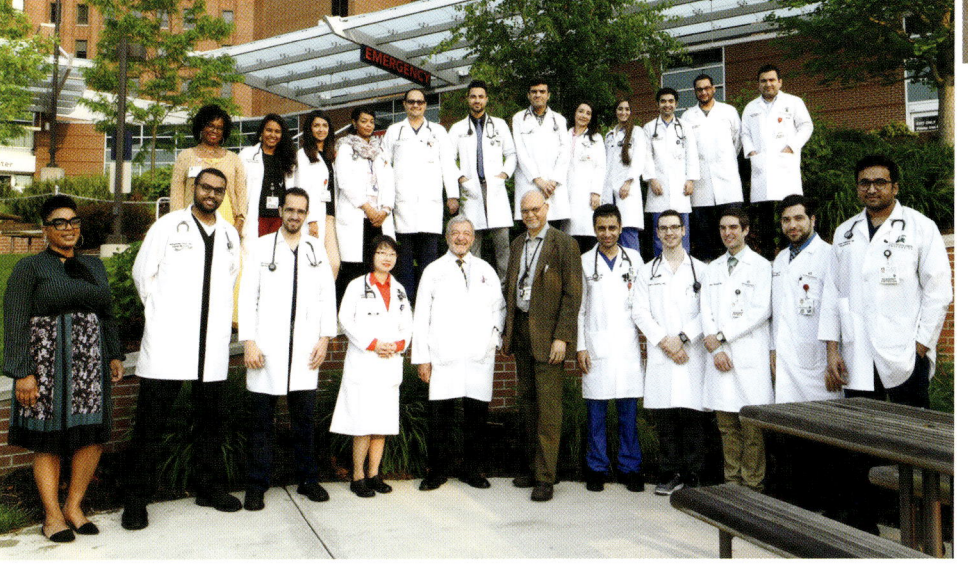

HMC residents with faculty. Top: Pediatrics, 2019; above: Internal Medicine, 2019.

requirements and to ensure institutional accreditation for medical education. We have full authority for all residency training program issues, including credentialing of resident physicians inclusive of visas, licensure, and certifications. Additionally, there are about 2,000 learners annually who receive their education at Hurley. HMC credentials all learners who rotate through the medical center," said Buterakos. He continued: "There have been a number of changes in the accreditation requirements since I started. The one change that created the biggest challenge and most anxiety has been acceptance of the Accreditation Council for Graduate Medical Education [ACGME] work hour rules. Resident work hours were capped at no more than 80 hours per week. It has remained controversial since its adoption, but it is a much-needed requirement to protect the safety of patients." In 2020, "Residency programs provide the sponsoring hospital with 24-hour physician coverage and maintain high-quality patient care by having teaching faculty on staff," said Buterakos. "Residency programs also benefit Hurley by bringing in full-time medical specialists who would not be there if they were not teaching opportunities."

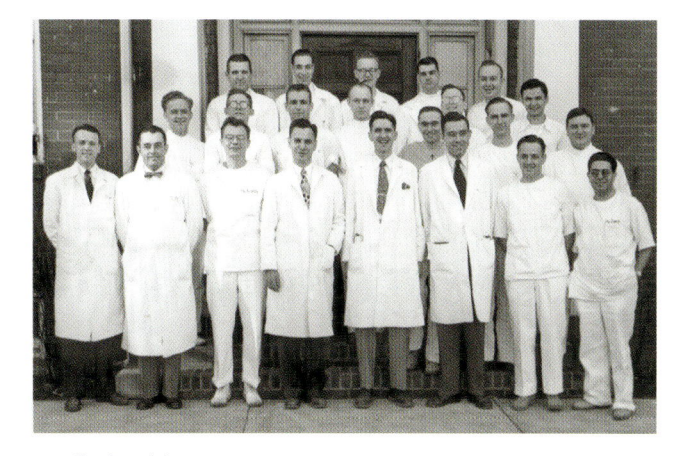

Medical residents, 1950

Graduate Medical Education – Medical Residency Programs

Interns at Hurley

Hurley Hospital began training medical interns in July 1919. Ira Odle, MD, was the first physician to complete a one-year internship at Hurley Hospital. Hurley accepted interns from 1919 until June 1983. Starting in July 1983, there were no longer internships—the term *intern* was used to represent a first-year resident. For many years, intern and resident positions were primarily held by males from American universities; it was not until the 1950s that interns and residents were accepted from universities outside of the United States and Canada. The first female interns at Hurley were Margaret Hatfield, MD, and Beatrice Lins, MD, who both completed their internships in 1927–1928. Female interns stayed in the nurses' home. According to Hurley records, until 1928, many of the internships were six to 12 months long. In July 1928, interns received training in surgery, medicine, obstetrics and gynecology, pediatrics, laboratory, isolation, X-ray, and outpatient.

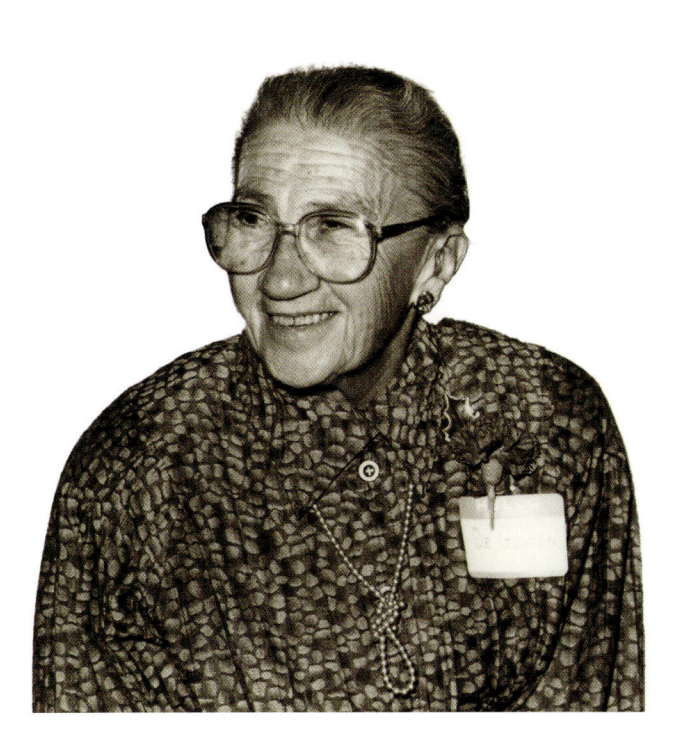

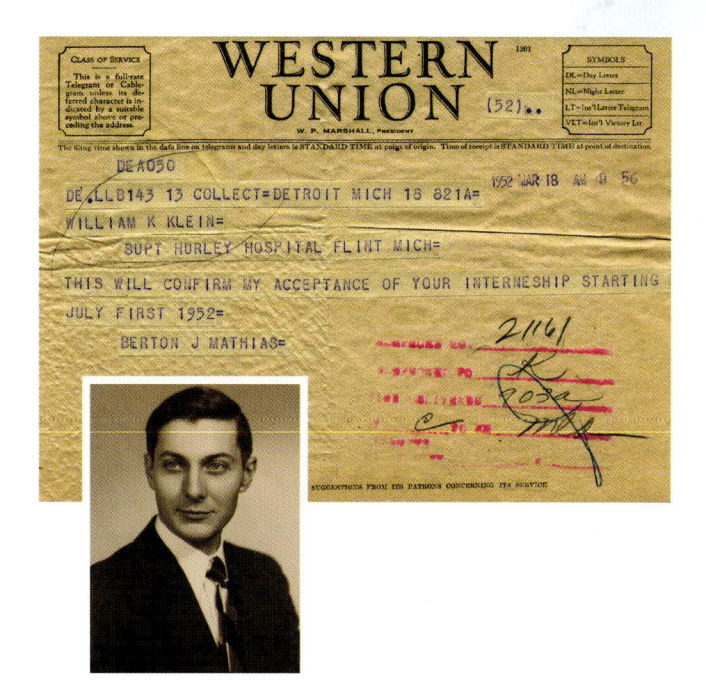

From an archived letter dated November 16, 1928:

We allow $25.00 per month and full maintenance [food and housing], exclusive of uniforms. We try to arrange so that each interne may have every other weekend (from Saturday noon until Monday morning) off, also allow a two week's vacation during the year. We are currently a 350 bed hospital.

From an archived letter dated May 17, 1946:

Hurley Hospital offers only rotating intern 12-month service. To be eligible for appointment to intern service, the applicant must be a citizen of the United States and a graduate of a Class A medical school. Internships are limited to men.

Evelyn Golden, MD

Evelyn "Effie" (Cohen) Golden was one of three women to graduate from the University of Wisconsin Medical School in 1936 and was the only female intern at Hurley Hospital from 1936 to 1937. For almost 50 years, Dr. Golden practiced medicine in Flint, specializing in women's health. She received numerous awards both during her life and posthumously. She was very active in the Flint community up until her death at the age of 91.

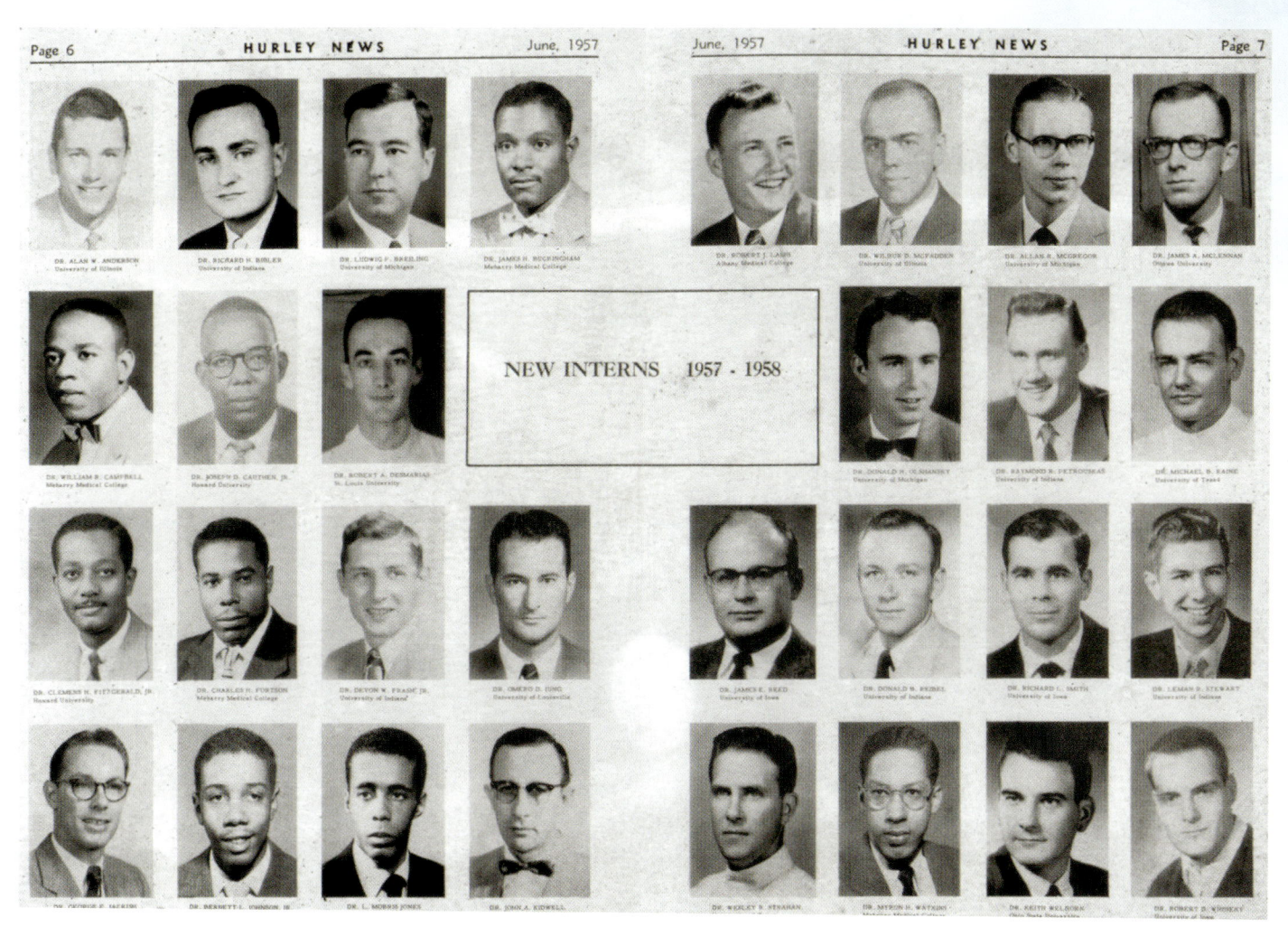

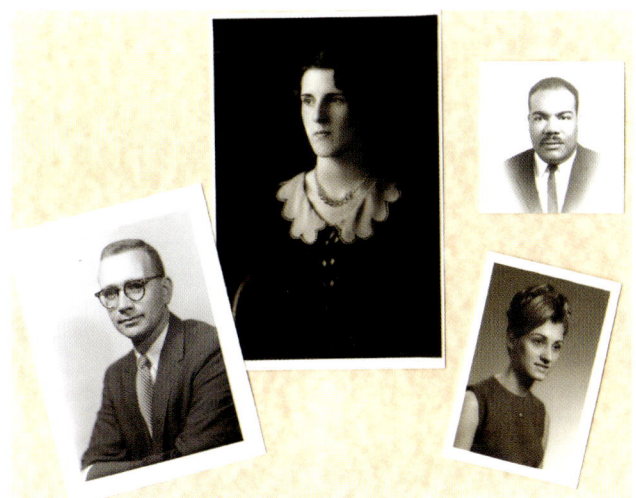

Residents through the decades (clockwise from the top): Bernice Stone, MD (Medicine, 1934–1936), William Roberson, MD (Ob-Gyn, 1964–1968), Joyce Fahrner, MD (IM, 1970–1974), and Paul Schroeder, MD (intern, 1952; IM resident, 1955–1958; IM Program Director, 1974–1978, Pinnacle Award recipient, 1998).

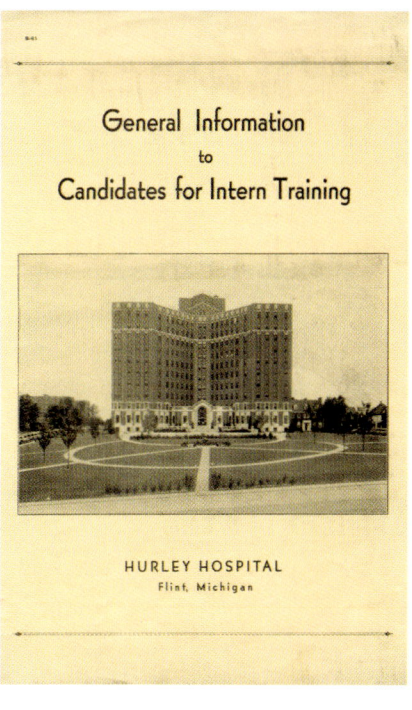

Hurley Graduate Medical Education Mission

To integrate medical education, research, modern medicine, and the mission of Hurley Medical Center to develop competent, skilled, ethical, and compassionate physicians who will meet the diverse needs of current and future patient populations, while cultivating lifetime skills for resiliency and wellness in the profession.

CHAPTER FOUR AN EDUCATION LEADER • 79

Hurley Residency Program

YEAR BEGUN	YEAR ENDED	RESIDENCY
1928	1985	Surgery
1929	Ongoing	Internal Medicine *(initially accredited on 8/8/1956)*
1930	1996	Pathology *(initially accredited in 1984)*
1933	1979	Radiology
1935	1936	Surgery/Pathology
1947	Ongoing	Obstetrics & Gynecology *(initially accredited on 3/5/1948)*
1950	1972	General Practice
1953	Ongoing	Pediatrics *(initially accredited on 11/7/1970)*
1970	Ongoing	Combined Internal Medicine/Pediatrics *(initially accredited on 7/1/2006)*
1970	1971	IM/Pathology
1975	Ongoing	Transitional Year *(initially accredited on 7/1/1983)*
1977	1986	Pedodontics *(name changed to Pediatric Dentistry in 1984)*

FELLOWSHIPS OFFERED AT HURLEY THROUGH THE YEARS

YEAR BEGUN	YEAR ENDED	RESIDENCY
1974	1982	Neonatology
1990	Ongoing	Psychology
2004	2020	Geriatric Medicine *(initially accredited on 7/1/2003)*
2008	Ongoing	Trauma
2013	Ongoing	Trauma Research

Surgery Residency: L. C. Snodgrass, MD, Hurley's first surgery resident, completed a seven-month residency from July 1, 1928, to February 1, 1929. During WWII, surgery was one of three primary residencies sought after. Records indicate that over the years, surgical residency training was from seven months up to six years. New residents joined the surgery residency every year from July 1945 until the residency ended in June 1985, except for 1936–1937. Program Directors: J. G. R. Manwaring, MD (1928–1929), G. Foster Kline, MD (1968–1969), and Alexander Nehme, MD (1979–1985, when the program closed).

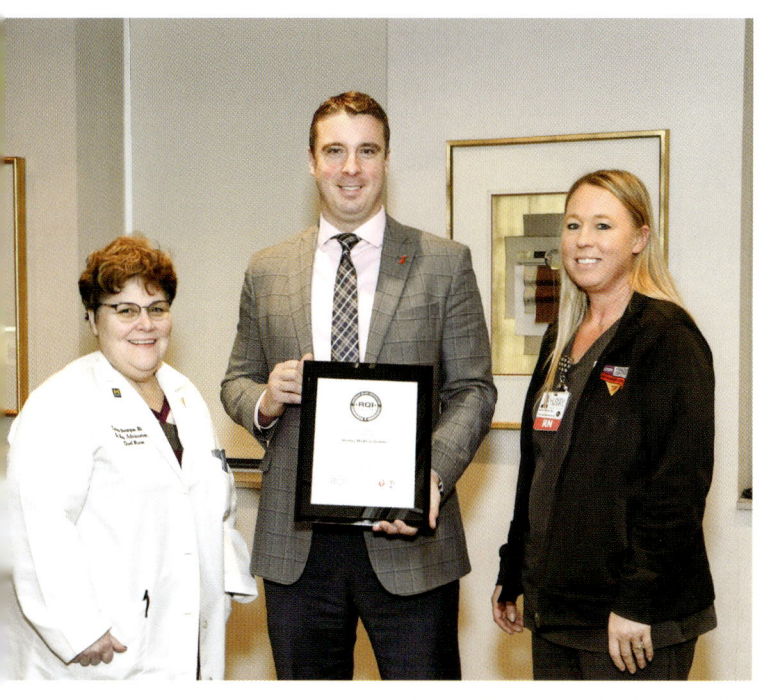

Hurley Recognized for Implementing Resuscitation Quality Improvement (RQI) Program

In early 2019, HMC was recognized by the American Heart Association and Laerdal Medical for implementing the RQI program and showing dedication to high-quality CPR. RQI refreshes CPR skills using mobile simulation stations instead of a classroom. HMC's contribution is reflected by a 97.25 percent compliance rate, leading to better patient outcomes. Left to right: Teresa Bourque, BSN, senior administrator, Nursing, Adam Cates, and Jennifer McDermitt, BSN, clinical nurse specialist.

Internal Medicine (IM)/General Practice Residency: George Case, MD, was the first internal medicine resident, from 1929 to 1930. Internal medicine is the longest, continual residency program at Hurley.

Director of Medical Service: W. H. Marshall, MD (1928–1930). Director, Department of Medicine: Glenn Drewyer, MD (1947 to at least 1965), Raymond Johnson, MD (1967 to at least 1972), Paul Schroeder, MD (1974–1978). Program Directors: Keith Champney, MD (1980–1982), Douglas Notman, MD (1982–1985), Robert Rosenbaum, MD (1985–1993), Barbara McIntosh, MD (1993–2005), Jeff Greenblatt, MD (2006–2009), and Ghassan Bachuwa, MD (2009–present). In 2021, the three-year IM program has 45 residents.

From an archived letter dated January 1947 regarding the medicine residency:

Hurley Hospital offers a program for graduate training in Medicine. This is a 3-year program. Two appointments are made each year for the 12-month period beginning July 1st. This period is spent at Hurley Hospital. At the end of the 12-month period the trainee who is considered the most qualified, automatically receives an extension of two years to his original appointment. The first year of this 2-year extension is spent in residence at the University of Michigan studying the basic sciences. The second year the trainee returns to Hurley Hospital.

From an archived letter from 1957 regarding the general practice residency:

The resident in General Practice will be assigned to the following services: 3 months pediatrics, 3 months medicine, 1 month trauma, 2 months obstetrics, 1 month psychiatry, including adult and children, 2 months in anesthesia with the afternoons spent in radiology and pathology – 1 month each.

Pathology Residency: The first pathology resident, Glenn Backus, MD, began his residency in 1930 and completed it in 1932. In January 1933, he was appointed chief pathologist and director of the Clinical Pathological Laboratories; it is unknown when he left that role. Records indicate that the next director of Pathology was E. M. Knights Jr., MD (1959 to unknown). The pathology residency was one of three core residencies at Hurley during WWII.

DID YOU KNOW | …in 1941 and 1942, the average cost of food for interns and residents was about $23.50 per month.

CHAPTER FOUR AN EDUCATION LEADER • 81

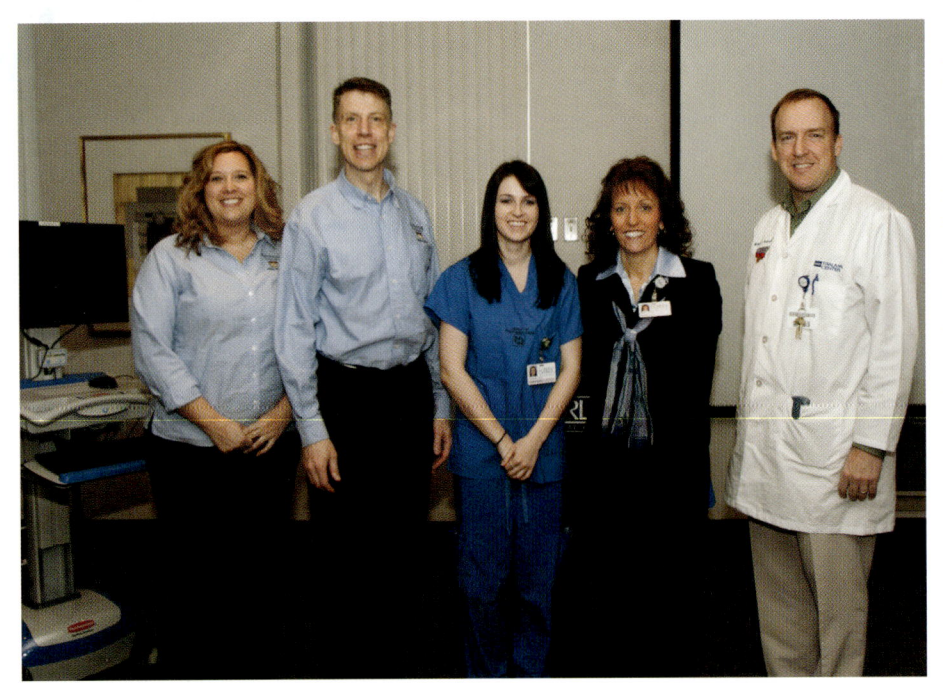

Joint Scribe Program – The First of Its Kind in the Country
In 2013, HMC and Kettering University unveiled the first joint physician-scribe program, offering support and training for medical professionals using the new electronic medical record (EMR) system. Scribes work closely with doctors to record patient information as they transition towards the computerized EMR. The program offers aspiring medical students an up-close view of working in the field of medicine. Left to right: Stacy Seeley, PhD, and Pat Atkinson, PhD, Kettering University; Alex Petit, Kettering scribe; Melany Gavulic, RN, MBA, president, CEO; and Michael Roebuck, MD, chief medical information officer.

Program Directors: Frank Hodges, MD (1978 until his death in 1981), and Willys Mueller Jr., MD (1981–1996, when the program closed).

Radiology Residency: Harold Woughter, MD, was the first radiology resident, from 1933 to 1934. The radiology residency was one of three primary residencies at Hurley during WWII. Hurley maintained this residency program from 1933 until 1979. In March of 1982, University Affiliated Hospitals of Flint, which was later changed to MSU Flint Area Medical Education (FAME), assumed administrative responsibility for the radiology residents, who rotated at all three local hospitals—Hurley, McLaren, and Genesys.

Obstetrics & Gynecology (Ob-Gyn) Residency: The Ob-Gyn residency began in 1947. Jack Thompson, MD, was the first obstetrics and gynecology resident, completing a three-year program in 1950. Records are unclear of program directors prior to 1980. Program Directors: Clinton Dowd, MD (1980–1996), and John Hebert III, MD (1998 to present). In 2021, the four-year Ob-Gyn program has 16 residents.

Pediatric Residency: Berton Mathias, MD, was Hurley's first pediatric resident, from 1953 to 1955. Program Directors: Robert Clark, MD (1966–1967), William Nicholls, MD (1967 to unknown), George Baker, MD (1972–1977), John Reid, MD (1977 to unknown), Thomas Marr, MD (1981–1984), Ralph Gordon, MD (1984–1991), John Tauscher, MD (1991–1992), Timur Sumer, MD (1992–1995), Melissa Hamp, MD (1995–2010), Mona Hanna-Attisha, MD (2011–2018), and Gwendolyn Reyes, MD (2018 to present). In 2021, the three-year pediatric program has 21 residents.

"Bachelors Quarters" for residents, built in 1969

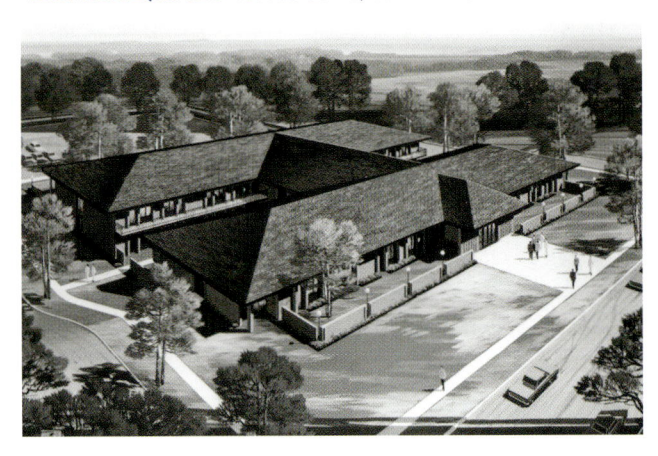

Combined Internal Medicine/Pediatrics (Med/Peds) Residency: Prior to being an ACGME-accredited residency in 2006, institutions that had both internal medicine and pediatric residencies could offer a non-accredited med/peds residency. Thomas Maggs, MD, was Hurley's first med/peds resident, from 1970 to 1971. Program Directors: Thomas Marr, MD (1982–1985), Ralph Gordon, MD (1985–1991), Melissa Hamp, MD (1991–1994), Timur Sumer, MD (1994–1995), Laura Carravallah, MD (1995–2014), Vijay Naraparaju, MD (2014–2019), and Adiraj Singh, MD, interim program director (January 2020 to present). In 2021, the four-year med/peds program has 12 residents.

Transitional Year Residency: The transitional year (TY) residency began in 1975. The TY residency provides a one-year, well-rounded clinical experience in internal medicine, obstetrics-gynecology, pediatrics, and other specialties as requested by the resident. Some residencies require completion of a TY program as a prerequisite to enter other residency training programs. Some physicians complete a TY residency to decide which specialty field they would like to pursue. Program Directors: Clinton Dowd, MD

E. Marshall Goldberg, MD, was a Hurley physician, researcher, and noted author who released his first nonfiction work, *Cell Wars*, nationally in 1988. Goldberg authored eight fictional novels, all medical mysteries, and wrote several episodes for the *Dr. Kildare* series in the 1960s.

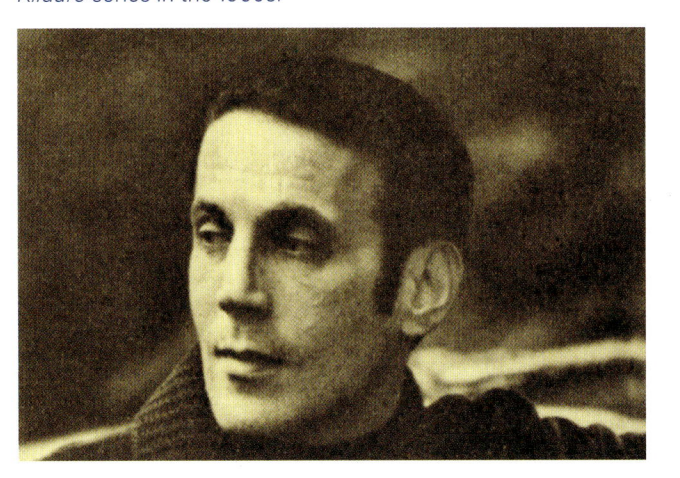

DID YOU KNOW | ...from 1961 to 1970, 60 percent of Flint's physicians had received all or part of their medical training at Hurley.

(1979–1983), Willys Mueller Jr., MD (1983–1997), and Ghassan Bachuwa, MD (1998 to present). In 2020, the one-year TY program has six residents.

Pedodontic/Pediatric Dentistry Residency: Daniel Klein, DDS, and Michael Chow, DDS, were the first two-year pedodontic residents, starting July 1, 1977; the program was renamed as the pediatric dentistry residency in July 1985. HMC Program Directors: Fred Bruner, DDS (1977–1984), and Daniel Carroll, DMD (1984–1991). In the following years, the program established affiliations with Mott Children's Health Center (MCHC) and the University of Michigan School of Dentistry (UMSD) to form a joint Hurley/MCHC/UMSD pediatric dentistry program.

Neonatology Fellowship: John Tauscher, MD, educational chief of Neonatology (1977 to unknown). Program Directors: Raymond Chan, MD (1979–1980), John Tauscher, MD (1980–1981), and Robert Meny, MD (1982–1984).

Psychology Fellowship: The fellowships include two separate options: rehabilitation (adult and pediatric) psychology and pediatric psychology. Program Directors: Michael Lechner, PhD (1993–2003), Eileen McKee, PhD (2003–2007), and Kirk Stucky, PsyD (2007 to present).

Trauma & Trauma Research Fellowship: In 1999, Farouck Obeid, MD, initiated an affiliation agreement with Henry Ford to have their trauma fellows complete a one-year trauma rotation at Hurley and a one-year critical care rotation at Henry Ford. In 2008, the one-year trauma fellowship established new affiliations with the MSU CHM surgery residency program and has been at HMC ever since. The one-year trauma research fellowship began in 2013. Program Directors: Farouck Obeid,

Michael H. and Robert M. Hamady Health Sciences Library

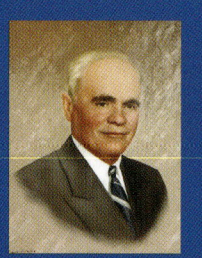

Since its beginning, Hurley's library has been a medical library of distinction, due, in part, from significant donations and support throughout the decades, but also because of HMC's reputation as a major teaching hospital, which shaped the repository over the years. "The Hamady Health Sciences Library (HHSL) is an integral component in graduate medical education at Hurley Medical Center," said Jennifer Godlesky, MLIS, Hamady Health Sciences Library manager. "We work closely with our medical faculty and resident physicians to not only provide the most current medical literature, but also teaching them how to navigate the world of health information and evidence-based medicine. The library collection contains about 1,000 print books and 58 print journal titles. Additionally, we provide access to over 1,500 textbooks and hundreds of scholarly journals online," noted Godlesky.

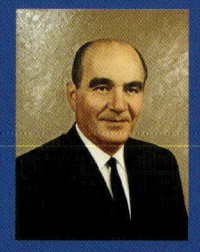

Michael H.   Robert M.

The foundation of Hurley's medical library began in 1938, when noted surgeon and one of the founders of the American College of Surgeons, Joshua G. F. Manwaring, MD,[1] donated 1,000 medical books to Hurley Hospital, which included rare, early editions of core medical books that are still part of the library collection today. At that time, it was open to the public under the direction of librarian Sarah Burgess.

The library was officially named the Michael H. and Robert M. Hamady Health Sciences Library when father and son CEOs, who founded Hamady Brothers, a large grocery store chain based in Flint, chose to leave a lasting legacy. In 1964, the Michael H. Hamady family made a generous donation, which established the comprehensive, full-service library. They made another significant donation in 1976, on behalf of Robert M., to establish a modernized audio-visual room, which turned it into one of the best medical libraries in the state. In 1968, Anthos (Anni) Hungerford, librarian, was hired to transform the library's standing.

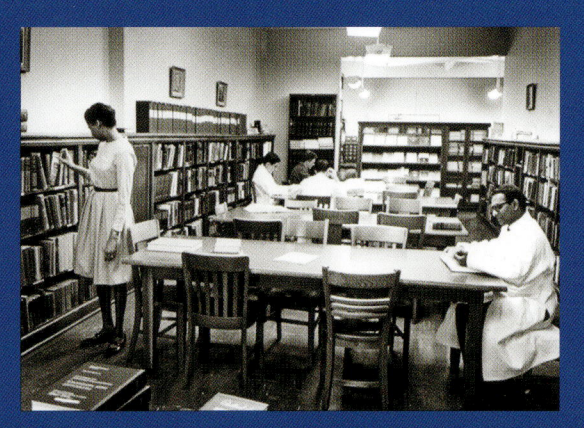

In 1974, the Edward Joseph portrait and collection of labor relations and management relations textbooks and tapes were donated to Hurley's library. Joseph was instrumental in shaping the medical center as we know it today. He served as president of the Hurley Board of Managers from 1969 to 1972 and was Hurley's legal counsel from 1974 to 1987.

The library was an essential study and research location for resident physicians and nursing students. Library staff have always sought an innovative approach to embrace and implement technological advances to aid in learning. "We were the first in the area to convert the card catalogues to an online catalogue, accessible through early desktop computer stations in the 1980s," said Sharon Williams, MLIS, retired library director, who worked for Hurley for 38 years and replaced the third library director, Martha Studaker.

"The library's responsibility is to provide the resources to serve and support the hospital's mission of 'Clinical Excellence – Service to People,'" adds Williams. "Another first, in 1980, was the establishment of the Community Health Information Library, where patients and their families could find out more about a particular disease/diagnosis or about health concerns. Hurley became known for providing lay-based health information material before it was available online."

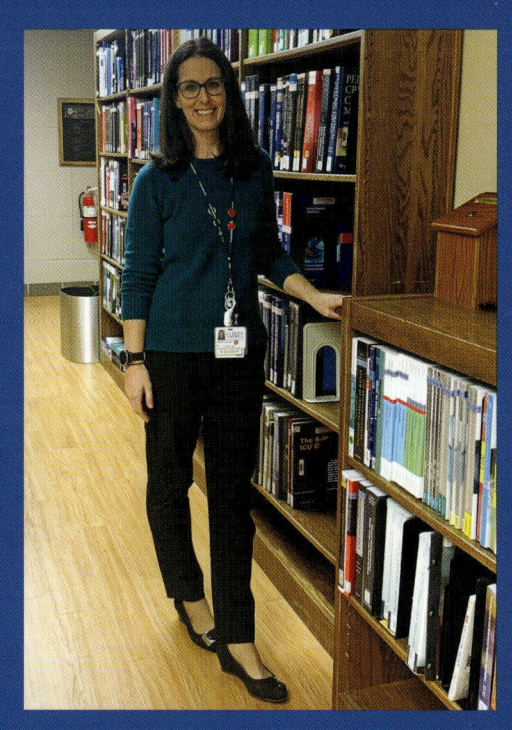

In November 2019, the medical library moved to the basement of the North Tower. Seen here is Jennifer Godlesky, MLIS, library manager.

"The library endowment fund was created in 1985 to help the medical library have access to the most up-to-date technology available. The endowment fund has helped the library purchase resources, including computers, scanners, databases with full-text medical textbooks and peer-reviewed journals, board review materials for our physicians, as well as iPads, iPods, and mobile device chargers," adds Godlesky. "The endowment fund has made it possible for the library staff to be creative in the delivery of library services and has helped us remain at the forefront of graduate medical education at HMC through the years." The Max R. Burnell Trust Fund helped to provide current information on gynecology, obstetrics, and perinatology.

The Hamady Health Sciences Library is a member of the National Network of Libraries of Medicine, an initiative of the National Library of Medicine, the National Institutes of Health, the US Department of Health and Services, the Medical Library Association, and the Michigan Health Sciences Library Association.

MD (1999–2008), James Wagner, MD (2008–2012), Michael McCann, DO (2012–2016), and Leo Mercer, MD (2016–present). In 2020, the one-year fellowship has one trauma fellow and one trauma research fellow.

Geriatric Medicine Fellowship: Haseeb Khawaja, MD, was the first one-year fellow, which began in 2004. Program Directors: Ghassan Bachuwa, MD (2004–2012), Myriam Edwards, MD (2012–2014), Amy Daros, DO (2014–2017), and Rasha Nakhleh, MD (2017 until the fellowship closed in 2020).

Duties and Responsibilities Changed Over the Years

From an archived letter dated May 17, 1946:

Hurley Hospital comes closer to an ideal internship than any hospital I know in the midwest. I say this for three reasons: 1) the enormous number of acute cases we see. Our bed capacity is close to 750 and the number of new admissions per year is in the neighborhood of 25,000 to 28,000; 2) our highly-organized teaching program, which makes a concerted effort to balance responsibility with teaching and puts service obligations at a minimum; 3) the combination of a full residency staff and a large visiting professorship series (80 per year) affords the intern excellent instruction on his difficult cases. I feel no qualms about assuring you that you will get to see and do as much as you possibly wish. The average patient load is 18 patients and we try to limit you to four work-ups during the day. The interns round with the house staff and the attending male four to five days a week. Private physicians are welcome to attend these rounds, but rarely do. The average call schedule is every third night for medicine, pediatrics and surgery; you work five 12-hour shifts a week in the emergency room and usually have weekends off. In OB it is on twenty-four and off twenty-four.

Wars and Their Impact on Graduate Medical Education

During World War II and the Vietnam War, internships and residencies were greatly reduced due to the calls to duty for the country. During World War II, the US War Manpower Commission dictated which residents could or could not continue their internship/residency and how many internship/residency programs throughout the United States could train at any given time. Clinical coverage was continually adjusted due to the constant changes being directed by the federal government. Many physicians left their residency early—either by enlistment or draft—to serve; some returned to complete their residency after their tour was completed. During these eras, many of the headshot photographs submitted with the internship and residency applications were of the physician in his military uniform.

World War II

Prior to World War II, internships and residencies began on July 1 of each year and were a minimum of one year. The attack at Pearl Harbor drastically altered residency programs around the United States. Internships were reduced from 12 months to nine months to meet the federally mandated quota, and to provide adequate clinical coverage; this 9-9-9 Program was initiated by the War Manpower Commission.

July 1941: There were seven interns and five residents

July 1942: There were two interns and six residents

1940–1944: Only internships and surgery, pathology, and radiology residencies were offered at Hurley

The federally mandated changes to residency programs during World War II allowed two physicians the opportunity to complete an internship and several residencies at Hurley Hospital:

Thomas Cox, MD
- Internship: July 1, 1940, to June 30, 1941
- Pathology Residency: July 1, 1941, to June 30, 1942
- Surgery Residency: July 1, 1942, to August 3, 1942 (left for the military)
- Surgery Residency: March 4, 1946, to December 31, 1949

Sydney Lyttle, MD
- Internship: September 1, 1944, to June 1, 1945
- Pathology Residency: June 1, 1945, to March 1, 1946
- Surgery Residency: March 1, 1946, to November 30, 1946
- Radiology Residency: February 16, 1948, to July 1, 1948

From an archived letter dated April 17, 1942:

The resident staff quota provides for one chief resident, six residents and ten internes. At this writing, the staff that is scheduled starting July 1, 1942 includes one chief resident, six residents and two internes. Up to this time, we have accepted internes only on a basis of twelve month appointments starting July of each year. You will note by the enclosed that this policy has been changed and for the duration of the war period, interne appointments will be made starting July, October, January and April. While contracts have not been completed we are anticipating six internes starting October 1, 1942, and hope that by January 1, 1943, we will again have a full quota of ten internes. We are making plans to accept two or three additional residents starting July 1, 1942, to help make up for the shortage of internes.

From an archived letter dated December 5, 1944:

The War Manpower Commission has established a quota for this hospital (Hurley) of 8 interns and 4 junior and/or senior residents. Beginning with the second Monday in January, 1945 and continuing the second Monday of each month until the quotas are filled, the Intern Committee will review applications for the 8 appointments of internships beginning April 1, 1945 and the 4 appointments of junior and/or senior residents beginning July 1, 1945.

From an archived letter dated July 21, 1952, sent to the chairman of the Michigan Volunteer Advisory Committee, Detroit, Michigan, regarding an intern application request:

Hurley Hospital is a large city hospital in a highly industrialized area, a good part of whose facilities are devoted to defense production. An acute general hospital of this type is subject to a large number of admissions as a result of industrial accidents. The intern in this hospital is a key part of the immediate medical service rendered to the patient. It is the intern who staffs the Emergency Room on a 24-hour basis, and the intern who covers the hospital night and day for medical emergencies and the immediate medical care. Our resident staff has been decimated by the demands of the armed services, and we have become more and more dependent upon the interns for medical coverage. It is our considered opinion, therefore, that this man is extremely essential not only to the operation of the hospital, but to the maintenance of the working population in the interests of defense production.

The Vietnam War

During the Vietnam War era, intern and resident applicants were required to include their "military status" as part of their employment application. Residents could be, and were, drafted for military service, regardless of their work status at the time. It was common for letters to be sent from Hurley to the US Selective Service attempting to justify its need for the residents and requesting permission to allow them to complete their residency at Hurley before being drafted.

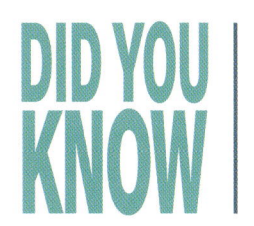

DID YOU KNOW …in 1980, HMC announced an innovative project for internal medicine residents to see patients in "model offices." Precipitated by internal medicine specialists, young doctors could experience a wide variety of patients in a private practice setting.

Wages through the Decades

The wage ranges below are listed by decades (lowest wage to highest wage) during the indicated periods. The highest wages typically represent wages for the most senior resident/fellow during that period. Where "up to" is noted, wage increases occurred during that period.

YEAR	ROLE	WAGES
1919 through 1929	Intern	$25 per month
1930 through 1939	Intern	$25 per month
Great Depression, 1928–1933	Resident	$41.60 per month
1940 through 1949	Intern	$25 per month
WWII, 1939–1945	Resident	$41.60 per month
1950 through 1959	Intern	$2,340 up to $3,000 per year
	Resident	$3,240 up to $5,100 per year
1960 through 1969	Intern	$3,000 up to $7,500 per year
United States' involvement in Vietnam begins in March 1965	Resident	$3,900 up to $9,000 per year
1970 through 1979	Intern	$7,500 up to $15,390 per year
United States' involvement in Viet Nam ends in April 1975	Resident	$8,100 up to $20,100 per year
1980 through 1989	Resident	$17,429 up to $24,134 per year
Internships no longer offered		
1990 through 1999	Resident	$26,246 up to $36,712 per year
2000 through 2009	Resident	$38,520 up to $58,369 per year
2010 through 2019	Resident	$47,046 up to $60,053 per year

Hurley School of Nursing – 86 Years of Excellence

Within a month of Hurley Hospital's opening in 1908, the board of managers established a training school for nurses. Mary Palma of Attica was the first student to apply for admission in January 1909. She started her two-and-a-half-year program in May 1909. Nursing students were not required to have a high school diploma at that time, classes did not start at the same time, and most of the students came from surrounding farm communities. The curriculum included housekeeping-type responsibilities, such as cooking, cleaning rooms, scrubbing floors, washing bandages, and making beds. By 1913, the course work had lengthened from its original two and a half years to three years, and completion of at least an eighth-grade education became a requirement for admission. Students spent 12-hour days and six and a half days a week in the clinical setting. The nursing students were supervised by hospital nurses and part-time instructors. The nursing director presided over the school while also living in the nurses' residence. Anna Schill was the first superintendent of Hurley Hospital, as well as the director of the nursing school from 1909 to 1921.

The fate of the graduating class of 1916 was caught up in a nation teetering on the edge of war. The United States entered World War I on April 6, 1917. During 1917 and 1918, Hurley divided its attention between the demands of

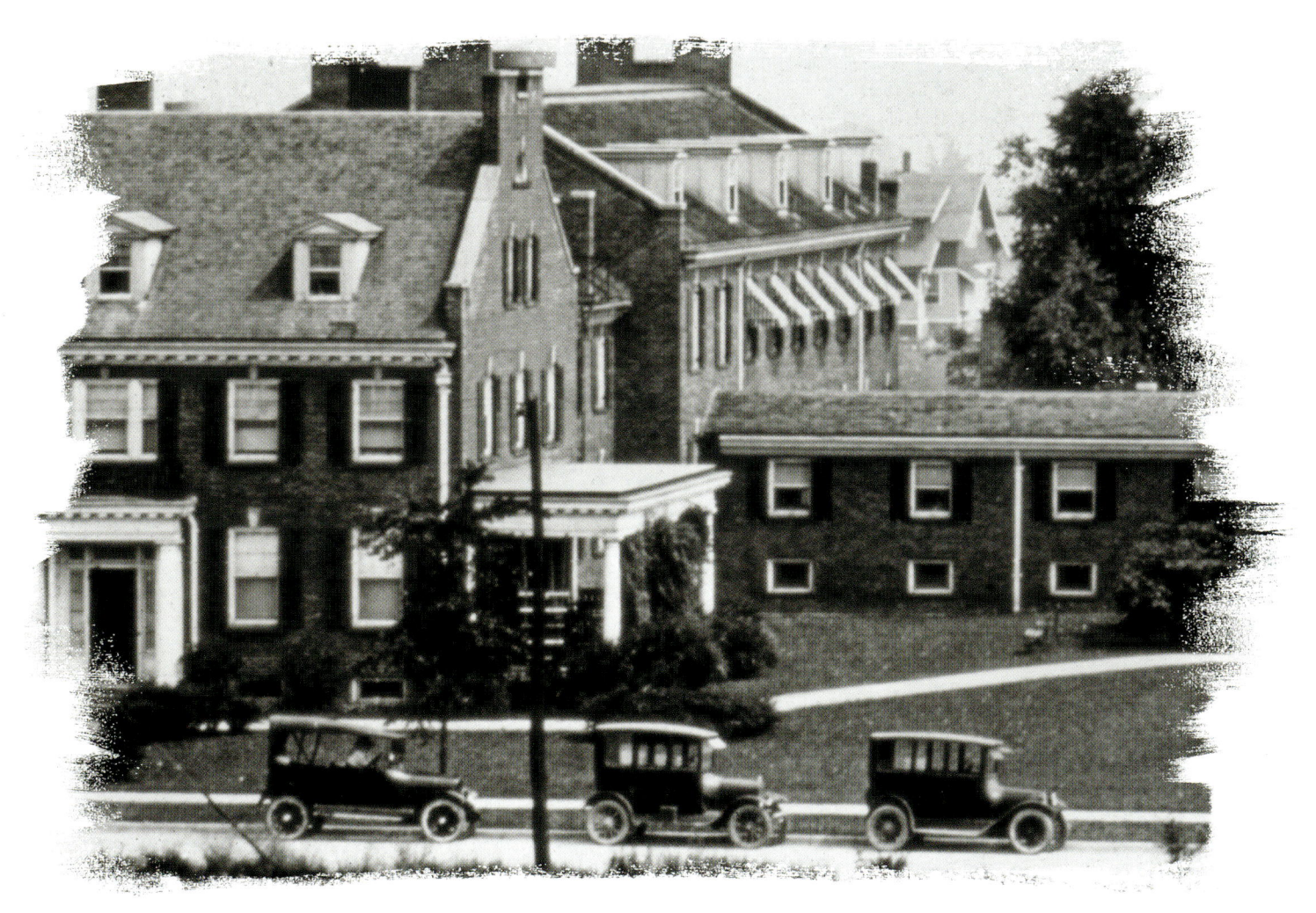

The first nurses' residence (left) was completed in 1912 at a cost of $13,000 and accommodated 30 students.

soldiers serving on the European front and the ever-escalating needs of civilians at home.[2] Telegrams and appeals for nurses arrived at a constant rate. Practical nurses could not be used by the armed forces, so the American Red Cross urged them to stay at home, while graduate nurses headed to the war front. The nursing shortage was felt everywhere, as one of every three graduate nurses was needed to meet the Red Cross' quota of 25,000.

As the war raged in Europe, the United States was being ravaged by a Spanish influenza epidemic. There were also brown-outs and power shortages that forced most of Flint to close down on a regular basis.[3] In Flint, when 95 new influenza cases were reported in one 24-hour period, city residents were asked, and later ordered, to wear gauze masks whenever they were in public, and all public gatherings in the Flint area were suspended. There was also a shortage of good, qualified, well-trained nurses.

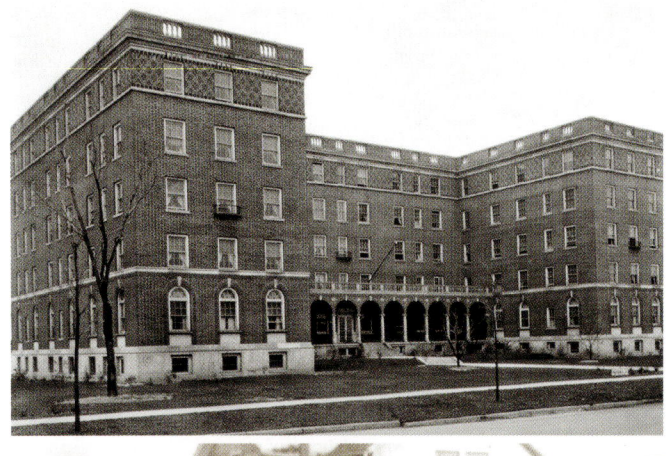

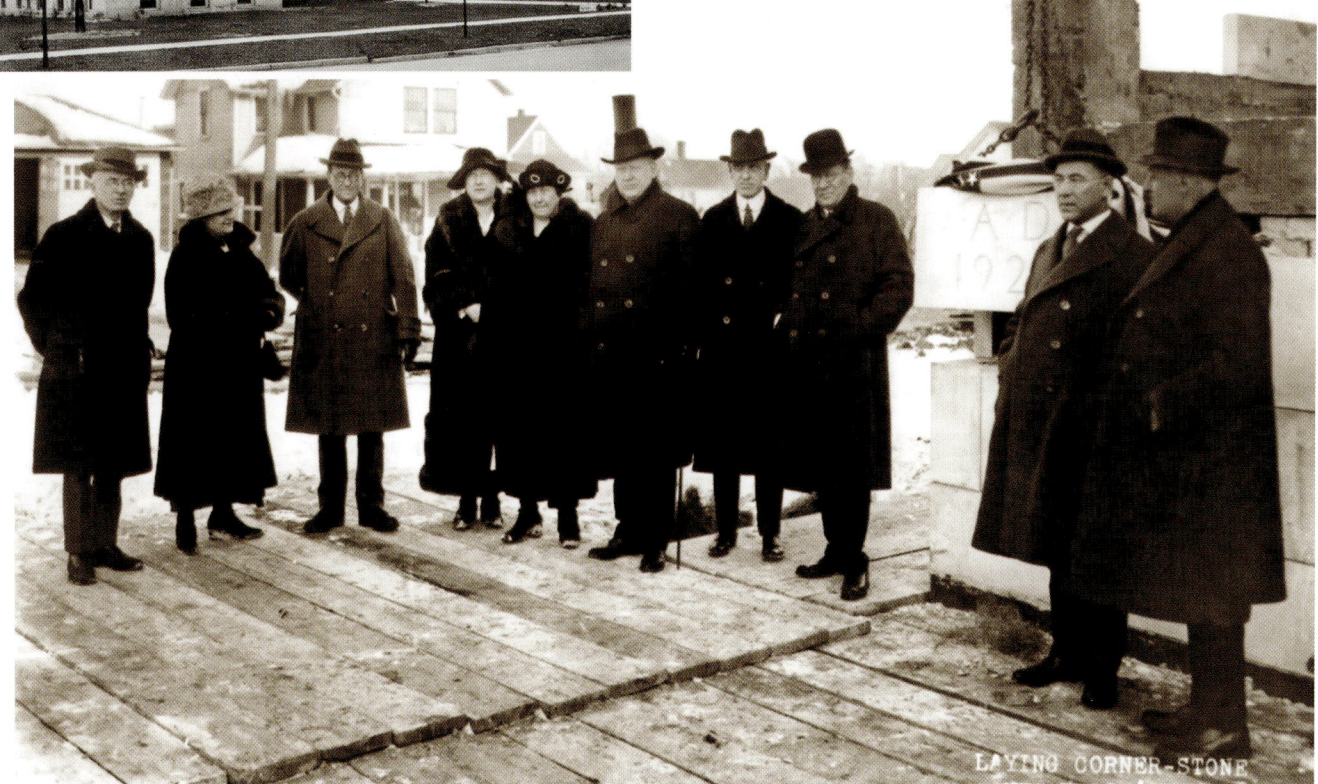

Laying the cornerstone for the new nurses' home (corner of Patrick and Sixth Streets) on February 24, 1924 (left to right): Board Treasurer James Martin, Assistant Secretary Florence Tucker, Mayor David R. Cuthbertson of Flint, Director of Nursing Mable Haggman, Hurley Hospital Superintendent Anna Schill, Reverend John Dysart, Board Secretary George Willson, and Board Members Dr. J. C. McGregor, Merliss Brown, and Board President Reinhard Kleinpell.

Inset: The New nurses' residence was completed in 1926. The school had its own gym and a tunnel leading to the hospital. One of the most popular features was its rooftop deck, where students could sunbathe.

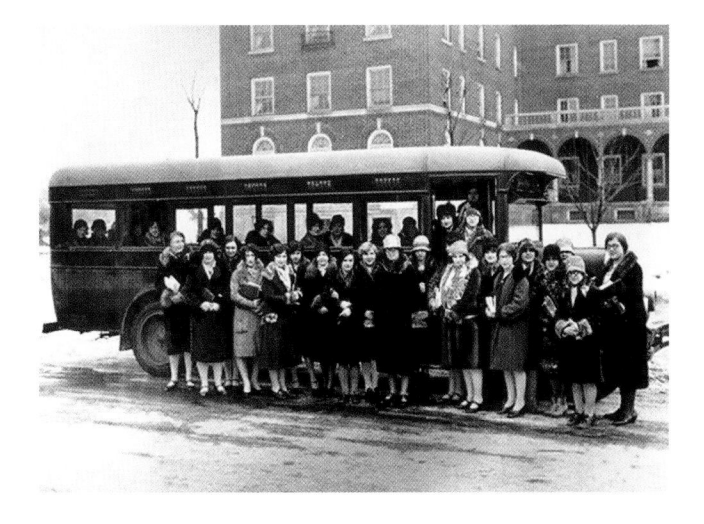

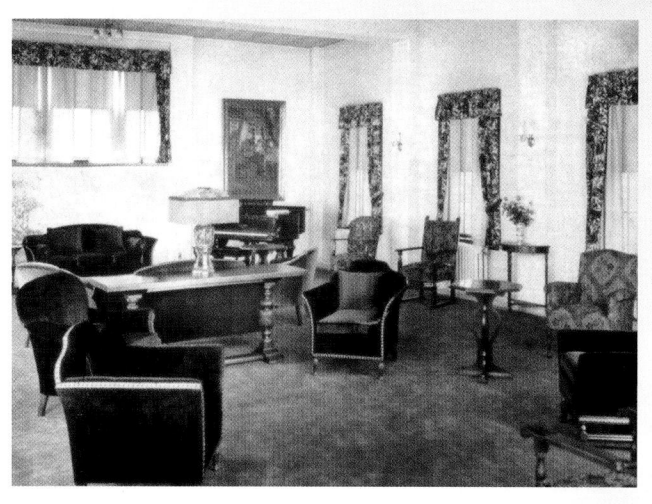

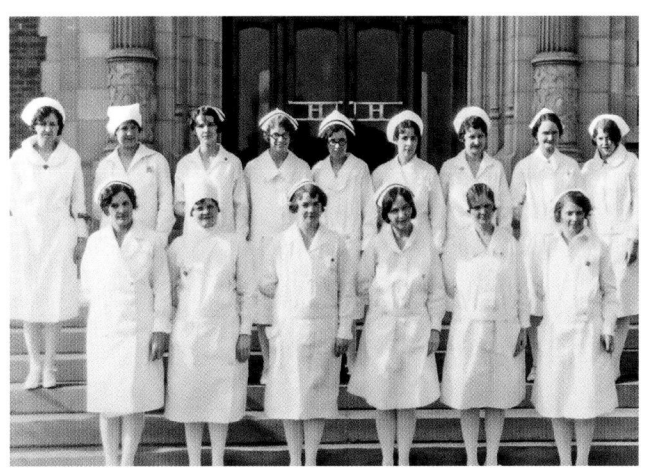

Nurses' lives, 1920s

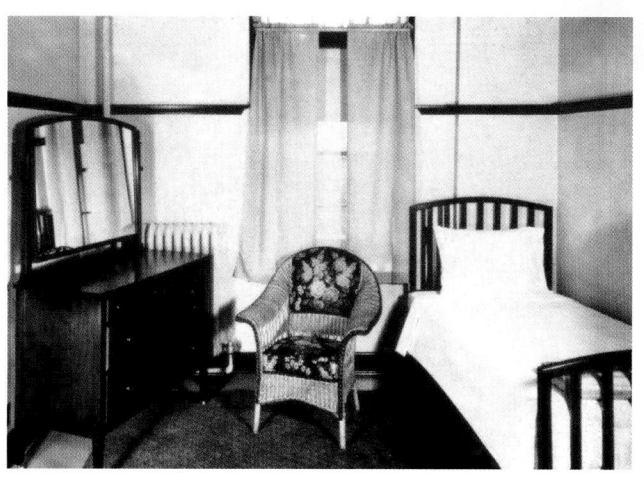

Interiors of new nurses' residence – the lounge and one of the bedrooms

By 1918, the prerequisites for admission to the nursing school were more defined: Candidates had to be women between the ages of 18 and 35, of average height and weight, and in good health. They had to provide credentials from their school showing good academic standing and the completion of courses. A letter of recommendation from a physician certifying mental and physical aptitude for the work was also required. Candidates needed to be proficient in proper English and grammar and able to write legibly, spell correctly, and have a working knowledge of mathematics.[4]

In 1922, Schill turned over the directorship of the school to Mabel Haggman. The nurses' residence was opened in 1925 and was considered to be one of the finest nurses' homes in the country. The five-story brick building held the dormitory, the living room, the tearoom, the library, the gymnasium, classrooms, and a domestic science lab. Seven years later, Mrs. Wilhelm Zeigler became the director of nursing, serving from 1929 to 1936.

The Great Depression hit the city of Flint hard, which had a ripple effect on the nursing school. Nurses worked for free room and board and an education. By 1932, a high school diploma had become a requirement; the school's focus was on teaching basic nursing care. Interns took blood pressure and started IVs, so nurses did not learn those techniques. By the end of the 1930s,

Sue Wright Award for Nursing Excellence

In 1984, Sue Wright was named Hurley's VP of Nursing, remaining in that position until her death in 2002. Throughout her career, she demonstrated excellence in patient care, clinical excellence, and nursing administration, and she was an advocate for nurses at Hurley. She was instrumental in developing the commitment for professional nurses at Hurley, as well as the University of Michigan-Flint/Hurley BSN program. Sue is remembered for her commitment, expertise, and leadership that inspired so many professional nurses at Hurley.

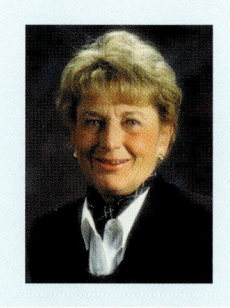

In Sue's honor, Hurley's nursing colleagues gather annually for the Sue Wright Award celebration to recognize exemplary nurses for being compassionate and caring, but also for going above and beyond for their patients, families, and co-workers. Nine nurses are nominated by their peers. The 2019 recipient was Carol Fechik, RN. Fechik has worked at HMC for 48 and a half years in various capacities, including interim nurse manager, assistant nurse manager, and ED staff nurse. According to John Stewart, "Carol is the consummate professional. She truly emulates all the characteristics of being a patient advocate, treating every patient with the same level of respect and expertise, whether they're presenting a medical emergency or if it's a behavior health patient in crisis, or a substance abuse patient needing our help."

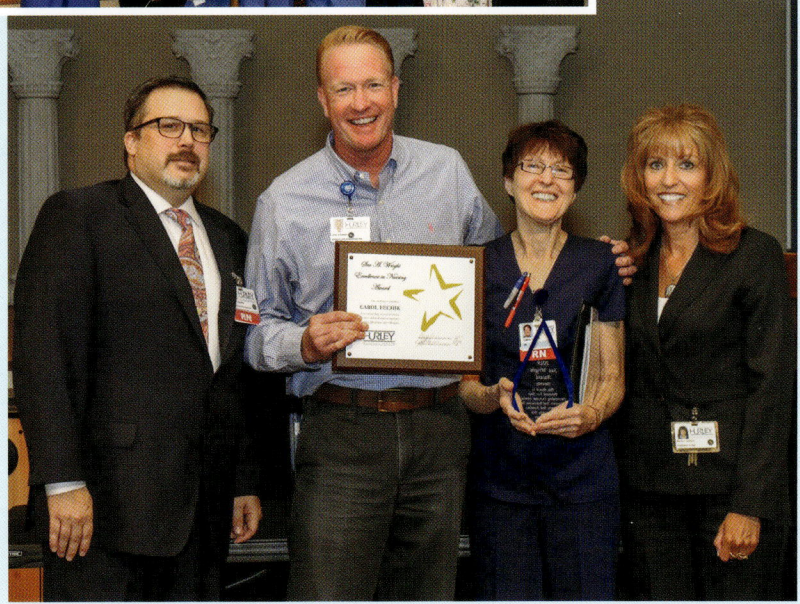

2019 Sue Wright Award Recipient
Left to right: Jeff Overman, BSN, administrator for Nursing Operations, John Stewart, BSN, Service Line administrator, award recipient Carol Fechik, RN, and Melany Gavulic, RN, MBA, president, CEO

Inset: The 2019 nominees for the Sue Wright Award for Nursing Excellence (left to right): Derek Samida, Jennifer Burmann, Terry Horton, Matthew Lamay, Mary Kirbitz, Carol Fechik, Michelle Beasinger, and Janet Lucas.

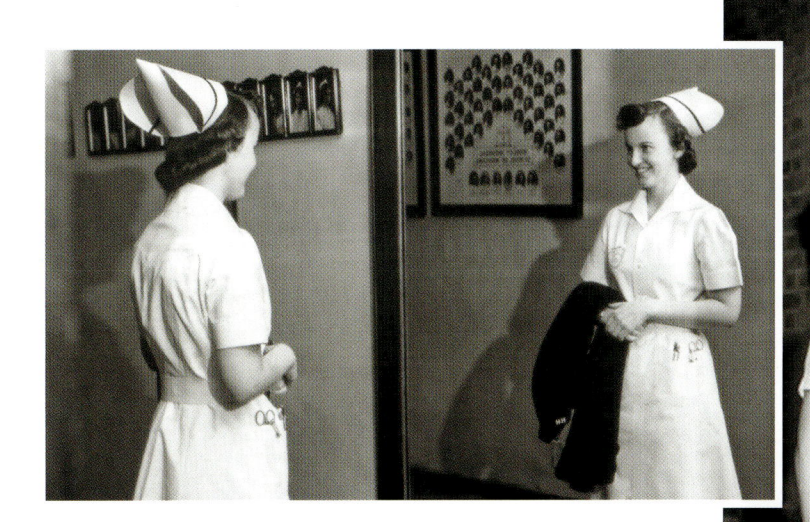

economic stability rebounded, and the new airlines industry sought registered nurses to be stewardesses. In 1940, the Nurses Training School was renamed The Hurley School of Nursing. The December 7, 1941, attack on Pearl Harbor signaled a new direction for nurses, as Hurley enrolled three nursing classes during World War II's Cadet Corps period. Mabel McNeel served as the director of nursing from 1936 to 1947.

In 1949, the school began to observe 40-hour weeks for students. Soon after, the school employed nurse instructors, whose primary job was to educate. In the 1950s, as a reflection that nursing was becoming more science-based, students began attending chemistry, anatomy, and physiology classes at what is now Mott Community College. The war was over, and nurses were in demand. Future nurses clubs and candy striper programs created a natural pipeline of nursing students and ready assistants in the hospital. In 1951, Hurley admitted Robert Esch, the first male student nurse. The first black students, Sharon Simpson (Wilson) and her cousin Wilma Watts (Brady), both graduated in 1956. In 1958, the School of Nursing became accredited by the National League for Nursing. Mrs. Ethel MacLennan served as director of Nursing from 1956 to 1968.

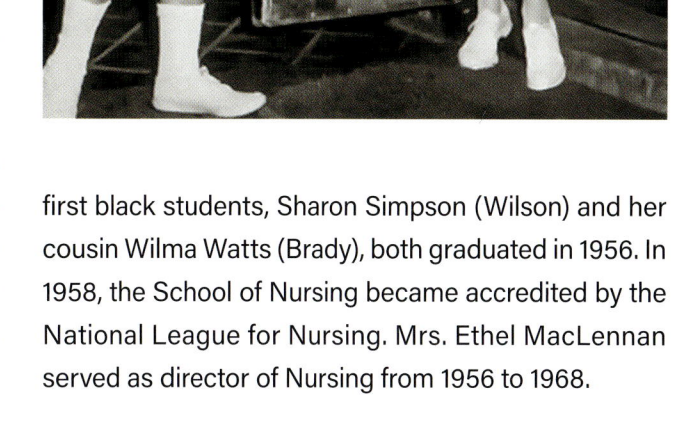

Through the 1960s, a nurse's role was primarily viewed as following doctors' orders and reporting to doctors. In 1964, a new, modern nurses' residence, which provided improved educational facilities, opened. In May 1969, the School of Nursing, with a fully accredited three-year diploma, had an enrollment of more than 300 students.

In the 1970s, the first-year pre-nursing courses could be taken at the college or university; second and third years were taken at the nursing school. Technology

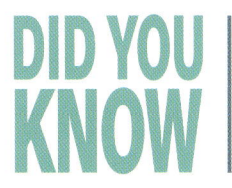

DID YOU KNOW | . . . the furnishings of the original nurses' home were donated by James Willson, MD. A piano was gifted by George Flanders, president of the Hurley Board of Managers.[5]

CHAPTER FOUR AN EDUCATION LEADER • 93

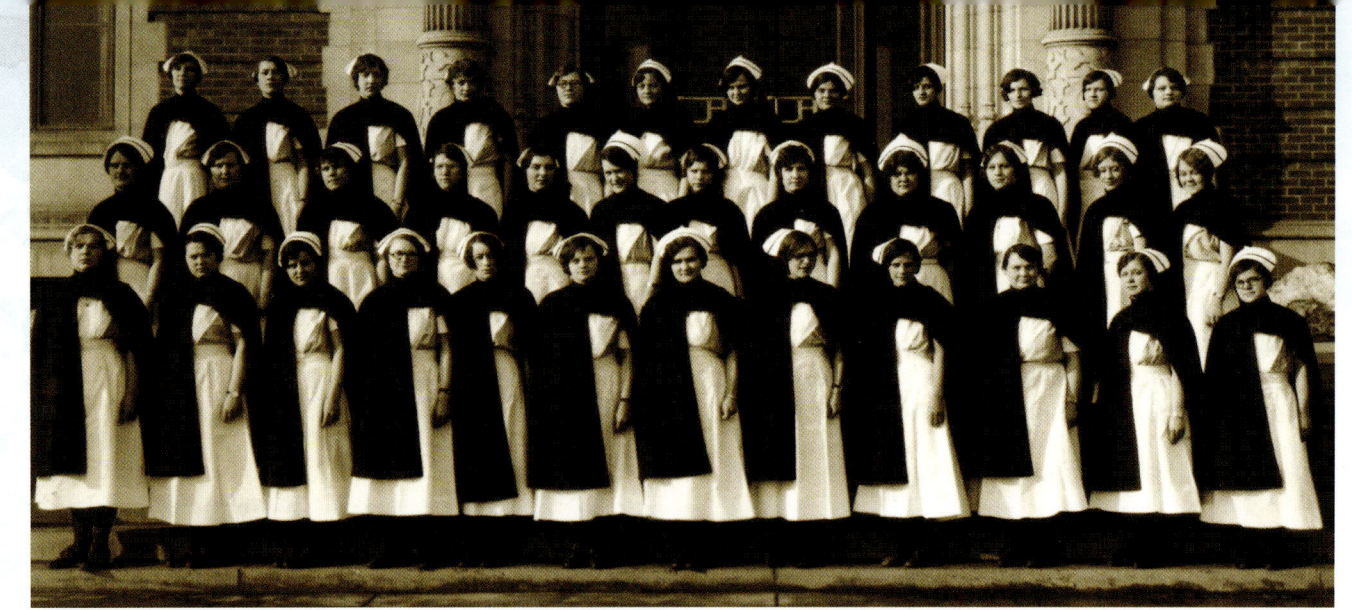

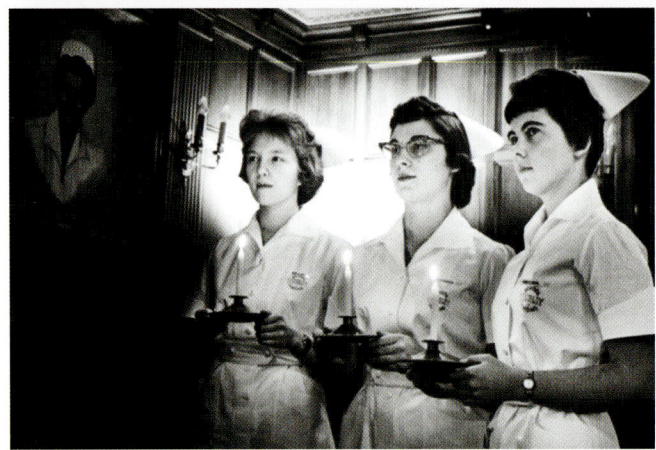

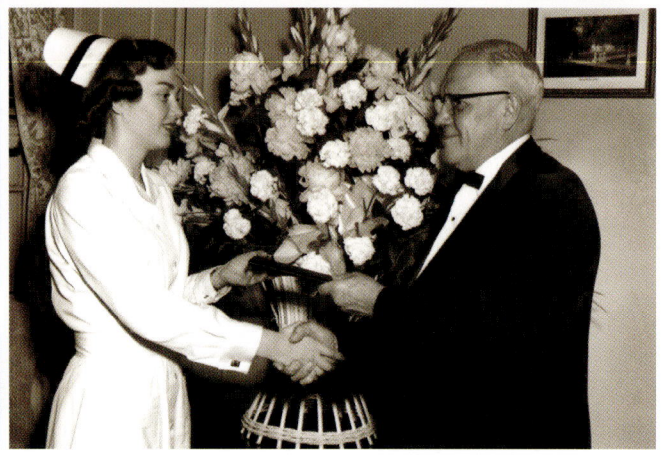

Top: Nurses' graduation, 1950s

Above left: A candlelight tradition during graduation ceremonies

Above right: Audrey Bretzke receives her nursing diploma from Earl Tallberg, president, Hurley Board of Managers, on May 28, 1954.

had exploded in medicine and was integrated into the nursing school curriculum.[6] This was also a time when nurses developed their own goals for patient care, a departure from just "following doctors' orders." Nursing training now gave more attention to underlying disease causes, such as poor nutrition, to assist in treatment and foster prevention. May E. Werrbach served as the director of Nursing from 1971 to 1982.

Throughout the 1980s, faculty kept up with computer technology, instructional videos, and lifelike nursing models for simulation learning, such as catheterizations, tracheotomy care, and dressing changes, and expanded the amount of college credit required. First-year students had to earn 29 credit hours. Nursing students spent about 32 hours a week in the classroom. Faculty qualifications also changed, with a master's degree in nursing sought. In 1982, Hurley was one of only three hospitals statewide accredited by the Michigan Nurses Association to provide continuing education classes. Between 1972 and 1982, 96 percent of Hurley nursing school graduates passed the state board examination for licensure on the first attempt.[7]

Nurses learned to develop their own care plans related to the patient's nursing diagnosis. Initially, some friction developed between doctors and nurses, which lessened over time. "New physicians look at nursing as a profession and realize we have the right to make some judgements," said Mary Jean Smith, Hurley School of Nursing director from 1983 to 1991.

In 1993, the 100th class graduated from the Hurley School of Nursing. In keeping with the nationwide

94 • HURLEY MEDICAL CENTER

trend toward four-year programs, the school admitted its last class in January 1994, which graduated in December 1995. The Hurley School of Nursing Alumni Association celebrated the official closing with a two-day event in October 1995. Alice Lorenz, RN, would serve as the last director of Nursing, from 1991 to 1995. More than 3,600 registered nurses graduated from HMC's diploma program. The HMC/UM-Flint nursing partnership, entered into in 1992, was designed to enhance both the teaching and the research of the university.

Nurses continue to play a vital role at Hurley. According to Teresa Bourque, BSN, chief nurse, who has worked at HMC since 1986, "There are over 900 nurses who work at HMC. According to a 2019 Gallup poll, for the 18th year in a row, nurses are the number one trusted profession."

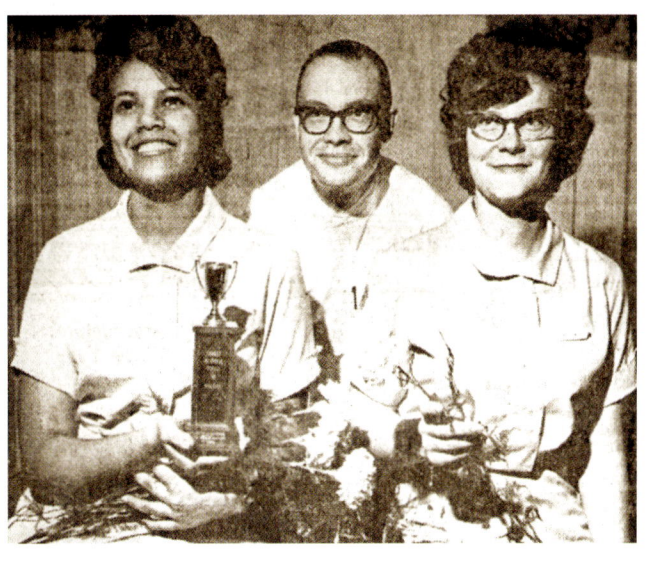

Nursing awards, 1964

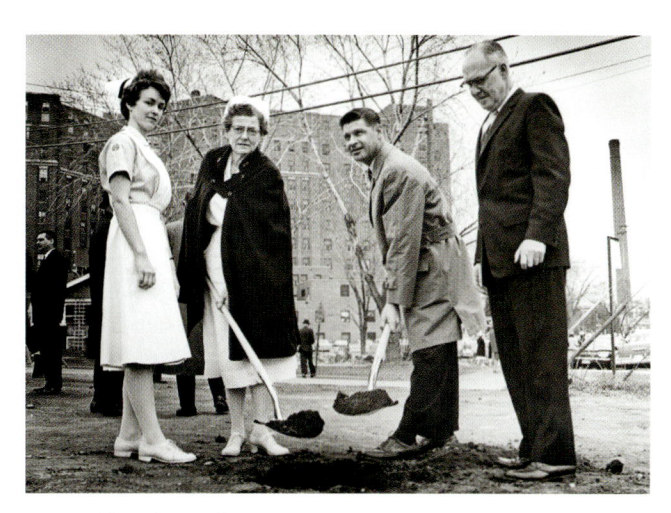

Ground breaking of new nurses' residence, 1964. Shown here is Ethel MacLennan (center left), director, Hurley School of Nursing, 1956–1968.

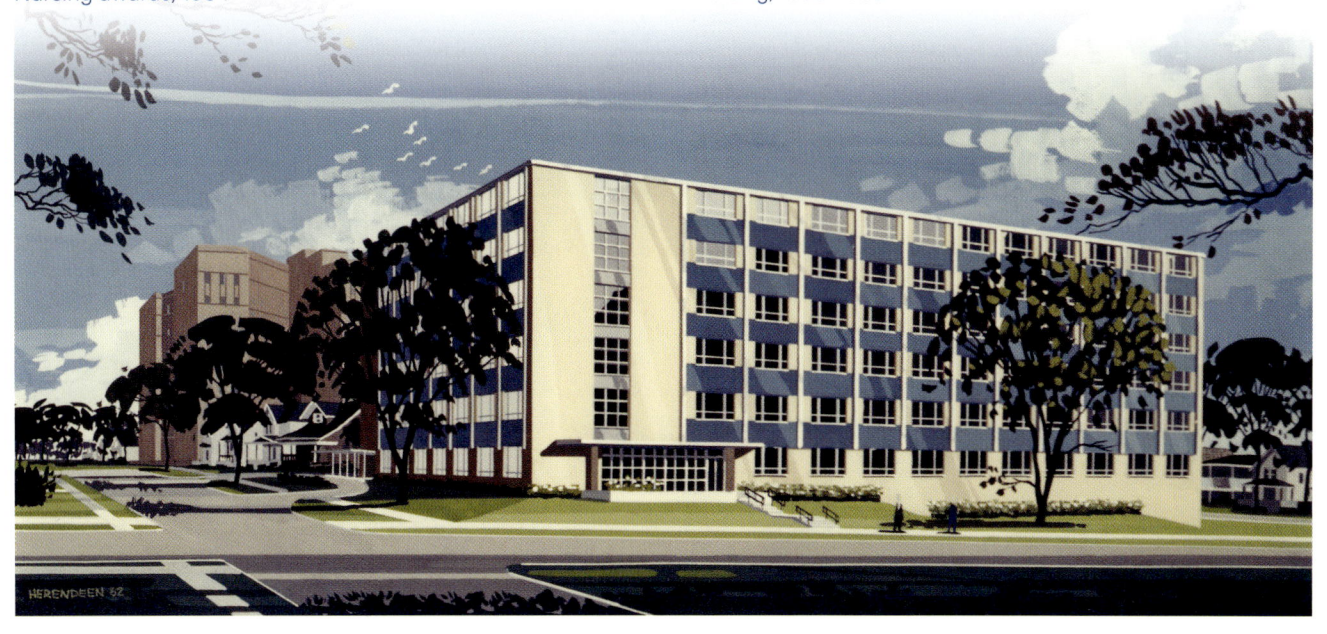

Artist's rendering of the new six-story (with a basement) nurses' residence, which housed 302 students and was built for $1,637,853. Furnishings were donated by the Industrial Mutual Association of Flint at a cost of $160,000.

CHAPTER FOUR AN EDUCATION LEADER • 95

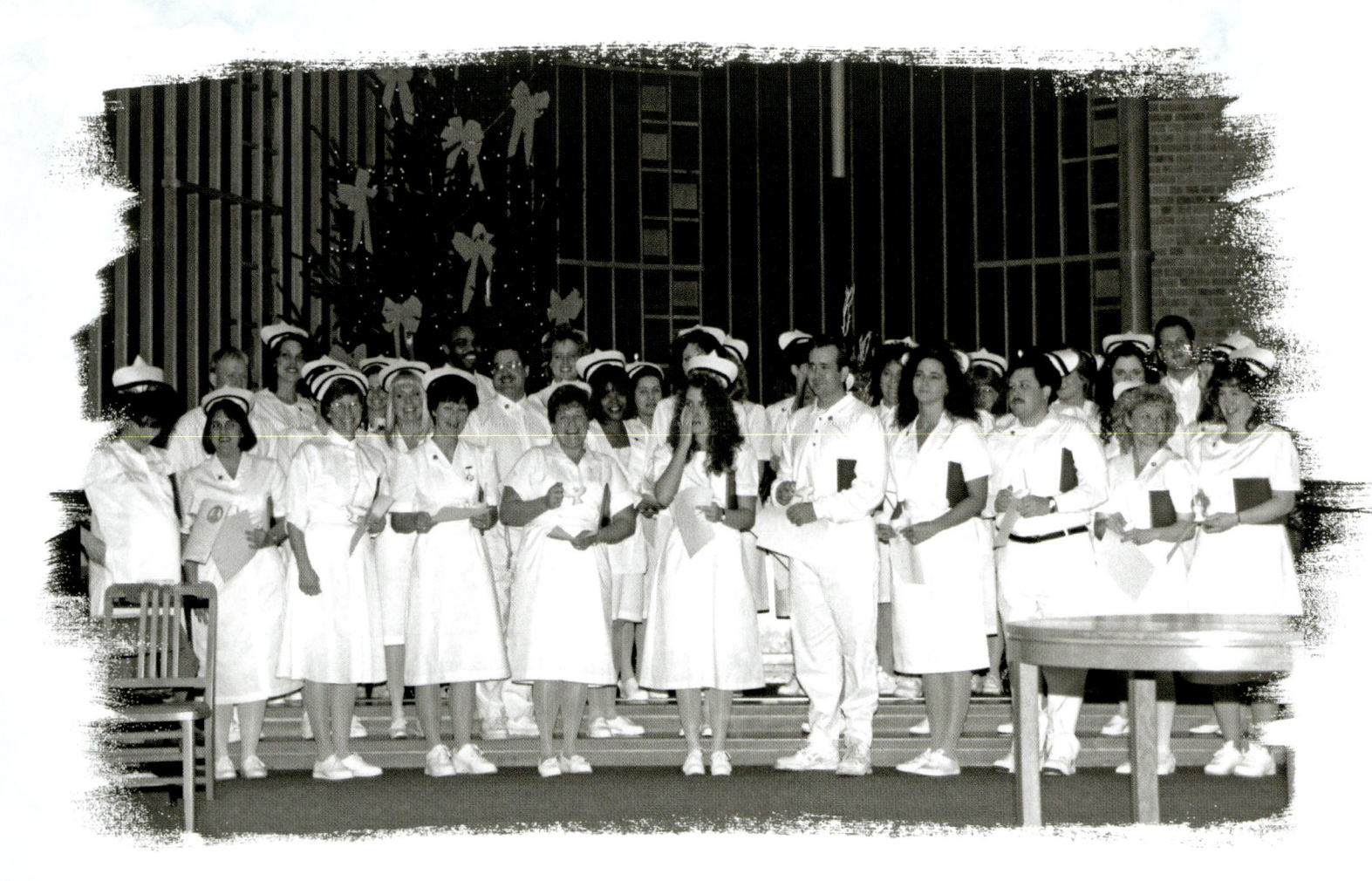

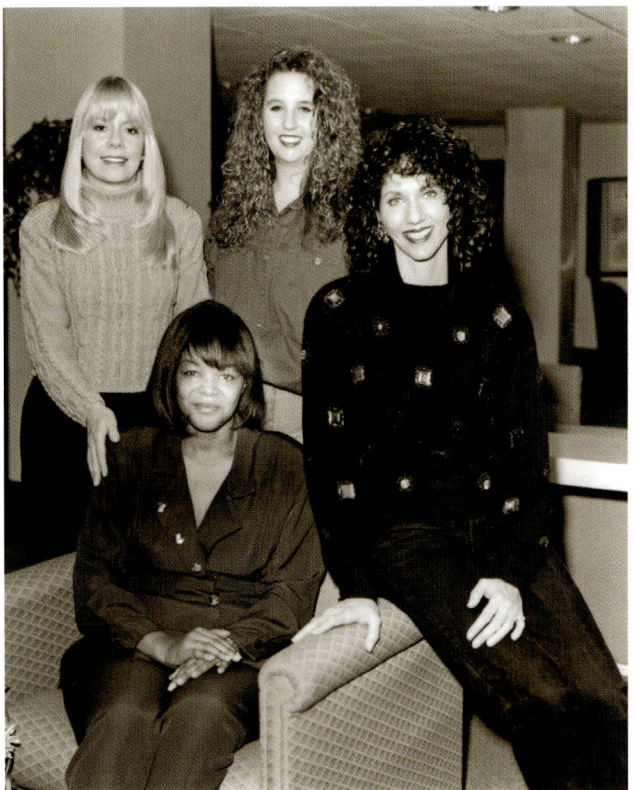

Members of the 104th and last diploma class of the Hurley School of Nursing, December 15, 1995

Left: Officers of the last graduating class of the Hurley School of Nursing, 1995 (left to right): Brenda Kehoe, secretary, Cynthia Hudson Adams, president, Amy Freeman, vice president, and Kim Hanson, treasurer.

School of Nursing 75th Anniversary, May 4–5, 1984

A dinner-dance and open house were hosted by the alumni association. Though the school had changed over the years, the mission remained: "To offer a program of theory and practice to develop mature individuals who can give quality, complete nursing care."[8]

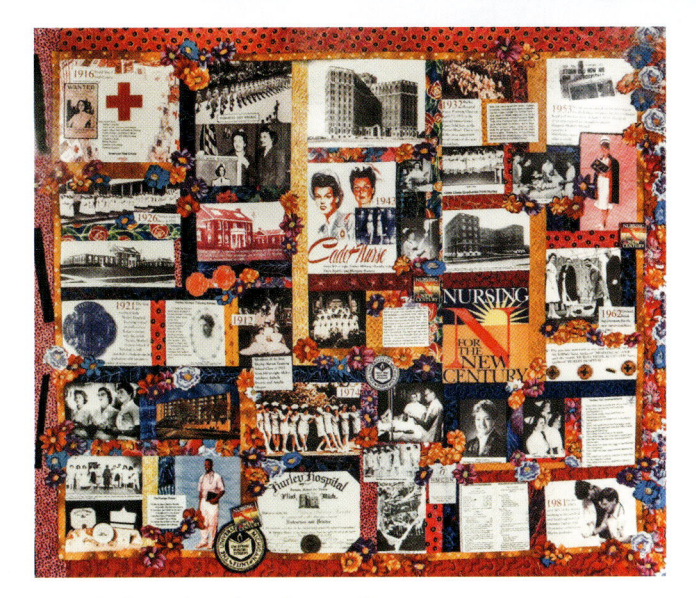

School of Nursing Alumni Annual Banquet, 1998
Three years after the Hurley School of Nursing graduated its last class, alumni held open house tours of the medical center and an art exhibit titled "Nursing . . . A Tapestry of Life." The centerpiece, a quilt, titled "Nursing for the New Century," was created by Mary Andrews, along with 13 multimedia pieces that described the caring provided by nurses.

Bourque says that technology has changed nursing. "Nursing is much more technical than it used to be. Before technology, a nurse manually calculated vital signs and IV drip rates; now, machines do the calculations for the nurse. Everything used to be recorded on paper, and now, all of the information is entered into an electronic record. Nurses have to watch that they don't lose the personal touch with their patients due to technology. The most rewarding aspect of being a nurse is when a patient you've cared for walks out of the hospital. It is when a nurse can spend more time with their patients."

In the late 1940s and early 1950s, Hurley's schools of radiologic technology, anesthesia, and medical technology began.

Hurley School of Radiologic Technology

According to early records, Carl Chapell, MD, began specializing in radiology, including radium therapy and X-rays, in 1907; he led Hurley's Radiology Department in 1916. By 1979, the East Tower expansion allowed for a greater commitment to the School of Radiologic Technology in order to meet the growing demands of the tri-county area. The new department moved into the lower level of the East Tower, with increased classroom space for the School of Radiologic Technology and radiology residents, 14 rooms for examinations and procedures, offices, an expanded viewing room, and a large vault for X-ray film storage. Robert Ormond, MD, took over as program director in 1971. Many Hurley physicians served as faculty for the Hurley School of Radiologic Technology, which has educated more radiographers than any other hospital-based program in the Flint area; the last class

In the foreground is the Maximar therapy unit GE 500-milliampere diagnostic X-ray machine used at HMC in 1938.

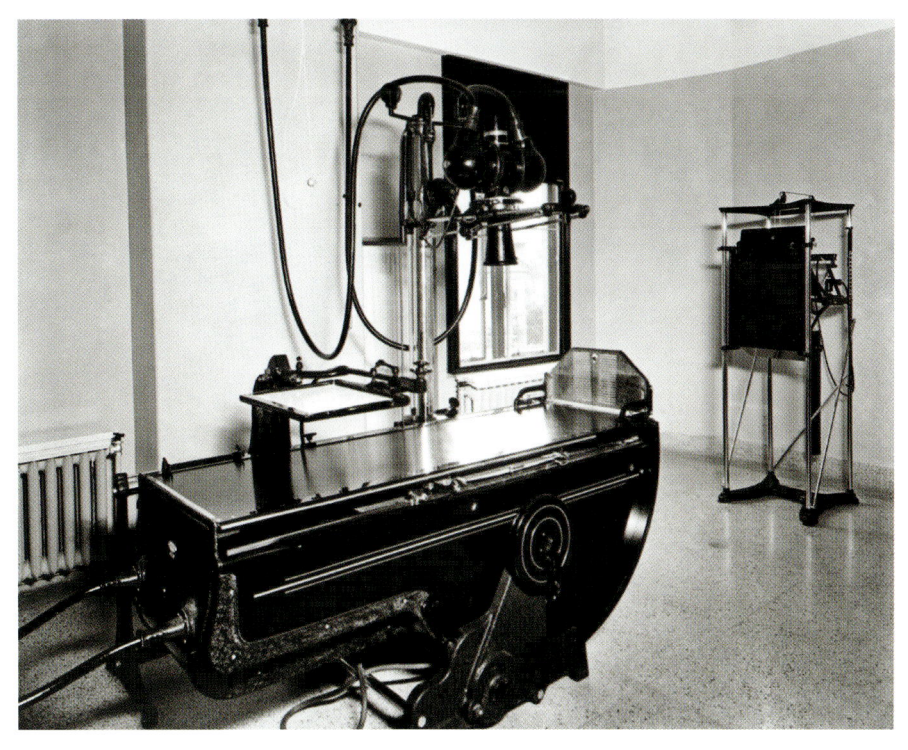

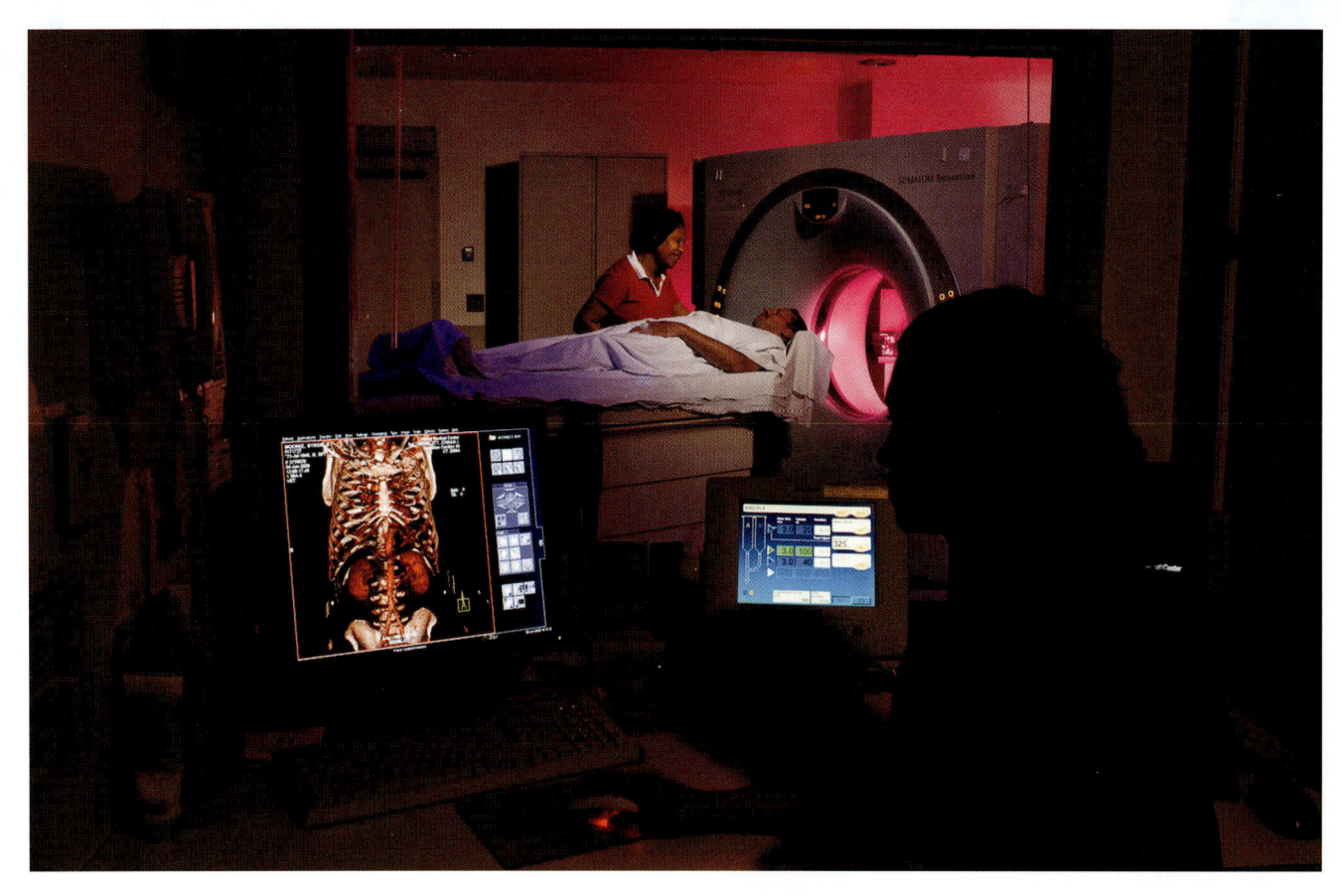

A 64-slice Siemens CT scanner

Right: Robert Ormond, MD, Radiology Department chair (1970–1989), who preceded AppaRao Mukkamala, MD

graduated in 2018. HMC continues to invest in the latest imaging technology and was the first hospital in Genesee County to acquire a 64-slice Siemens CT scanner; they also installed the first MRI system within a Genesee County hospital.

Hurley School of Medical Technology

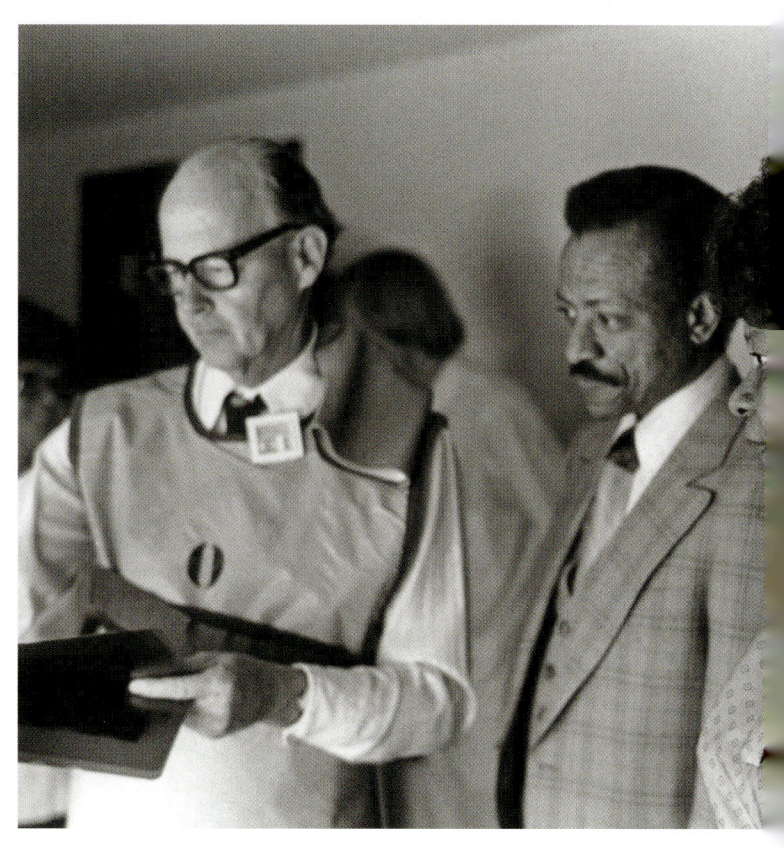

Hurley School of Medical Technology was established around 1948. According to 2000 graduate Tom Downs, MT, coordinator of Chemistry and Special Chemistry, "The goal of the school is to graduate professional, entry-level medical technologists of the highest caliber by providing knowledge and technical skills needed to render efficient and effective service in supplying medical staff with the diagnostic data essential to delivering quality patient care." Between 1963 and 2019 (no records could be found prior to 1963), 456 students graduated from the school; the last class of five graduated in 2019.

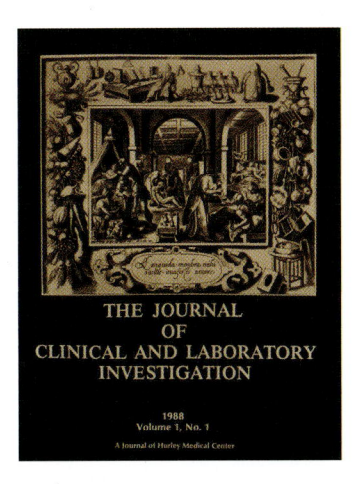

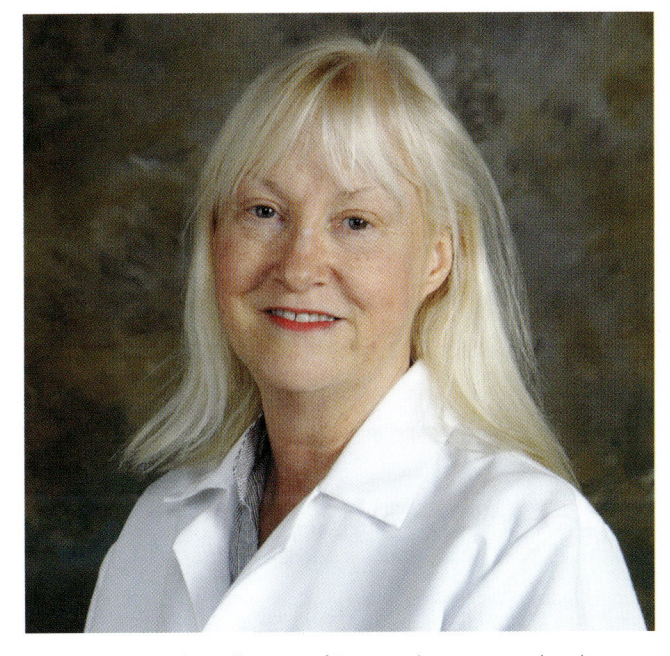

D. Kay Taylor, PhD, director of Research, oversaw the rigorous process required for the designation as a Center of Research, which was accomplished in September 2003. The center, with its academic, administrative, clinical, and community programs, encompassed six residency programs of more than 100 resident physicians, three fellowships, and 50 or more third- and fourth-year medical students.

Top: As a teaching hospital associated with MSU, U of M, and Henry Ford Health Systems, Hurley experts conduct hundreds of research projects each year. These works have been published in numerous prestigious medical journals. Funded through grants, private financial support, and by HMC, research not only contributes to local health initiatives, but also to the health of all Americans.

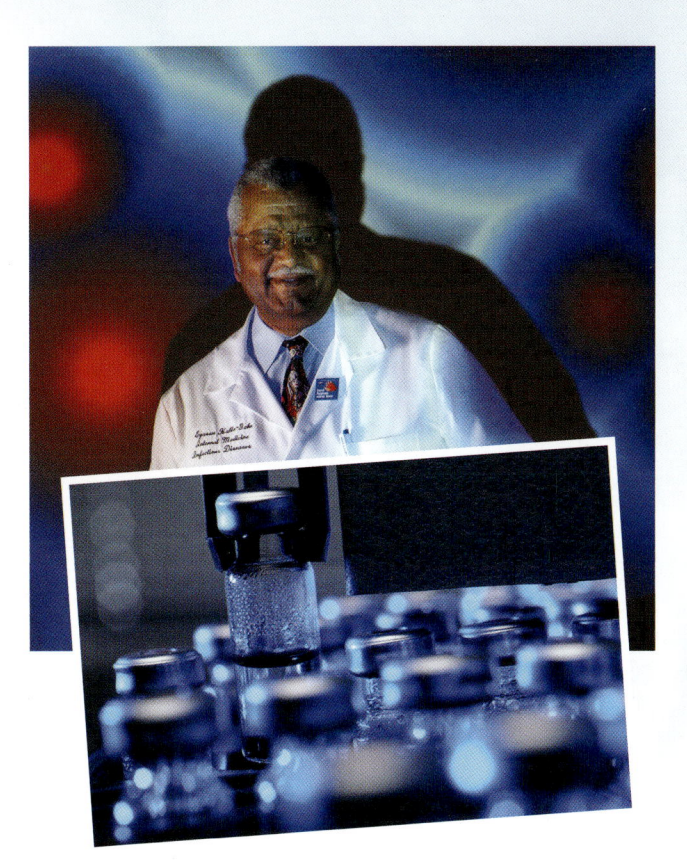

Top: Eyassu Habte-Gabr, MD, FACP, FIDSA, director of Infectious Diseases, and professor of medicine at HMC/MSU CHM, authored *Antimicrobial Resistance: A Global Public Health Threat*, among other books.

Hurley School of Anesthesia

In May 1950, Hurley Hospital established the Hurley Hospital School of Anesthesia as a diploma program to alleviate a shortage of trained nurse anesthetists. The 12-month program received full accreditation by the American Association of Nurse Anesthetists, thanks to the dedication and determination of Director Helen Vos, CRNA. The curriculum was expanded to 18 months in the 1960s and to 24 months in the 1970s, at which time it was renamed Hurley Medical Center School of Anesthesia.

HMC and the University of Michigan (UM)-Flint partnered in March 1981 to advance the program to a bachelor of science level. Although financial constraints caused the school's closure in 1988, it re-emerged in 1991 as the UM-Flint/HMC Master of Science in Anesthesia Program. Program Directors: Francis Gerbasi (1991–2002), Lynn Lebeck (2002–2012), and Shawn Fryzel, CRNA (2012–2018).

Hurley Helped in the Fight Against AIDS

Acquired immune deficiency syndrome (AIDS) was first identified in 1981. HMC was one of five Michigan alternate test sites, checking blood for presence of HTLVII antibodies within people who may develop or carry AIDS. "The medical center is prepared, but not panicked," a distinction stressed by Willys Mueller Jr., MD, HMC Pathology director and director of the American Red Cross Wolverine Region. "There is no need to ostracize AIDS victims, but high-risk people should take personal measures to reduce their chances of contracting the disease."[9] Infectious disease specialist Eyassu Habte-Gabr, MD, served as the HIV specialist for the Academy of HIV Medicine. Dr. Habte-Gabr was the 2005 Hurley Pinnacle Award recipient.

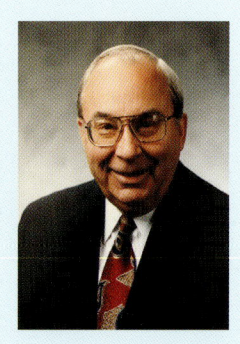

Willys Mueller Jr., MD, HMC Pathology Director

Teaching Special Operations Combat Medics

In 2012, the US Army contacted Hurley to see if they were equipped to provide adequate clinical experiences (traumas, burns, births, surgeries, etc.) to train special operations combat medics (SOCM). Representatives from the US Army visited HMC numerous times over several months. In May 2013, Hurley, as well as the Genesee County Sheriff's Office paramedics, began a partnership to provide pre-hospital (sheriff's office paramedics) and hospital clinical experiences. Debi Wright, GME, program coordinator and HMC employee for over 44 years, was invited to be Hurley's liaison. Wright said, "I was honored to be offered the HMC liaison position for the SOCM program. Any way that I can serve these young soldiers for the sacrifices they make for our country is a great privilege." The SOCM course is a 36-week program of instruction that teaches army and navy enlisted service members who hold—or are designated for assignment to—a special-operations medical position. The course qualifies participants as highly trained combat medics with the necessary skills and abilities to provide initial medical and trauma care and aptitude to increase team survivability. Since many missions are in areas with limited access or ability to evacuate to more definitive care, the overall goal for SOCM is to provide care for the wounded for up to 72 hours. Students graduating from the SOCM course are certified as national registry paramedics. Hurley is one of four US civilian institutions to train SOCM students.

Time Capsules

In August 2010, construction workers discovered two concrete cornerstones containing time capsules near the original West Tower hospital entrance. One was dated 1907—just before Hurley Hospital opened—and the second was dated 1907–1927; by 1927, Hurley had built two additional wings. The time capsules' contents were opened in 2011 at Flint's Sloan Museum at the "A Moment in Time" celebration. The 1907 capsule contained James J. Hurley's biography, his will, a copy of the proceedings with the bequest, and a copy of the proceedings to create the hospital board, along with their names.[10]

Volunteering at Homeless Shelters

According to Eyassu Habte-Gabr, MD, "Every spring since 2012, Hurley residents volunteer their time at Carriage Town Ministries, YWCA, and My Brother's Keeper homeless shelters in Flint to offer access to flu shots, vaccinations, health screenings, and risk assessments (smoking, hypertension, diabetes, STDs, etc.)." Each client is given a health passport on which residents record their blood pressure, weight, and important health details. Staff from the Hurley Diabetes Center educate attendees about the risks of diabetes and how to avoid becoming pre-diabetic.

Internal medicine resident Subhadra Mandadi, MD, gives medicine to a local woman.

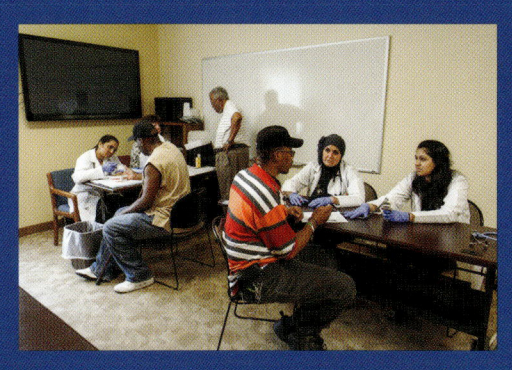

Eyassu Habte-Gabr, MD (center back), talks to Michele Bernreuter, Diabetes Program manager.

NOTES

1. *New York Times*, obituary, July 10, 1935, p. 1, column 3.
2. Sally Jessup, *Hurley School of Nursing 1909-1995: 86 Years of Excellence*, (Flint, Michigan: 1996), p. 9.
3. Ibid.
4. Ibid., p. 10.
5. Edwin Wood, *History of Genesee County, Michigan: Her People, Industries and Institutions* (Indianapolis: Federal Publishing Company, 1916), p. 801.
6. Hurley Foundation, *Inside Report* Volume 1 (1994), p. 13.
7. Hurley Foundation, *Inside Report* (January 1982), p.2.
8. Becky O'Grady, "School of Nursing changes with profession," *Inside Report* (Winter 1984), pp. 5-6.
9. Hurley Foundation, *Inside Report* (Holiday Edition 1985), p. 13.
10. Wood, *History of Genesee County, Michigan*, p. 801.

"We should never underestimate the value of residency training programs and the impact on patient care. By providing a culture of learning, residents and teaching faculty are continuously expanding their clinical knowledge and expertise to provide the best possible care for our patients."

—JIM BUTERAKOS
Chief Academic Officer and DIO

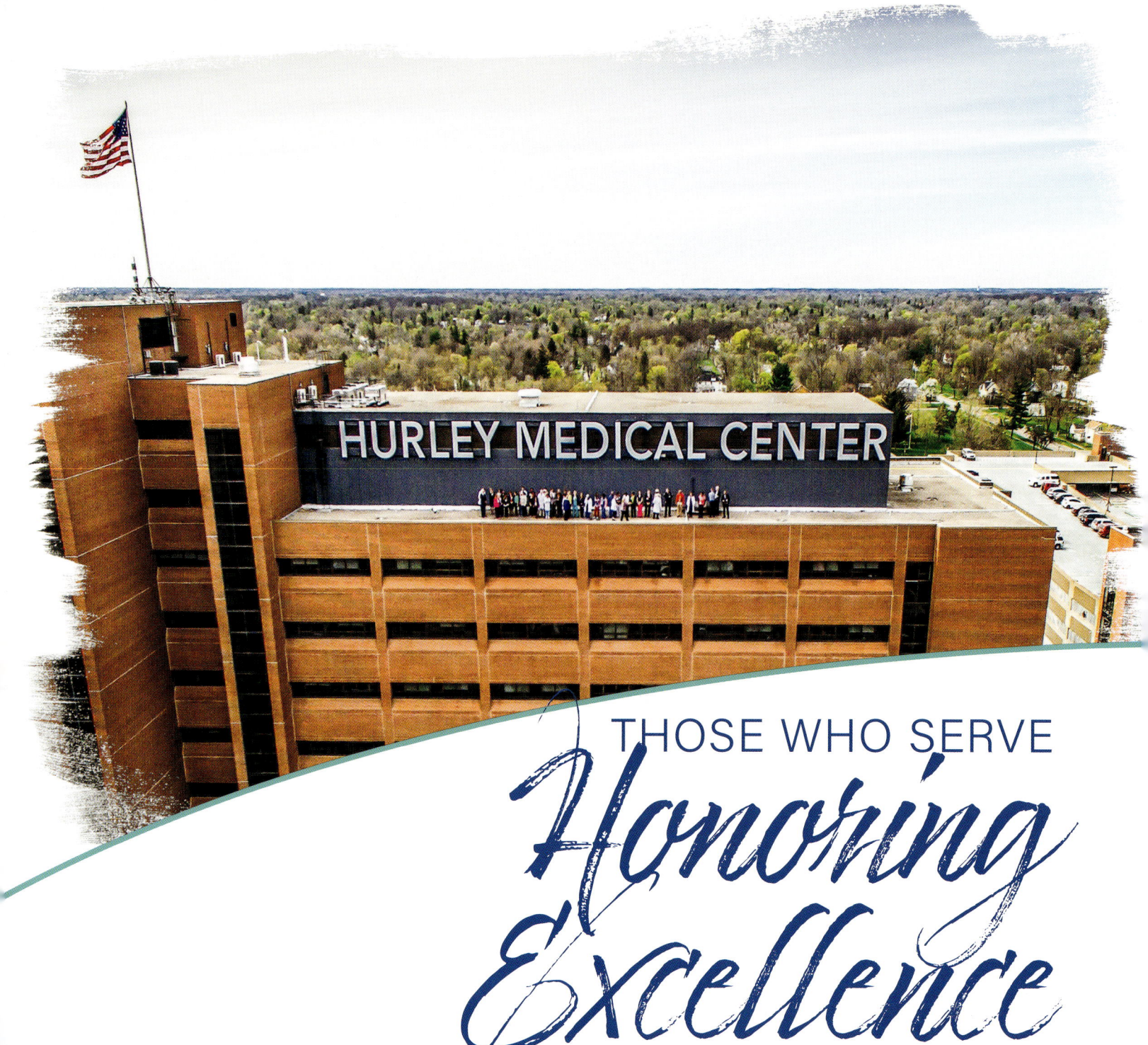

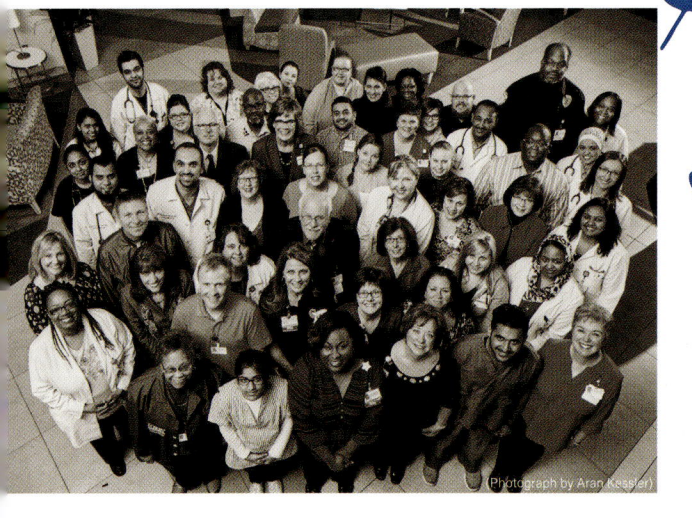

THOSE WHO SERVE
Honoring Excellence
CHAPTER FIVE

*T*hroughout Hurley's history, people have distinguished themselves by willingly exceeding the demands of their professions and, in doing so, honoring excellence. Hurley is one of the largest employers in Genesee County, employing approximately 2,700 people in a myriad of positions. The corporate culture is one of high morale. Many multigenerational families consider HMC as their working home and, in many cases, the place that they love to give back and volunteer their time.

(Photograph by Aran Kessler)

Leadership at the Top

An institution is only as good as its leaders, and Hurley is no exception. Those who have served as president and chief executive officer give generously of their time to multiple constituencies, while guiding the medical center forward.

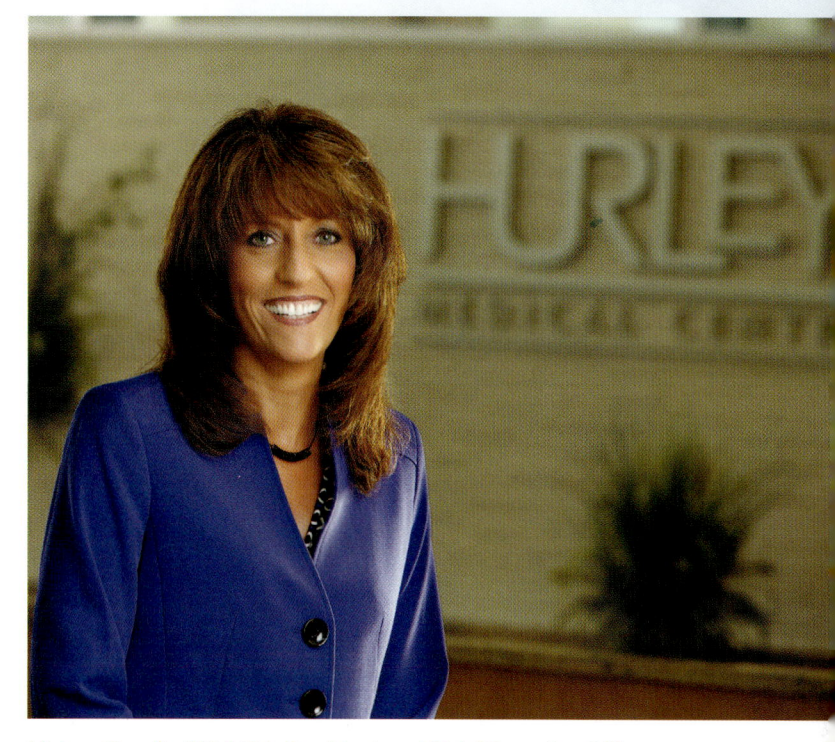

Melany Gavulic, RN, MBA, president, and chief executive officer (CEO), was appointed to this position in April 2012. Prior to this, Gavulic served as interim president and CEO, as well as senior vice president and chief operating officer, where she was responsible for operations, nursing, and all patient care services. Gavulic has a wealth of health care experience, serving in leadership roles within HMC for the last 21 years. She set her sights on a career in health care while working as a health career volunteer at HMC during her junior and senior years of

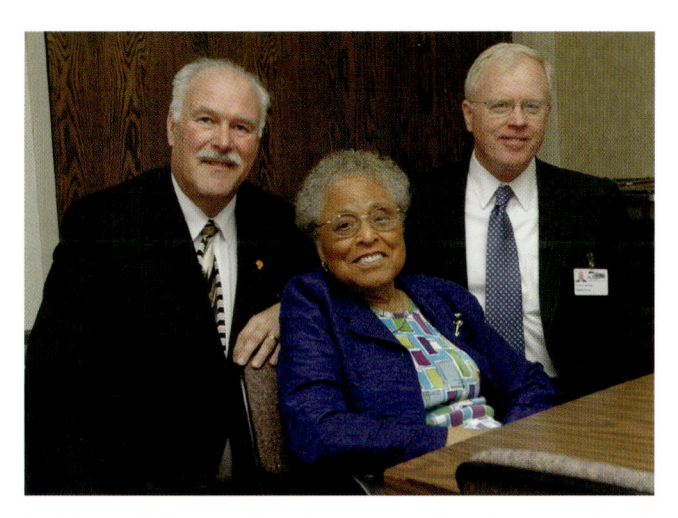

Melany Gavulic, RN, MBA, President, and Chief Executive Officer

high school. As a results-oriented professional, with a proven track record of collaborative working relationships with physicians, staff, colleagues, and external customers, she has been successful in developing and facilitating teams that have positively impacted quality outcomes, demonstrated performance improvement, enhanced the delivery of services, and created effective community partnerships. Gavulic received her BS degree in management systems from Kettering University in 1991 and an associate degree in nursing from Mott Community College in 1997; she received her RN license in 1997 and an MBA from Baker College of Graduate Studies in 2005.

Left to right: Richard Warmbold, Hurley Foundation president, with Claudia Tarver, RN, Hurley's first black nurse administrator, and Patrick Wardell, CEO. Tarver was hired by Hurley Hospital in 1951 and left in the 1960s to become a public health nurse for Flint. According to Samuel Dismond Jr., MD, who considered Tarver a pioneer, "She didn't have many peers or mentors, because there just weren't many." He also credits Tarver for opening the door for his rise in becoming the first black chief of staff. "You knew she was in charge. But she was good with people. I think that people respected her. People were glad to say they knew her," said Dismond.

Patrick Wardell served for six years as president and CEO, from 2005 to 2012, and presided over the 100th anniversary celebration in 2008. During his tenure, Wardell took Hurley from a $10 million deficit to financial stability. Under his leadership, HMC received the designation as a children's hospital and the creation of a new, $30 million emergency department.[1]

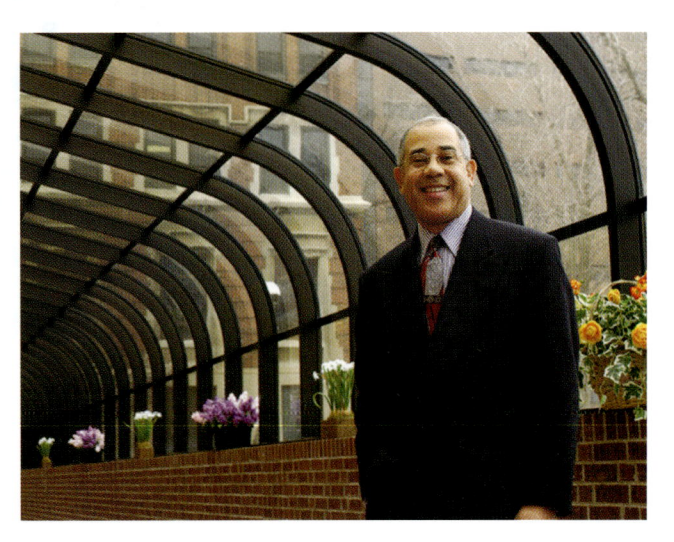

Julius Spears Jr.

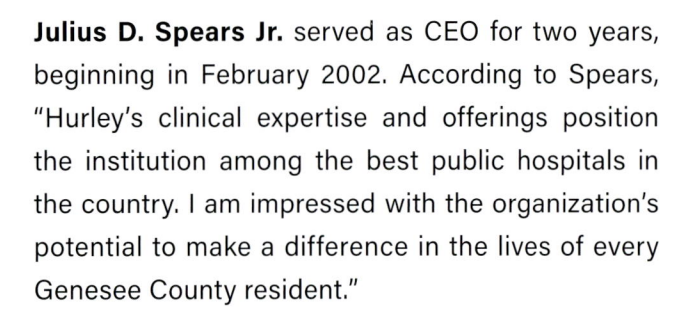

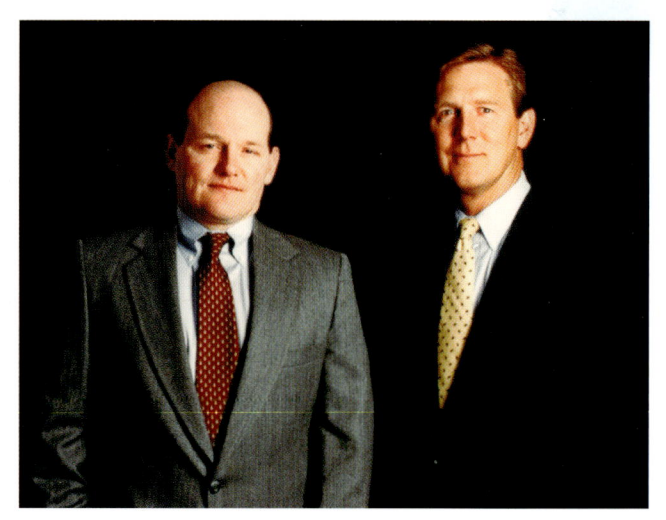

Glenn Fosdick and Phillip Dutcher

Julius D. Spears Jr. served as CEO for two years, beginning in February 2002. According to Spears, "Hurley's clinical expertise and offerings position the institution among the best public hospitals in the country. I am impressed with the organization's potential to make a difference in the lives of every Genesee County resident."

Glenn A. Fosdick was named CEO in August 1996 after serving as interim CEO after Phil Dutcher left HMC. From 1992 to 1996, he served as HMC's COO, responsible for operational services. He was credited with taking a $6.7 million loss in 1992 to a profit of more than $10 million in 1995. Fosdick oversaw reductions in operating costs, improved cooperation with HMC's unions, reorganization of the medical center's leadership structure, implementation of a 30-bed rehabilitation unit, acquisition of a 222-bed nursing home, and development of a Continuous Quality Improvement Program. "No one can predict the changes in health care ahead," said Fosdick. "But I will make one prediction. With the spirit of partnership, service, and community outreach we have created here, Hurley will not only meet those challenges, but will remain Flint's leading medical center."[2] Fosdick left in 2001.

Phillip Dutcher was believed to be one of the youngest hospital CEOs in the nation when he accepted the top job in May 1981, after serving as interim CEO since the fall of 1980. Dutcher started his HMC career in 1975, as installation director for HMC's new electronic computer system. He then advanced into hospital administration as an assistant director and then associate director in 1979. A majority of his time was spent overseeing the newly constructed North Tower building, which housed surgery suites, the Obstetrics Department, the newborn nursery, laboratory services, the ER, medical and pediatric clinic space, physical therapy, and Sterile Services Departments. Dutcher is credited with opening the Hurley Health and Fitness Center and the Hurley West Flint Campus ambulatory centers, developing Hurley Home Care Services, and for the cooperative partnership with the University of Michigan-Flint (nursing and physical therapy). He also established the Joint Union Management Policy Committee (JUMP). Dutcher's focus remained on achieving significant financial performance and inspiring those who trained under his leadership, who have now moved on to serve as CEOs or in senior positions in health care organizations. Dutcher served as CEO from 1981 until August 1995, when he left HMC.

Richard Schripsema, hospital director from 1974 to 1980, led HMC through a $22 million expansion and renovation program that resulted in community-driven fundraising, advisory committee participation, and fully accredited graduate medical education programs that aggressively recruited from the best American and Canadian medical schools. Hospital occupancy rates consistently topped 90 percent. "Richard Schripsema is responsible for converting Hurley from an outdated hospital into a thriving medical center," said Keith Champney, MD, director of Medical Education at that time. "The impact he has made will be felt for a hundred years."[3]

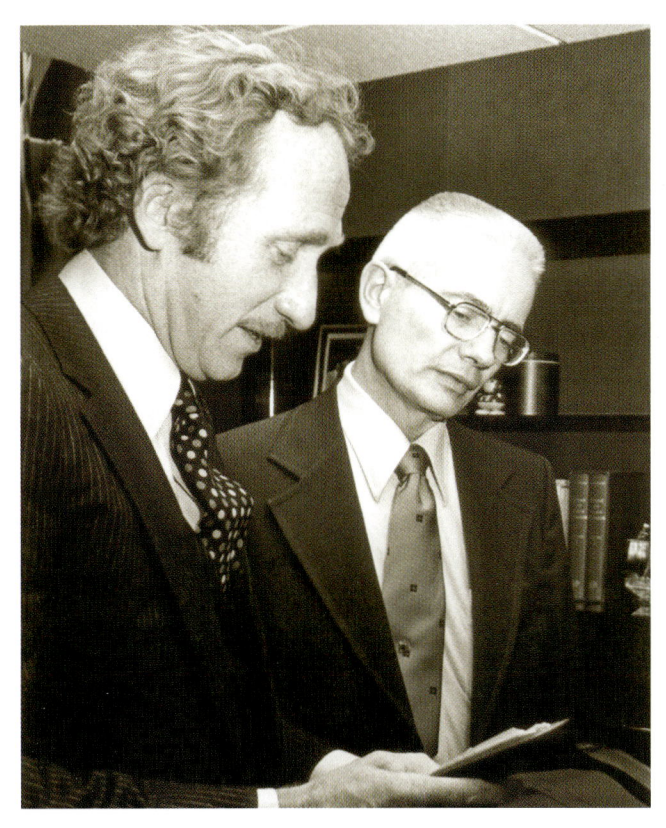

Richard Schripsema and Charles Thompson, MD

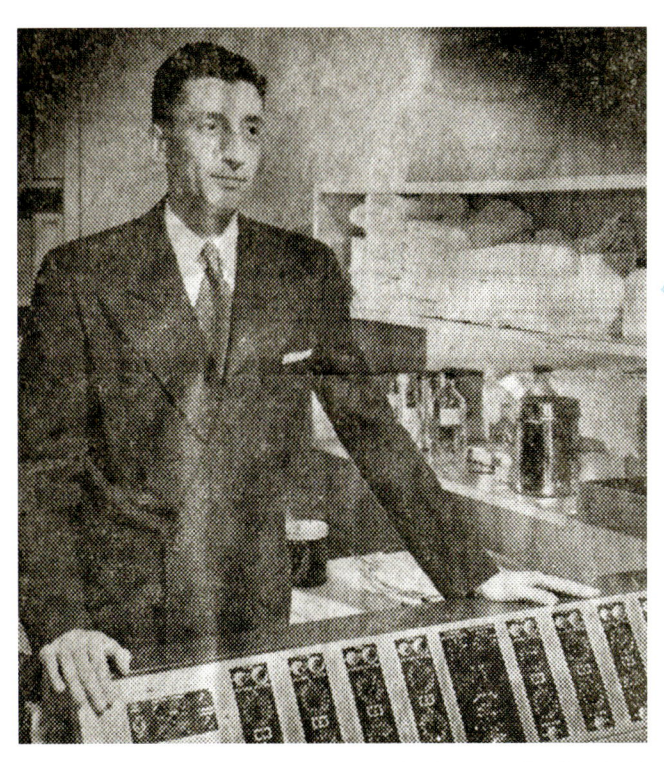

Ralph Hutchins, superintendent, stands by the controls of Hurley's electroencephalograph, a machine that detected disorders of the brain, on November 7, 1954.

First Board of Hospital Managers

An ordinance creating a board of hospital managers was adopted by the Flint Common Council on July 24, 1905. Mayor D. D. Aitken appointed the following citizens: George L. Walker (until May 1, 1906), William Martin (until May 1, 1907), Edward Black (until May 1, 1908), J. Dallas Dort (until May 1, 1909), and Charles Lippincott (until May 1, 1910). The first recorded meeting of the board was held at the Union Club room on September 23, 1905. Charles Lippincott was elected president, William Martin, treasurer, and Edward Black, secretary.[4]

CHAPTER FIVE THOSE WHO SERVE – HONORING EXCELLENCE • 105

Hurley's Chief Executives, 1908–2021

- Melany Gavulic, President & CEO, 2012 to present
- Patrick Wardell, President & CEO, 2005–2012
- Andrea Price, Interim President & CEO, 2001–2002 and 2004–2005
- Julius D. Spears Jr., President & CEO, 2002–2004
- Glenn A. Fosdick, President & CEO, 1995–2001
- Phillip C. Dutcher, President & CEO, 1980–1995
- Richard C. Schripsema, Hospital Director, 1974–1980
- Milton Saks, Hospital Director, 1964–1974
- Donald Walchenbach, Hospital Director, 1961–1964
- Stephen Lott, Hospital Director, 1957–1961
- Edward Gilgan, Hospital Director, 1956–1957
- Ralph C. Hutchins, Superintendent, Hospital Director, 1953–1956
- William K. Klein, Superintendent, 1947–1953
- W. W. Buss, Acting Superintendent, 1947
- Ralph Hueston, Superintendent, 1936–1947
- Dr. T. R. Ponton, Acting Superintendent, 1935
- Frank D. King, Superintendent, 1927–1935
- Dr. Byron E. Biggs, Acting Superintendent, 1927
- Louis Teffeau, Superintendent, 1926–1927
- Anna M. Schill, Superintendent, 1910–1926
- Alice M. Gregg, Superintendent, 1909–1910
- Mary B. Hall, Superintendent, 1908–1909

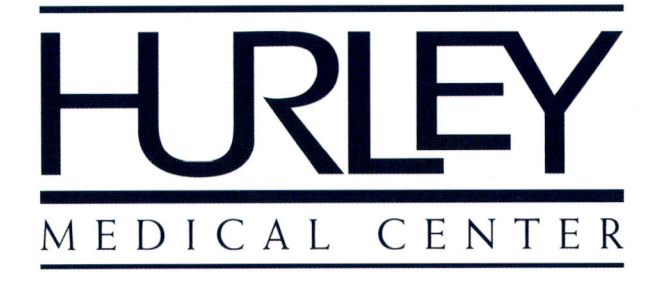

Hurley Medical Center Board of Managers

Hurley's board of managers has played a key role in maintaining Hurley's mission over the years. The first board was composed of five members, but it was increased to seven members by an amendment to the Flint City Charter. It was then expanded to eleven when board members determined that more people were needed to sufficiently represent the people of Flint. Today, fifteen Hurley leaders represent a wide cross section of the larger community, such as the law, education, the UAW union, state government, the NAACP, medicine, religion, industry, small businesses, and volunteers.

Hurley Medical Center Board of Managers (2020)

- Jason Caya
- Jessie Collins
- Charlotte Edwards
- Corinne Edwards, EdD
- Christopher Flores
- Marilyn Fuller, RN
- Frances Gilcreast
- DeAndra Larkin
- Reverend Herbert Miller
- Brian Nolan, MD
- Reverend Daniel Scheid
- Harriet Scott
- Philip Shaltz
- Marsha Strozier Wesley, RPh
- Brenda Williams

All members of the board of managers further the causes of Hurley. Some have made significant contributions, and the following people are only a few.

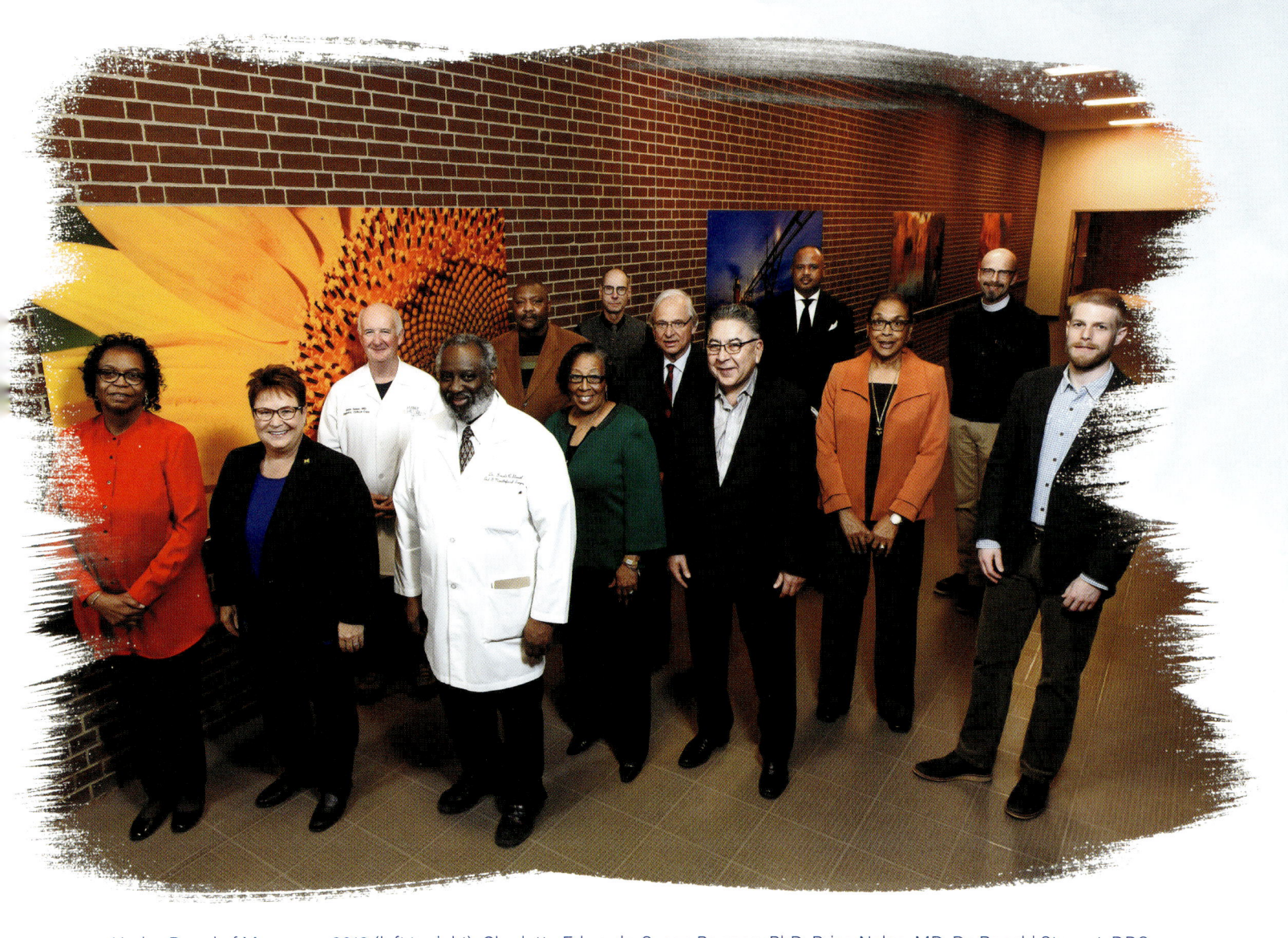

Hurley Board of Managers, 2018 (left to right): Charlotte Edwards, Susan Borrego, PhD, Brian Nolan, MD, Dr. Ronald Stewart, DDS, Jessie Collins, Frances Gilcreast, Philip Shaltz, Carl Bekofske, Christopher Flores, Reverend Herbert Miller, Harriet Scott, Reverend Daniel Scheid, and Jason Caya

Zolton Papp served for 42 years on the board (1945–1987), including two terms as president. He said that he "wanted to serve Hurley after reading a newspaper article about a woman who gave birth in a taxi, as she was turned away from a hospital due to lack of money." Furthermore, "I wanted to make sure nothing like that ever happened again," said Papp. "I went to the [Flint] city council with my concerns and interests for the community and was appointed to the Hurley Board of Managers." Papp, a retired pharmacist, was

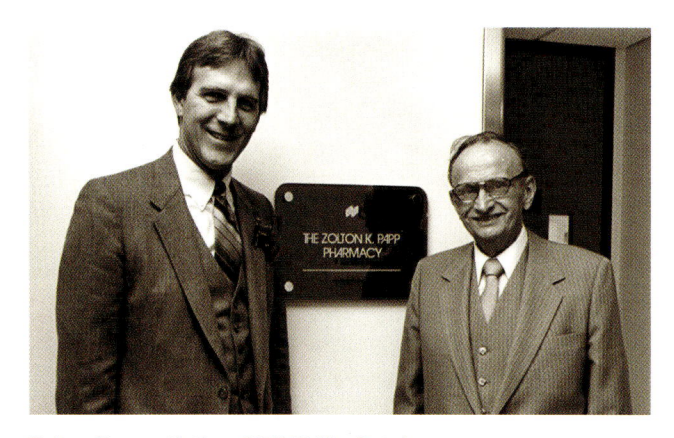

Zolton Papp with then CEO Phillip Dutcher

CHAPTER FIVE THOSE WHO SERVE – HONORING EXCELLENCE • 107

honored for his service when they named the Hurley pharmacy for him. "I'm being honest when I say that I love every brick in that building," said Papp.[5]

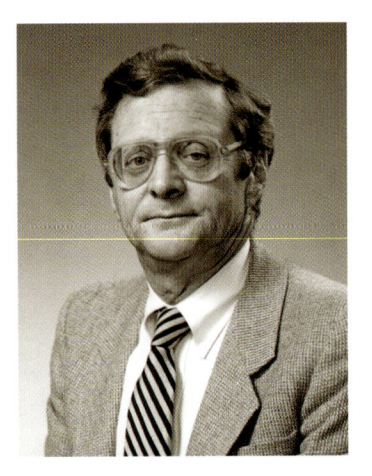

Charles White, a Flint attorney who joined the board in 1960, was honored as the second-longest-serving member of the board of managers in 1996 for his 35 years of service. A five-time president of the board, his leadership helped guide HMC through over three decades of growth into a respected regional medical center. He played an integral role in 1979's "The New Face of Hurley" project, was instrumental in having the School of Nursing built, improved the parking situation by buying property for new lots, and led the opening of the Hurley Health and Fitness Center.

Charles White

Ronald Warner, retired manager of the former Chevrolet manufacturing plant, joined the board in 1968. "Hurley has always been willing to reach out and meet the needs of the community and will continue to be a leader," predicted the longtime supporter, who helped raise funds for "The New Face of Hurley" in the late 1970s. "The medical center's caseload increased when corporate fringe benefits made health care more affordable," he recalled. "The board

Ronald Warner

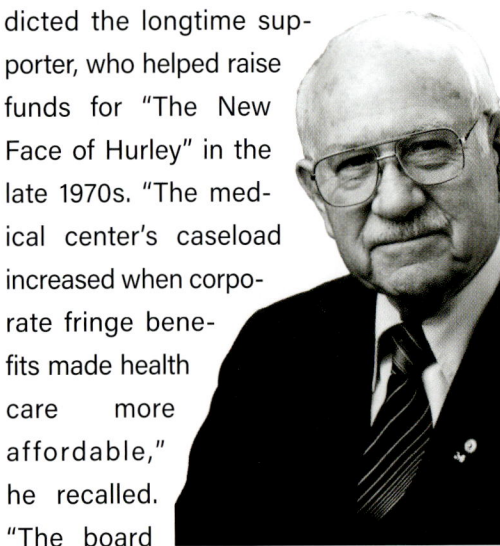

recognized that the intensity of change, called for change in management, and sought additional personnel. These changes provided the base from which we could reach out into the community."[6]

Elizabeth "Libby" Wright, a prominent Flint-area realtor, was the first female president of the board of managers (1980) and the first board president to take office after the completion of the East Tower expansion in 1979, the hospital's largest building project.

Leadership at Its Best

Directly reporting to Hurley's CEO, Melany Gavulic, are a group of vice presidents who represent the main reporting structure of HMC, guiding the employees and managing the strong corporate culture.

Cass Wisniewski, MBA, CPA
Senior Vice President (VP) and Chief Financial Officer (CFO)
Wisniewski has been with HMC for 19 years, and CFO since 2012. "I have been in health care finance for more than 40 years. I am not a clinician but feel that I offer guidance from a financial perspective to make sure clinicians have what they need and that Hurley continues to exist at a high level."

"Our corporate culture starts at the top with our CEO, Melany Gavulic," said Cass Wisniewski. "She has put together a good team. They are not silo thinkers, but support decisions after they are made."

Michael Burnett, MSW, MBA
VP, Service Line Development, and Chief Strategy Officer
Burnett has been with the medical center since 2003. Burnett oversees growth and partnership initiatives associated with HMC's 11 service lines: behavioral medicine, cardiac, emergent services, geriatrics, internal medicine, musculoskeletal, oncology, renal and transplant, trauma and surgical services, vascular,

and women and children's services. Included within his scope of responsibility is positioning strategies for health care reform for population health management and physician alignment. Burnett also leads the Hurley Foundation in its role as a support to HMC.

Amy Benko, PharmD
VP, Patient Care Services
Benko has been working at HMC for more than 20 years. She started as a pharmacy intern, from 1990 to 1994. She returned in 1999 as pharmacy clinical coordinator, introducing clinical pharmacy services to the critical care and trauma teams by rounding and working closely with doctors and nurses to monitor critical patients. She was promoted to Pharmacy director in 2007. In 2012, Benko became VP of Patient Care Services, where she maintains the pharmacy management responsibilities, as well as oversees the operations of the laboratory, radiology, operating room, anesthesia, nursing, facilities, nutrition services, and environmental services. Department heads report to Benko from a quality, safety, operational, efficiency, budgetary, and regulatory perspective. "It's the people that I work with that make my job most rewarding, because Hurley is a unique place; employees like to excel. Our collective heart is for caring about people, and we have a lot to give. Many take on extra work, and we don't mind it because we consider it to be giving back. We are responsive and quick to help each other. We are truly a tight-knit group."

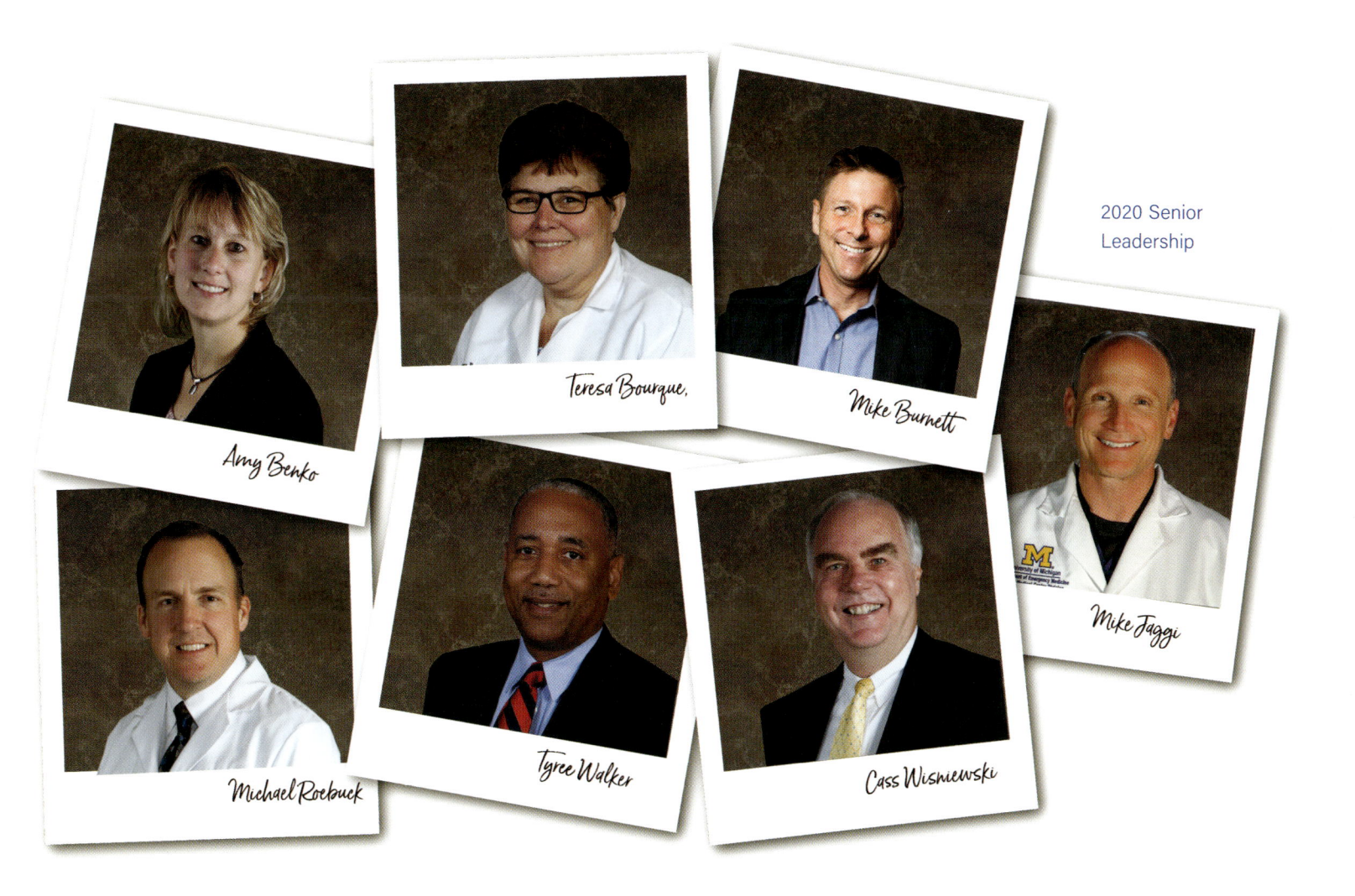

2020 Senior Leadership

Amy Benko

Teresa Bourque

Mike Burnett

Mike Jaggi

Michael Roebuck

Tyree Walker

Cass Wisniewski

CHAPTER FIVE THOSE WHO SERVE – HONORING EXCELLENCE • 109

F. Michael Jaggi, DO
VP, Chief Medical Officer (CMO)
Dr. Jaggi finished his combined internal medicine/emergency medicine (IM/EM) residency at Henry Ford Hospital in Detroit in 1996. At that time, the U of M EM department and HMC had just formalized a relationship for the university to provide emergency services at HMC. Dr. Jaggi joined the team at Hurley in July of 1996, working in the ED, as well as providing IM staff service. "The relationship with U of M has created a pipeline of clinicians and researchers that are dedicated to the mission of Hurley: 'Clinical Excellence – Service to People.' This permeates through the ranks, and people feel good about what they are doing." When Jaggi started in Hurley's ED, they were treating just over 50,000 patients a year. "That volume has steadily grown, and in 2013, [they] treated over 100,000 ED patients."

Michael Roebuck, MD
VP, Chief Medical Information Officer (CMIO)
Dr. Roebuck has been serving as Hurley's CMIO since 2012; he is also an assistant professor of emergency medicine at the U of M Medical School. Dr. Roebuck joined the HMC medical staff in 1998 to work in the ED. He says, "The most rewarding part is being part of the transformation of medicine, which has occurred over the last 10 years during the implementation of electronic health records."

Tyree Walker, MS
VP, Human Resources (HR)
Walker began his HR career at HMC, from 1982 to 1995. He served as a labor relations assistant, personnel analyst, employment manager, and assistant personnel director. He returned to HMC in October 2014. According to Walker, "What I find most rewarding is to work alongside the many dedicated and hardworking people who serve the health care needs in our region. We have a great team at Hurley."

Teresa Bourque, RN, BSN
Chief Nurse, Senior Administrator, Nursing
Bourque began her career at Hurley in 1986, holding various clinical positions at Hurley, including ICU nurse for over 10 years, Hurley Home Care nurse, nurse case manager, nurse manager, director of Case Management, and Service Line administrator for critical care. She believes that working in different positions throughout the organization has allowed her to care for patients in many different ways. The most rewarding aspect of her work is knowing that the staff make a positive difference in patients' and families' lives every day.

Medical Excellence

Medical Staff Officers, 2019–2020
Chief of Staff: Elmahdi Saeed, MD, MBBS, FAAP, FACP
Vice Chief of Staff: Muhammad Jabbar, MD
Secretary: Paul Musson, MD
Members at Large: Michael Roebuck, MD; Elfateh Seedahmed, MD; Basim Towfiq, MD
Allied Health Members at Large: Sherry Bowman, ANP-BC; Melanie Krznarich, PA-C

Chief of Staff: Elmahdi Saeed, MD, MBBS, FAAP, FACP
Known as Dr. E. Saeed—to differentiate him from his brother, Dr. S. (Seif) Saeed—earned his medical degree from the University of Khartoum in Sudan. He completed his combined internal medicine/pediatrics residency at HMC in 1991. Dr. E. Saeed was a Pinnacle Award recipient in 2007. He has been an associate professor of medicine and an assistant professor of pediatrics at

MSU since 1991. Dr. E. Saeed provided steady and strong guidance during his time as chief of staff, always handling issues in his own quiet manner with the utmost of respect for anyone involved. He was always approachable, and many staff members felt comfortable sharing a variety of topics with him, as his contemplative nature provided reassurance.

Over the decades, many have contributed to HMC's reputation for medical excellence. While others have been mentioned in previous chapters, unfortunately, we cannot mention everyone who has played a vital role. Here we acknowledge physicians of distinction that have left an indelible mark on their years of service, for which we will be forever grateful.

F. Michael Jaggi, DO, FACP, FACEP, Director, Emergency Services, CMO, Clinical Assistant Professor, University of Michigan
Dr. Jaggi has made outstanding contributions to Hurley's Emergency Department and to Hurley as a whole. Hurley's CMO was honored with the 2019 Michigan Medicine Dean's Award in recognition of medical school faculty and staff who demonstrate exceptional accomplishment in the areas of teaching,

F. Michael Jaggi, DO

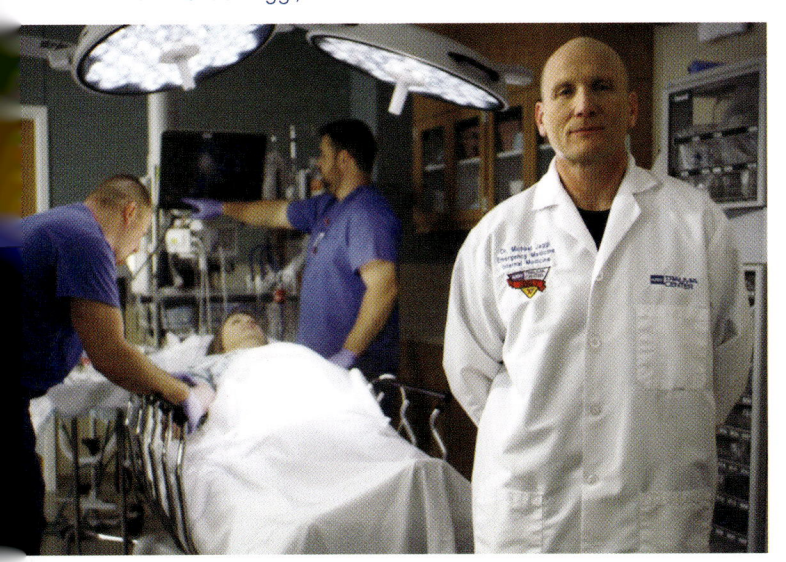

Chiefs of Staff, 1944–2021

2021–	Khalid Ahmed, MD, MRCP, FACP
2013–2020	Elmahdi Saeed, MD, MBBS, FAAP, FACP
2009–2012	Jitendra Katneni, MD
2001–2008	Brian Nolan, MD, FAAP
1995–2000	Samuel Dismond Jr., MD
1971–1994	Charles Thompson, MD
1969–1970	R. James, MD
1965–1968	A. Sirna, MD
1959–1964	L. Shantz, MD
1956–1959	L. Bateman, MD
1944–1946	Arthur D. Kirk, MD

research, clinical care, community service, innovation, and administration. He was the Gift of Life recipient of the 2019 Hospital Executive Leader Champion Award and the 2002 Hurley Pinnacle Award recipient. "In his time at Hurley, he has helped so many patients and families give their final gifts. He's been known to drop—even vacation—to help with a case so that donors and their families are served," said Dorrie Dils, CEO, Gift of Life. Dr. Jaggi is a clinical assistant professor, Department of Emergency Medicine (U of M), and clinical assistant professor, Department of Internal Medicine (MSU CHM).

Susumu Inoue, MD, FAAP
Dr. Inoue, former director of Pediatric Hematology/Oncology, has been studying and treating cancer since 1969. During his distinguished career, his tireless devotion to patients and his ideas on treatments resulted in significant contributions in both research and his commitment to education. He served as a

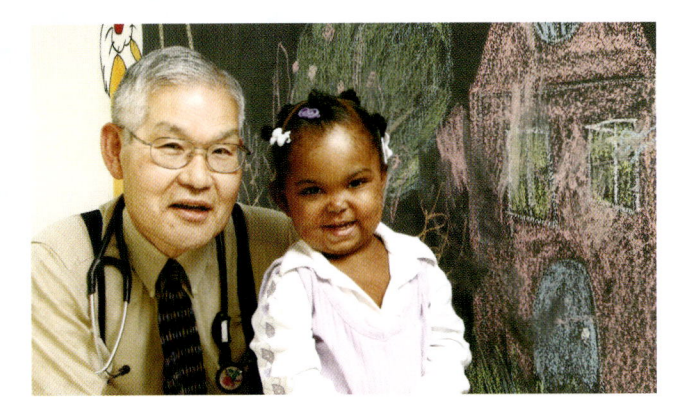

Susumu Inoue, MD, FAAP

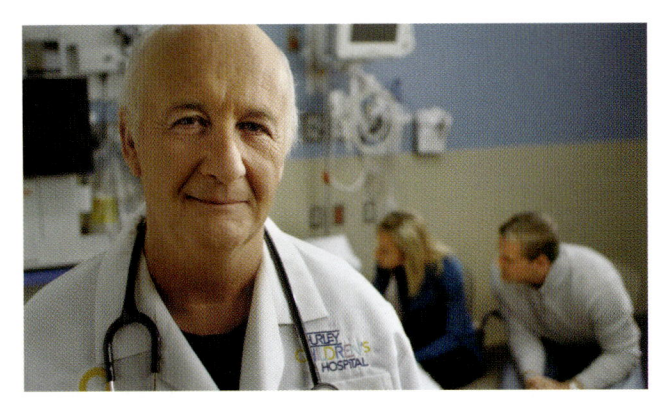

Brian Nolan, MD, FAAP

professor of pediatrics/human development at MSU CHM and clinical professor of pediatrics at Wayne State University School of Medicine. He made strides with his ongoing involvement and efforts to stem hemophilia, sickle cell, and pediatric AIDS. His clinical leadership in healing children has provided numerous miracle stories through the Children's Miracle Network. Dr. Inoue was the 2006 Hurley Pinnacle Award recipient.

Brian Nolan, MD, FAAP
Dr. Nolan is a Level II pediatric trauma physician who has worked for HMC for a total of 44 years, starting as a pediatric resident from 1976 to 1979. He completed two fellowships, pediatric intensive care and neonatology, at Detroit Children's Hospital, which took three years. "I am originally from Ireland, and after medical school, I did a rotating internship in medicine and surgery," said Nolan. "I am very happy with my decision to come to the United States to start my pediatric residency. I have no regrets. It is very rewarding to take care of children." Nolan is currently the director of Pediatric Critical Care and is certified in child abuse pediatrics, neonatal-perinatal medicine, pediatric critical care, and pediatrics. He was chief of staff from 2001 to 2008, and he is currently serving on the Hurley Board of Managers. He was clinical director of Pediatrics from 2009 until 2020, when Mahesh Sharman, MD, assumed the role. Dr. Nolan was the Hurley Pinnacle Award recipient in 2010.

Raouf Mikhail, MD, FACS, FRCS(C), Associate Clinical Professor of Surgery, MSU
After completing his surgery residency training from 1976 to 1981 at HMC, Mikhail went on to train as a

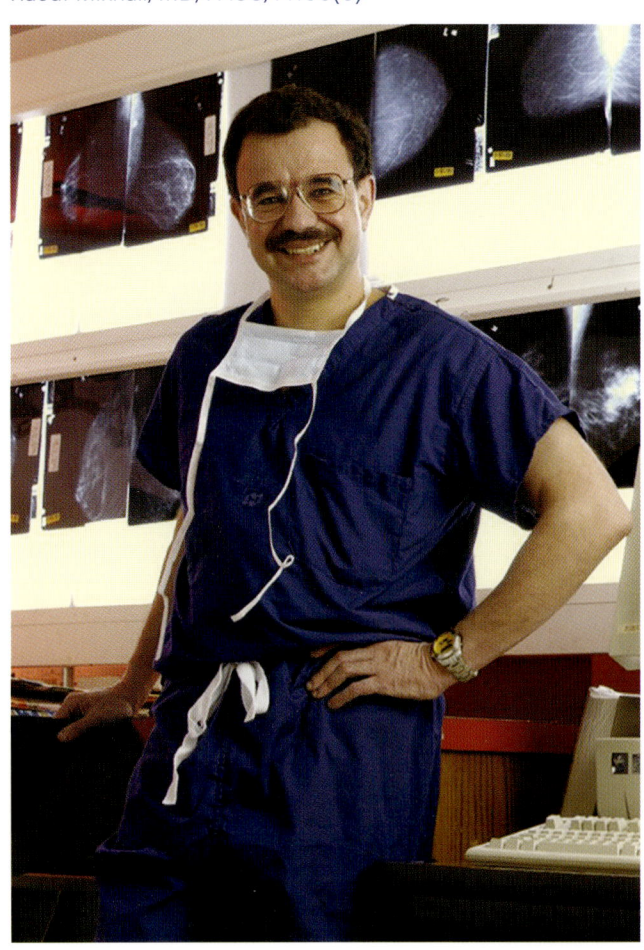

Raouf Mikhail, MD, FACS, FRCS(C)

112 • HURLEY MEDICAL CENTER

fellow in head and neck surgery and surgical oncology at the world-renowned MD Anderson Cancer Center in Houston, Texas. He returned to HMC and assumed the position of director of Oncology and associate clinical professor of surgery at MSU from 1985 to 2020. During his tenure, the hospital received continuous accreditation from the ACS as an approved cancer center. Mikhail sought to add gynecological oncology, surgical oncology, and pediatric oncology to Hurley's services. Mikhail is particularly proud of transforming HMC into a Center of Excellence for Breast Cancer Care, having had the hospital become an approved center by the Commission on Cancer for breast cancer care with NAPBC accreditation. Dr. Mikhail was the Hurley Pinnacle Award recipient in 2003.

Farouck Obeid, MD
As the Hurley Pinnacle Award recipient in 2004, Dr. Obeid was recognized for his distinguished career as a surgeon, which spanned more than 27 years, providing care for more than 1,600 trauma and burn patients annually and assisting in more than 1,000 bariatric surgeries. Dr. Obeid was instrumental in HMC receiving its initial Level I Trauma Center designation by the ACS.

Samuel Dismond Jr., MD
Dr. Dismond was affectionately known as the "Voice of Hurley" due to his easily recognizable and commanding voice, combined with his passion for Hurley. Whenever he walked into a room, his charismatic energy seemed to uplift everyone in his presence. In January 1995, he was the first African American physician to be voted Hurley's chief of staff, serving in that role until 2000. "One of the things that I hope to accomplish is to help our staff physicians be in step with Hurley's efforts toward courtesy and cultural diversity. The practice of medicine has become burdensome, complicated, and very demanding as we move into areas of managed care, high litigation, and patient satisfaction surveys. The field of medicine is changing more rapidly than ever. As chief of staff, I hope to help colleagues cope with these changes, understanding fully that our basic commitment is to our patients and their families." Dr. Dismond served on the Hurley Board of Managers from 1998 to 2012, serving as board chairman from 2005 to 2007. "I was secretary of the medical staff for a few years. Charles Thompson, MD, was chief of staff for 23 years, and when he retired, I took over from him." Dr. Dismond was the recipient of the Hurley Pinnacle Award in 2000. He passed away in 2021.

Dr. Dismond's leadership and patient care were supported by Janice Dismond, RN, his office manager and wife. The team worked together in private practice from 1985 to 2012. Dr. Dismond retired in August 2012 at 80 years old, after 50 years of service to Flint-area families. "When patients tell Dismond they are sad to see him go [retire], he tries to respond with a little humor. 'I say to them "Well I've given you 50 years of time. How much do you want?" That makes them smile,' he said."[7]

Members of the neuro/ortho/surgical team in 1995. Left to right: Margie McClain, nutrition services; Doris Dutcher, volunteer; Marilyn Rembert, medical records clerk; Michelle Pastue, RN; Belinda Jones, nursing assistant; and Samuel Dismond Jr., MD.

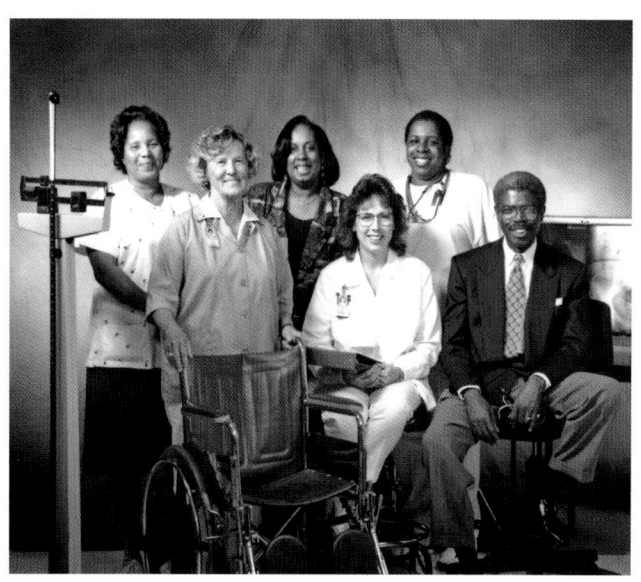

Khalid Ahmed, MD, MRCP, FACP, 2021–2022 Chief of Staff

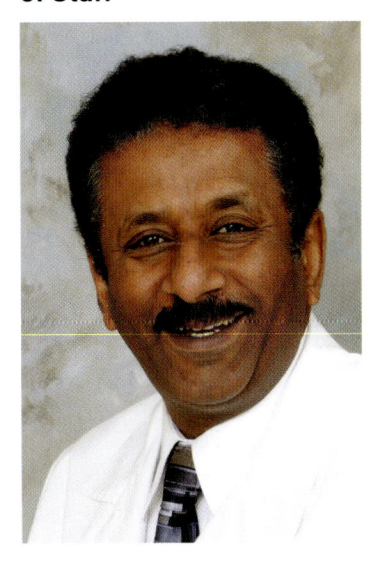

Khalid Ahmed, MD, MRCP, FACP

Dr. Ahmed has served in many leadership roles throughout his thirty-plus-year career with Hurley. Having completed his internal medicine residency in Hurley's program, Dr. Ahmed was immediately drawn to our mission. His service in private practice within the community has always led to a strong partnership with Hurley, ensuring that patients have access to the care that they need. Dr. Ahmed serves as clinical associate professor of internal medicine at MSU-Flint. Dr. Ahmed has served in many leadership roles, starting during his residency as president of the Housestaff Association, and later in his career serving as chair of Internal Medicine, clinical director for Internal Medicine, and vice chief of staff. As recently as January of 2021, he was elected by the medical staff as chief of staff. Dr. Ahmed was the Hurley Pinnacle Award recipient in 2012.

Donna Fonger, BSN, MSN, AND

Fonger joined Hurley in 1963, straight out of nursing school. She served Hurley in many capacities—as a staff nurse on the medical floors, the neurovigil unit, and the ED. She served as a nursing supervisor for over 10 years, providing unwavering support to the clinical team. She spent 16 years as nurse manager for the Oncology Unit. She was selected as the 1982 employee of the year by HMC for her nursing expertise, diligence, and empathy. According to Margie Murray-Wright, "When Donna lost her courageous battle with cancer, we knew she needed to have an indelible footprint at Hurley. It is the bench that sits in the elevator alcove on 9E, the oncology unit, which allows for quiet repose for grieving families. For being Donna Fonger meant giving more, caring more, knowing more, and expecting more . . . quite simply, the 'more' that Donna touched our hearts, it made us better. Her unrelenting message, which resonated with all the patients, staff, and physicians, is the reason she deserves honor. She was persistent, steadfast, diligent, and insightful. She combined a keen analytical ability and critical thinking with an attribute I refer to as 'heart.' This combination was a catalyst for many contributions, which led to systematic change and quality improvements. Donna was a nurse's nurse."

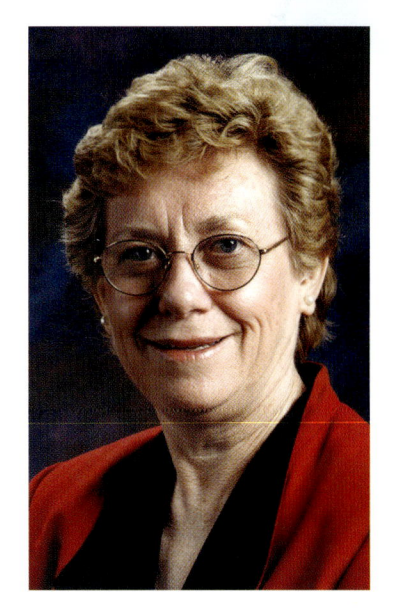

Donna Fonger, Nurse of Distinction

Basim Towfiq, MD, Michael Jaggi, DO, CMO, and Ghassan Bachuwa, MD, MS, FACP

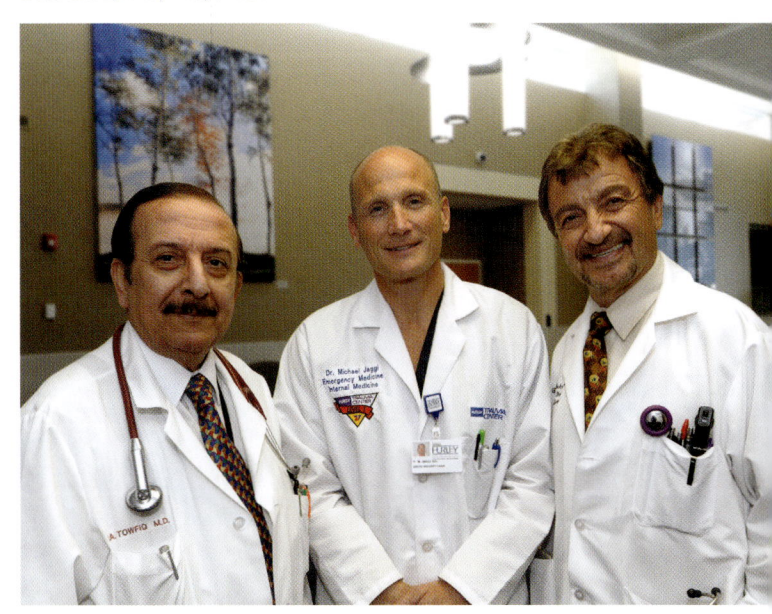

Multiple Generations at HMC

So many family members have joined the ranks of staff at Hurley that there are too many to feature. Here, we highlight a few of the physicians after whom the second generation followed in the footsteps of their elders, or husband and wife physicians who have both served at Hurley.

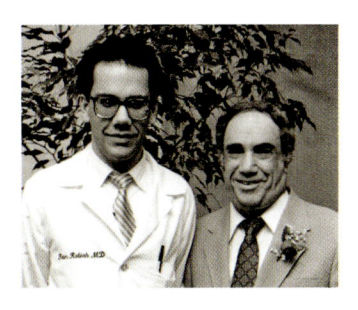

Fouad Rabiah, MD, thoracic surgeon, retired in 1989 after 25 years, but not before he saw his son **Peter Rabiah, MD,** finish his transitional-year residency at Hurley. The elder Rabiah was the first board-certified thoracic surgeon in Flint to insert a cardiac pacemaker, the first to ligate patent ductus arteriosus, and he pioneered the first rib resection for thoracic outlet syndrome. His son chose ophthalmology.

David Congdon, MD, completed both a Hurley internship (1961–1962) and a pathology residency (1962–1966). He was a Hurley pathologist from 1966 until his retirement in 1991. **Douglas Congdon, DO,** also completed a pathology residency at HMC (1987–1991). He had plans to specialize in radiation therapy, but he took his father's advice and chose a year's residency in pathology. He hired in as an associate pathologist on July 1, 1991—the same year his dad retired—and assumed the role of director of Pathology on July 23, 2018. "Once I got into pathology, I liked it," he said. "It's scientific; you can look at something and know what it is."

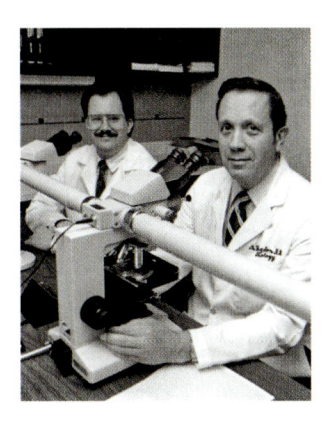

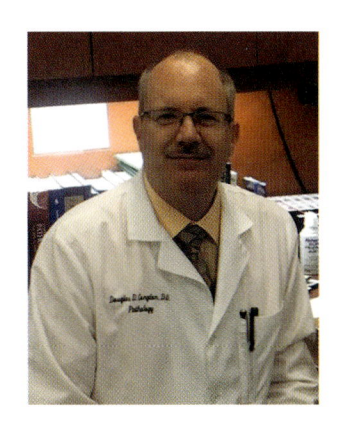

Larry Young, MD, and Omari Young, MD (See page 72 in Chapter 3)

Jitendra Katneni, MD, FACP, completed an internal medicine residency at Hurley (1987–1990). His son, **Srikar Katneni, MD,** a Hurley NICU grad, began the same residency program at Hurley 32 years later. Dr. J. Katneni served as chief of staff from 2009 to 2012.

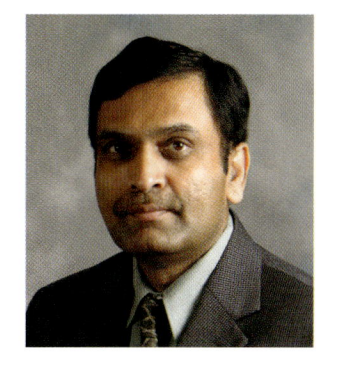

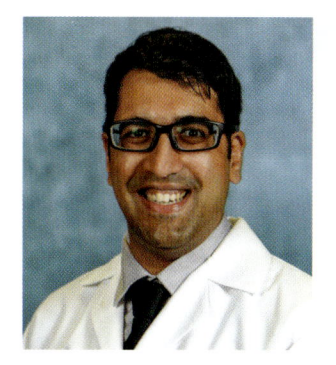

Mahesh Sharman, MD, director of Pediatric Critical Care at Hurley's Children's Hospital, completed Hurley's pediatric residency in 1997, and his wife, **Punam Sharman, MD,** completed a combined internal medicine/pediatric residency in 2002. In honor of their 30-year wedding anniversary, M. Sharman gave the gift of a lifetime to his wife of 30 years. In 2018, his gift was revealed: he had sponsored a private pediatric room in the new 11 West Tower pediatric hospital.

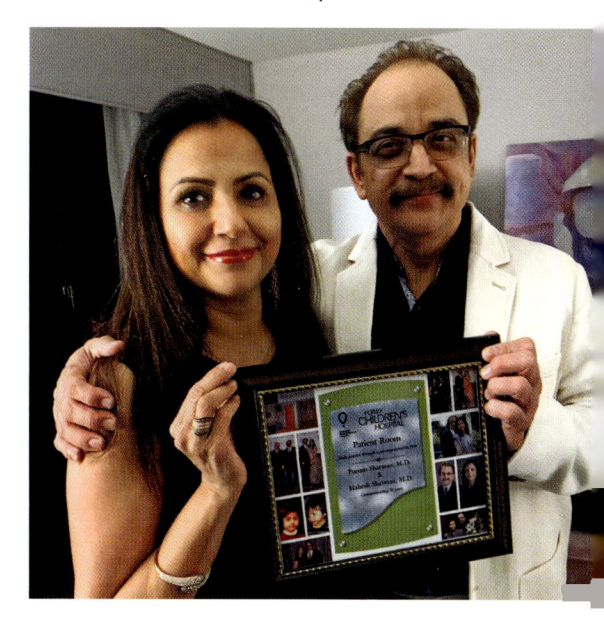

CHAPTER FIVE THOSE WHO SERVE – HONORING EXCELLENCE • 115

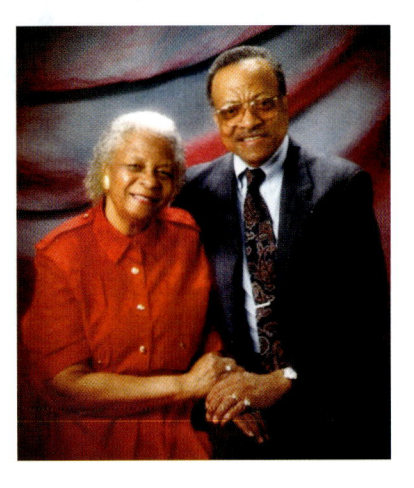

Billie Lewis, MD, completed his internship (1959–1960) and surgery residency (1960–1964) at Hurley. **Vivian Lewis, MD,** the first African American female physician to work at Hurley Hospital, completed an internship (1959–1960) and a pediatric residency (1961–1963) at Hurley. Both were active participants in Hurley programs to promote professional development, patient service, and community focus. Dr. V. Lewis was the first president of the Genesee County Medical Society to be both female and African American. She served as a board member on the Hurley Foundation Board for many years. In 1996, she was honored with the Governor George Romney Lifetime Achievement Award. She received a Hurley Pinnacle Award for her excellence in caring in 1997. In 1998, she was recognized by the American Medical Association as one of the "Fifty Most Positive Doctors in America."

Clinton Dowd, MD, an obstetrician-gynecologist, and **Sharon Dowd, MD,** former director of the Outpatient Hematology-Oncology Clinic. Dr. C. Dowd served as the program director for the obstetrics and gynecology residency from 1980 to 1996.

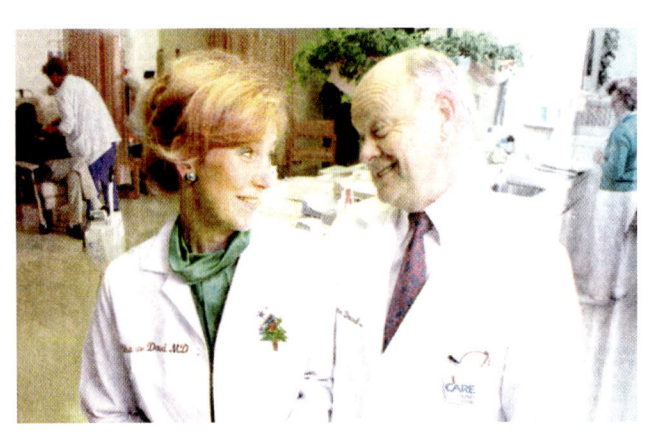

Quality Care through a Physician Hospital Organization (PHO)

During the 1980s and 1990s, Health Maintenance Organizations (HMOs) contracted with employers to provide health care coverage for their employees. In 1994, Hurley formed a PHO; Daniel George was president and CEO. "We worked with physicians to offer the right clinical care, at the right time, in the right setting, at the right cost, to achieve the best clinical outcomes," said George. "Hurley's was a model PHO in that we had 270 participating physicians, 55,000 covered lives, and our sophisticated, physician-led, clinical model successfully balancing quality care with cost." The PHO dissolved in 2007, and participating physicians and the hospital assumed independent negotiations with health insurance carriers, which continues to this day.

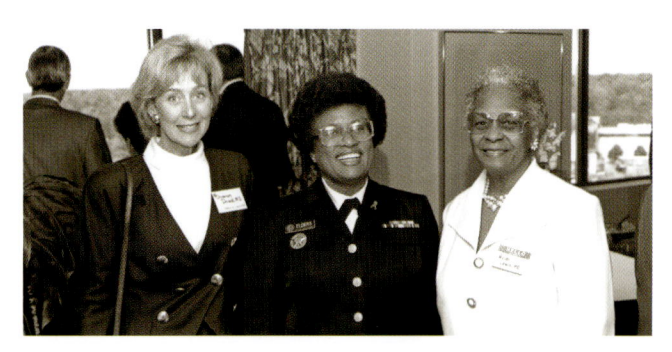

Several famous figures have visited HMC. In 2001, Vice President Al Gore and Senator Joe Lieberman toured the pediatric unit. Renowned surgeon and author Ben Carson, MD, joined Flint's celebration of African American heritage in 2000. James Brady, former White House press secretary and vice chairman of the National Brain Injury Association, visited HMC in 1997. Surgeon General Vice Admiral Joycelyn Elders, MD, pediatrician, and public health administrator, visited HMC in 1993. Elders is pictured with Vivian Lewis, MD, and Sharon Dowd, MD.

Dedicated Spaces

Paul F. Reinhart Emergency Trauma Center

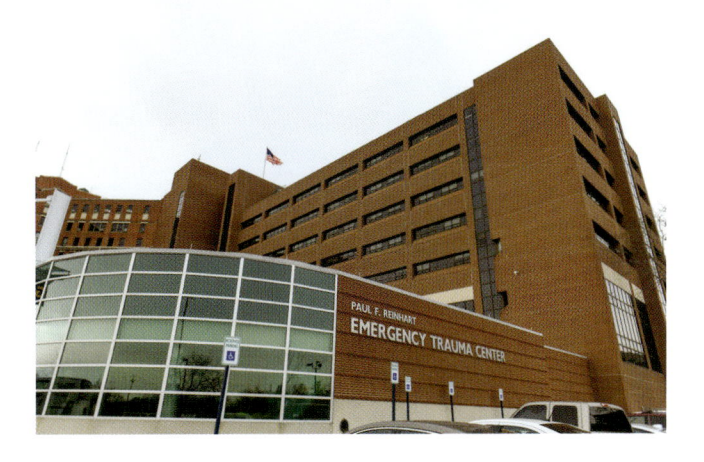

Farouck N. Obeid Trauma Bay

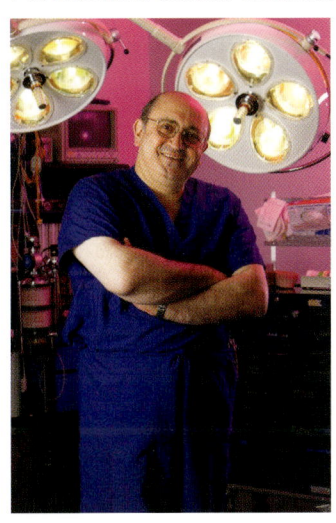

Hospital administrators pushed for the trauma bay to be named in honor of Farouck Obeid, MD, because he was instrumental in HMC obtaining its initial Level I Trauma Center status. Unfortunately, Dr. Obeid passed away in 2008 before the trauma bay was completed.

Dr. R. Roderic Abbott Medical Education Center

In 2019, Hurley Foundation unveiled a new education center in honor of R. Roderic Abbott, MD, a selfless oncologist who never took a salary and returned all patient payments back to Hurley. Abbott was the director of Medical Education in the 1960s and served as the first chairman of the Hurley Research Committee. "Dr. Abbott respected everybody. We learned a lot of things from him, not just medicine, but how to be a person," said Jitendra Katneni, MD. Margaret Setter-Abbott, MD, wife of the late Dr. Abbott, followed that sentiment: "He truly was selfless in what he did. Everyone was his friend, and that meant so much to him." Abbott was honored with the Dr. Clement A. Alfred Humanitarian Award in 1995 for his leadership and significant contributions to the advancement of family planning through education, medical service, and public advocacy. The education center provides enhanced technology conferencing and training in seven sponsored rooms, all to further the vision of "leaders in transforming health through academic and clinical excellence, and expanding access to innovative care," according to education center fundraising committee chair Dr. Katneni.

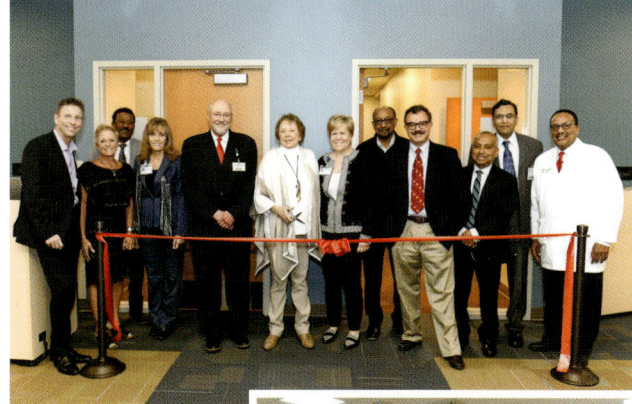

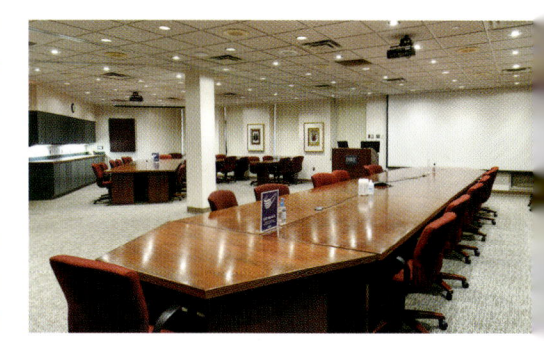

Charles W. White Conference Center

HMC honored the second-longest-serving member of its board of managers by dedicating its conference center in 1996 as a permanent tribute to the 35 years of selfless contributions by attorney Charles W. White. White also served on Hurley's School of Nursing Advisory Board and helped structure the joint four-year nursing degree program with the University of Michigan-Flint. The Charles W. White Conference Center is located off of Hurley's West Tower Lobby.

Max. E. Dodds, MD, Comprehensive Cancer Care Center

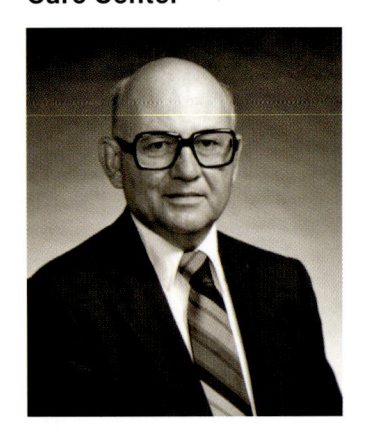

Dr. Dodds was Oncology director in 1953. "During the 1980s, Dr. Dodds provided the leadership necessary for Hurley's cancer care program to expand and be recognized throughout the area, state, and nation," said Hurley director Phillip C. Dutcher. According to cancer surgeon Raouf Mikhail, MD, FACS, FRCS, "Dr. Dodds was responsible for starting and developing Hurley's cancer center into the comprehensive program it is today." Dr. Mikhail trained under Dr. Dodds during his surgical residency and considers him to be his mentor. "He was truly my hero," said Dr. Mikhail. "He is the person that made me interested in the field of surgical oncology and is the main reason why I returned to Flint from Houston, to complete his mission. He was a very calm man, and a gifted surgeon. He was the doctor of doctors, and the leader of the surgical community in Flint for three decades." The naming of the Max. E. Dodds Comprehensive Cancer Care Center took place in 1990.

Merliss Brown Auditorium
On October 24, 1928, as part of the million-dollar expansion, Hurley Hospital's first auditorium (the only one of its kind in the state) was officially dedicated as the Merliss Brown Auditorium. The auditorium was named for Murdock Merliss Brown, a GM factory worker for 45 years, who willed $300,000 to Hurley after serving for 50 years on the board of managers.

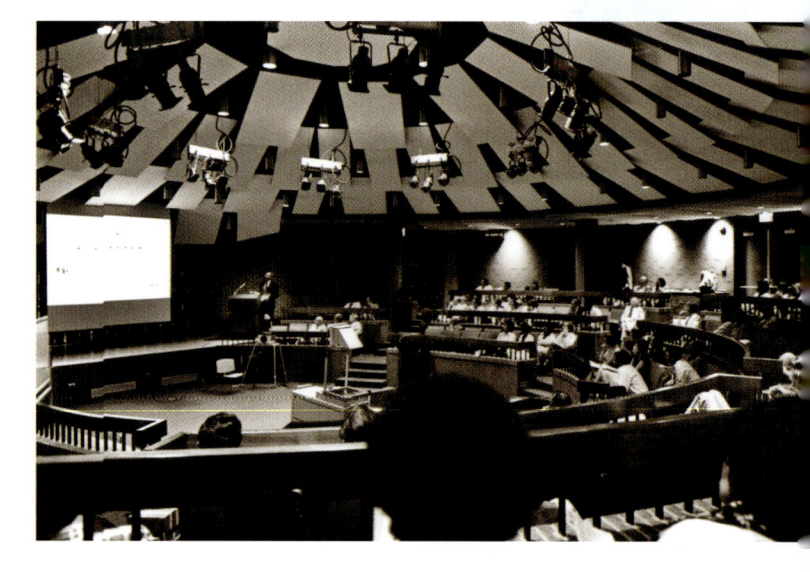

Brown was credited with securing funding for the new hospital. The theater-style space had a sizable stage and upholstered seating for 300. The acoustics and décor were top of the line and featured a physician's area with a library, the auditorium, and amphitheater operating rooms.[8] In 1983, in honor of Hurley's 75th anniversary, a new auditorium was constructed and again named for Merliss Brown. Over the years, he gained the titles of "Philanthropist in Overalls" and the "Father of Hurley Hospital." Brown started on the board in 1920, was president of the hospital board from 1928 to 1929, and then served as secretary until 1970. In 1955, he was honored by Hurley Hospital for 35 years of service on the board.[9] In 1969, the city commission appropriately chose National Hospital Week in May to appoint him to his eighth consecutive seven-year term on the board so that he could reach a solid half century of service, even though he passed in 1969.

Zolton K. Papp Pharmacy
Named in 1983 in honor of Zolton Papp, retired pharmacist, who took intense personal interest in Hurley and helped plan Hurley's 5,000-square-foot pharmacy, which was considered a showcase among institutional facilities and one of the largest in the nation when it opened in May 1981. The 24-hour operation could process 1,800 medication orders per day.

Frank V. Hodges Laboratory

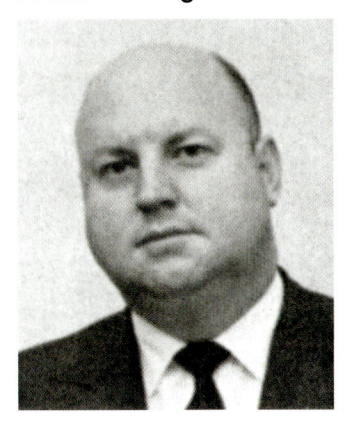

In 1982, HMC's laboratory was officially dedicated to the physician who was chief of Pathology from 1963 until his death in 1981. Dr. Hodges is credited with developing the laboratory into the largest, most automated, and most technical lab in the tri-county region. More than 1.5 million lab procedures are performed each year to aid in the diagnosis and treatment of diseases. Dr. Hodges was also noted for encouraging medical education and scholarly research. He was instrumental in organizing HMC's Annual Research Forum for resident physicians and medical students.

Franklin V. Wade Regional Burn Unit

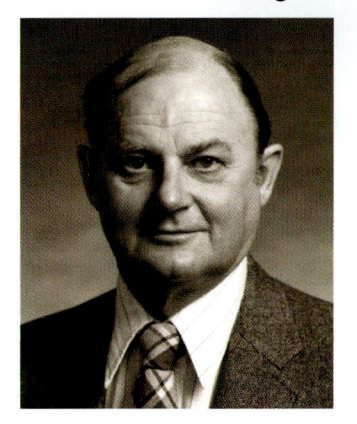

Hurley's prestigious burn unit, the only one in the area, was named in honor of Franklin V. Wade, MD, chairman of Hurley's Department of Surgery in the 1980s. He became the first director of Trauma Services in 1981. He devoted his time to trauma and surgical care, and to trauma service education to emergency field personnel through the newly established emergency telemetry system.

Sumathi Mukkamala Hurley Children's Center

On August 11, 2015, the Sumathi Mukkamala Hurley Children's Center opened above the Flint Farmer's

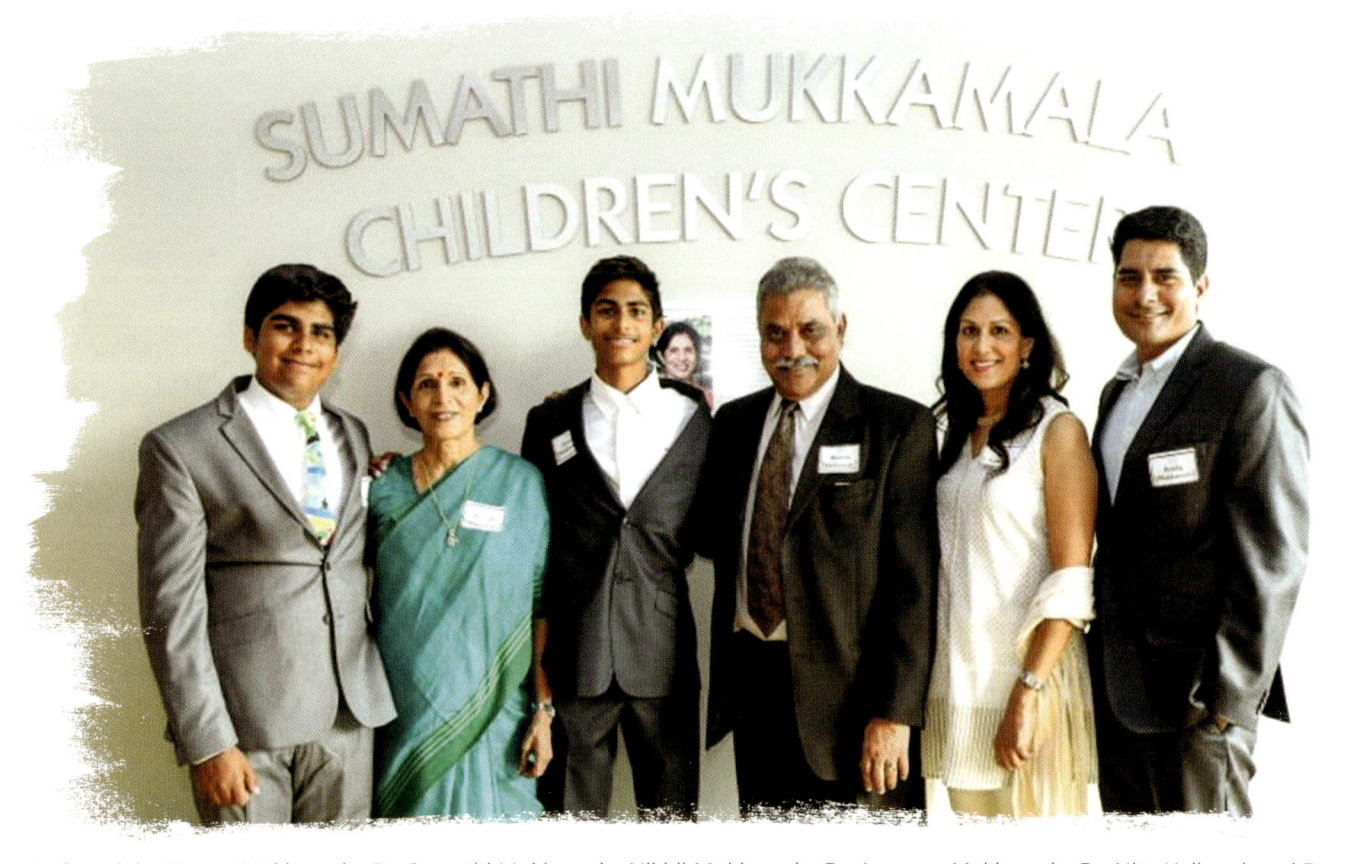

Left to right: Deven Mukkamala, Dr. Sumathi Mukkamala, Nikhil Mukkamala, Dr. Apparao Mukkamala, Dr. Nita Kulkarni, and Dr. Srinivas (Bobby) Mukkamala

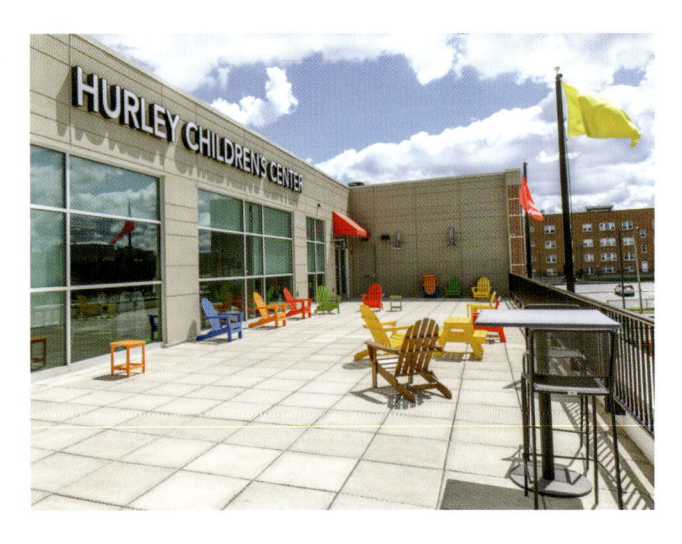

Market in downtown Flint. It was proudly named in honor of Sumathi Mukkamala, MD, who has dedicated her life to caring for children. She completed an internship from 1972 to 1973 and a pediatric residency from 1973 to 1976 at Hurley before practicing pediatric medicine for 20 years in Flint. Dr. Sumathi's husband and fellow Hurley graduate, AppaRao Mukkamala, MD, donated funds for the construction of this facility to honor his wife. Dr. AppaRao Mukkamala, chair of Hurley's Radiology Department and clinical professor of radiology at MSU College of Human Medicine, was the former chair of the Hurley Board of Managers (2009). Dr. A. Mukkamala was a Hurley Pinnacle Award recipient in 2009. He served as a Michigan delegate to the American Medical Association (AMA) for four years, starting in 2007.

Charles A. Thompson, MD, Education Center

Charles Thompson, MD, was chief of staff at the medical center for 23 years, stepping down in 1996 to devote more time to his private practice. His dedication and commitment to his patients and families were trademark values that distinguished him as an exemplary physician and human being. He was the Hurley Pinnacle Award recipient in 2000. The Thompson Education Center opened inside the Hurley Children's Center at Flint Farmer's Market in August 2015 as a learning area for students, instructors, and physicians to utilize, develop, and enhance clinical skills for the future, while recognizing Dr. Thompson's devotion to education and passion for Hurley.

Michael H. and Robert M. Hamady Health Sciences Library

(See sidebar in Chapter 4)

Phillip C. Dutcher Center

Dedicated on April 30, 1996, the Phillip C. Dutcher Center (named for Dutcher, HMC director/CEO from 1981 to 1995) is located within the "Bachelors Quarters" (or staff residence) building and was primarily used for large group events, such as new-employee orientation, employee training sessions, continuous quality improvement (CQI) awareness, and cultural diversity training courses. A photograph of the building is found on page 82.

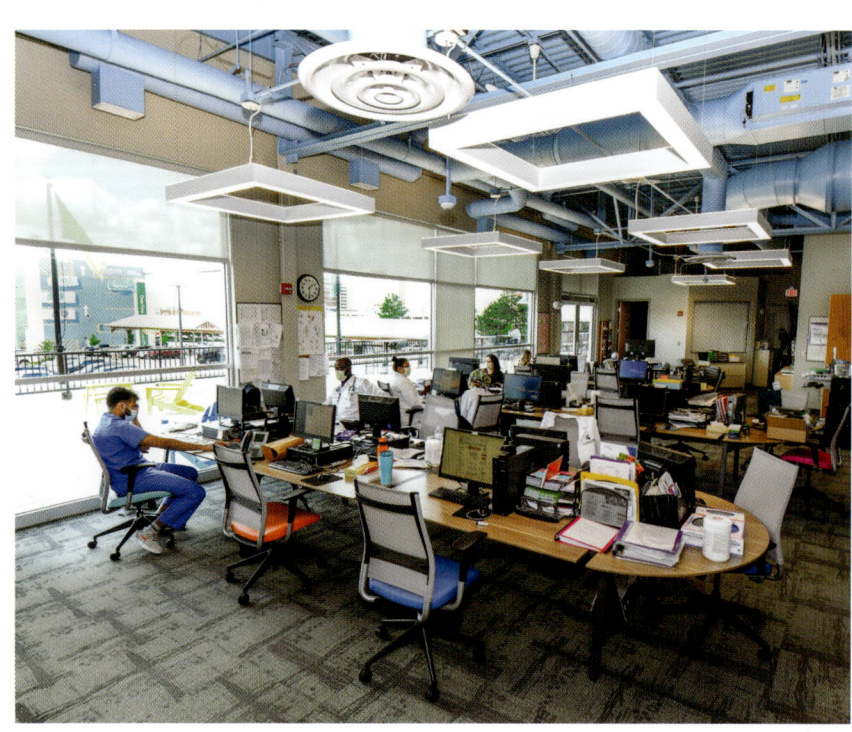

EMPLOYEES HAD A GOOD TIME DURING EMPLOYEE APPRECIATION WEEK JULY 20-24, 2020.

(HLM) Committee, composed of Hurley management leadership and union leaders from the 10 unions representing Hurley employees. Tyree Walker, vice president of Human Resources, has been the chair of the committee since 2018. According to Walker, "It helps to keep the doors open with ongoing dialogue and communication, as the committee offers a collaborative format where issues of concern can be discussed and resolved. Our aim is to improve the work environment of our employees and the value of services for our patients."

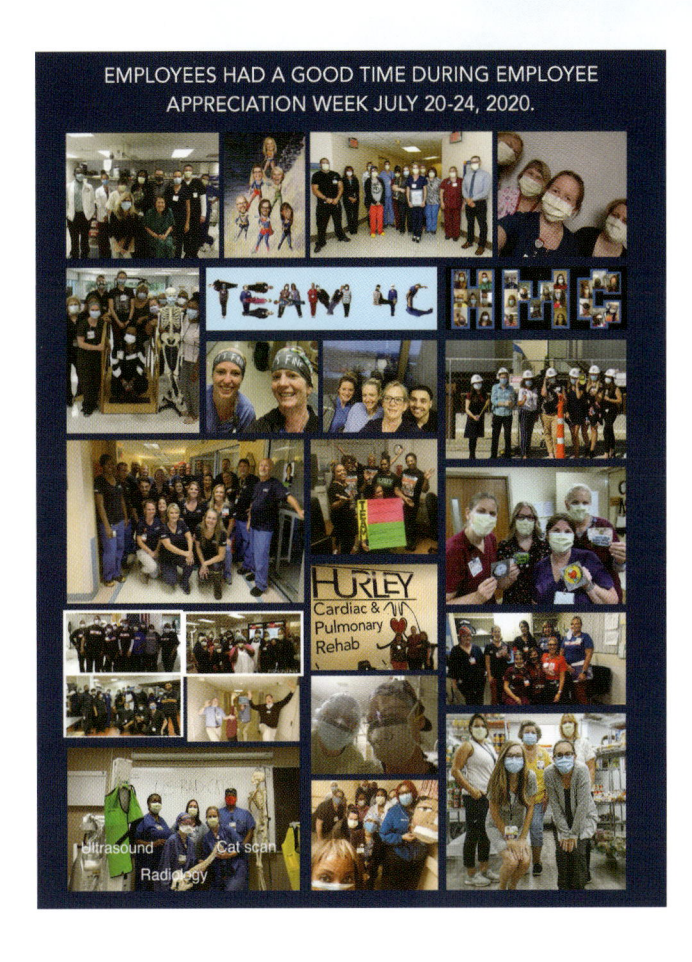

A Great Place to Work

It is one thing for HMC to transform health throughout the region, but as the fourth-major employer in the city of Flint, HMC also advocates for staff wellness and community action. HMC not only attracts some of the best and brightest trainees from around the world, but it is also proud of its multicultural environment and opportunities. Not only is the patient population one of the most diverse in the state, but the nurses, residents, faculty physicians, and many other employees also represent a wide variety of nationalities, which is a great honor to the rich history of the organization.

Joint Union Management Policy Committee

The Joint Union Management Policy (JUMP) Committee was formed in 1987 under the direction of Phillip Dutcher to foster a cooperative approach to medical center issues and to serve as an ongoing relationship-building vehicle for the staff. In early 2011, JUMP became known as Hurley Labor Management

HMC Community Connections – Serving the Public through Good Deeds

There are many examples of how the Hurley staff comes together to help out their community. Here are just two, which benefit the children and families of Genesee County. Every fall when school resumes and temperatures drop, an "ALL HURLEY" e-mail is sent out requesting new shoes and new or like-new coats for elementary-school-aged kids in Flint schools. The Hurley family *always* comes through!

- **Shoes That Fit:** Every year, more than 500 pairs of kid shoes are donated by generous HMC employees to the kids of Doyle-Ryder, Durant-Turri-Mott, and Neithercut Elementary Schools in Flint. This project offers dignity through a new pair of shoes.

- **Coats for Kids:** 178 new and gently used children's coats, plus hats and gloves, were donated by HMC staff in winter 2019 for kids in our community.

CHAPTER FIVE THOSE WHO SERVE – HONORING EXCELLENCE

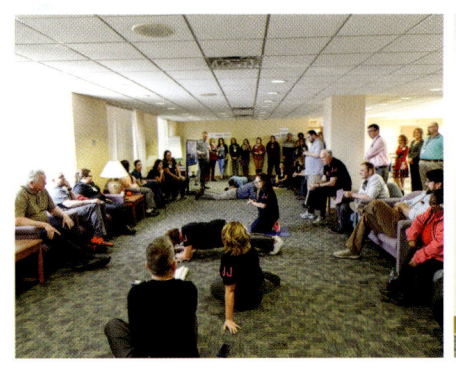

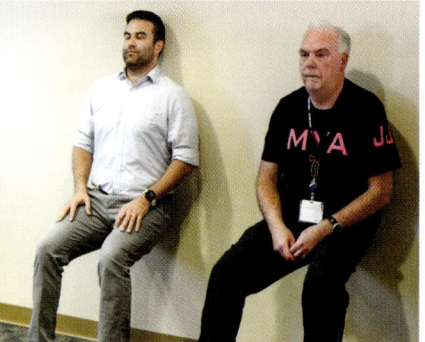

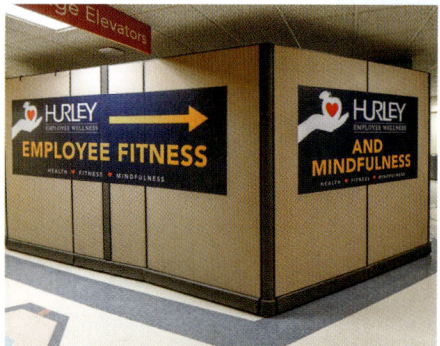

Left: In early 2020, the IT and Finance Departments competed in a wellness challenge. The IT Department won the wall-sit competition, while the Finance Department won the plank competition and held a slight win in the weight-loss competition.

Middle: Hurley CFO Cass Wisniewski (right) created the interdepartmental competition and competes in the wall sit with Nicholas Lecea in 2020.

Employee Wellness – The Importance of Improving Emotional Health

HMC is a big proponent of staff wellness and has spearheaded programs since the 1970s. While many HMC employees are directly responsible for the health care and well-being of their patients at HMC, all employees are encouraged to maintain their own health and wellness so that they can continue working at their optimum pace. The Hurley Health and Fitness Center (HHFC), the only medically based fitness facility in Genesee County, opened its doors in 1991. HHFC was a popular resource for individuals that wanted to stay fit, as well as an outpatient cardiac rehabilitation center for patients. It was later transitioned to private ownership. HMC's wellness department offers many options: chair massages, on-site exercise classes, and wellness challenges among many other timely pieces of wellness support. HMC installed two on-site gyms for employee use. Additionally, HMC's patient relations/spiritual care department offers courses, such as success over stress (SOS) and code lavender, that provide employees or groups with emotional support during stressful or traumatic events. In 2020, the employee-wellness web portal was updated; employees now have access to a variety of health and wellness topics.

NOTES

1. Sarah Schuch, MLive, January 25, 2012, https://www.mlive.com/business/mid-michigan/2012/01/patrick_wardell_president_ceo.html.
2. Willys Mueller Jr., MD, *Perpectives* Vol. 1 (1996), p. 6.
3. Hurley Foundation, *Inside Report* (December 1980), pp. 4–5.
4. Edwin Wood, *History of Genesee County, Michigan: Her People, Industries and Institutions* (Indianapolis: Federal Publishing Company, 1916), p. 806.
5. Hurley Foundation, *Inside Report* (Winter 1988), pp. 12–13.
6. Ibid., p. 14.
7. https://www.mlive.com/news/flint/2012/10/flint_family_physician_dr_samu.html.
8. C. B. (Colonel Bell) Burr and Michigan State Medical Society, *Medical History of Michigan* (Minneapolis and St. Paul: Bruce Publishing Company, 1930), pp. 616, 617.
9. *Hurley Tower* Vol. 22, no. 7 (August 1969), pp. 7–8.

DID YOU KNOW ... in 2000, Hurley staff sent a giant Valentine's Day card to those serving in the Afghanistan War. The 28-foot colorful heart grew into a seven-page booklet with more than 1,000 signatures, letters, hand-drawn pictures, and touching messages of thanks!

MRS. FRANKLIN D. ROOSEVELT
55 EAST 74TH STREET
NEW YORK CITY 21, N. Y.

December 29, 1961

Dear Miss Eckenrode,

I was most interested to hear about your project to provide funds to send an employee of the Hurley Hospital to the S.S. HOPE hospital ship for a 4 months' service period.

I think it is a wonderful undertaking and I congratulate you on your initiative. I am sure your project will arouse great enthusiasm and engender much positive help. I wish you every success in this fine venture.

Very sincerely yours,

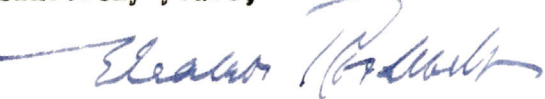

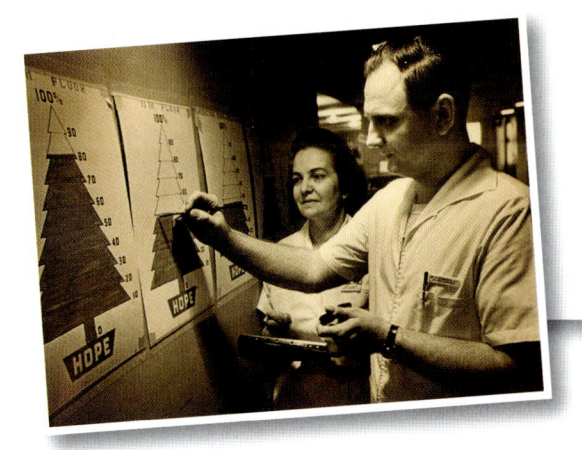

Eleanor Roosevelt

Help Hurley Help Hope – 1962 Staff Fundraising Campaign

The campaign, held December 1961 to January 15, 1962, raised money to send a Hurley employee on a four-month tour aboard the USS *Hope*. The goal to raise $3,000 to finance an employee's salary for four months turned into $6,108—enough to send two employees. The giving spirit was an all-out effort from Hurley's employees, medical staff, board of managers, students, hospital volunteers, the general public, and even a few Hurley patients. Some employees made payroll deductions of 10 cents, 25 cents, 50 cents, or one dollar per week for the entire year of 1962. Eighty-four percent of Hurley employees contributed. Twenty-three employee applications were received. Project Hope reviewed all applications and chose Richard Hennessy, X-ray supervisor (April–August), and Janet Paulson, RN, and nurse instructor (August–December). The two served aboard the ship while it was docked in Trujillon, Peru, providing health care to the Peruvian people. Letters of thanks were received from both the White House and former first lady Eleanor Roosevelt. Flint's mayor proclaimed March 16, 1962, "Hurley Hospital Employees Day." This big mission of love and support meant a lot during an era of international unrest.

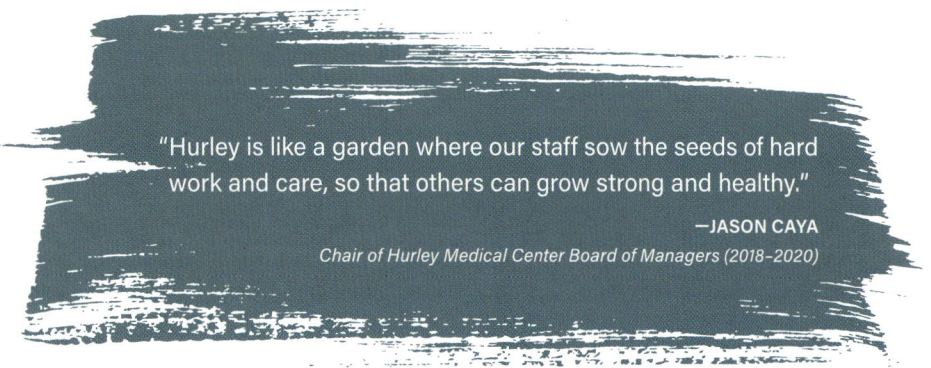

> "Hurley is like a garden where our staff sow the seeds of hard work and care, so that others can grow strong and healthy."
>
> —JASON CAYA
> *Chair of Hurley Medical Center Board of Managers (2018–2020)*

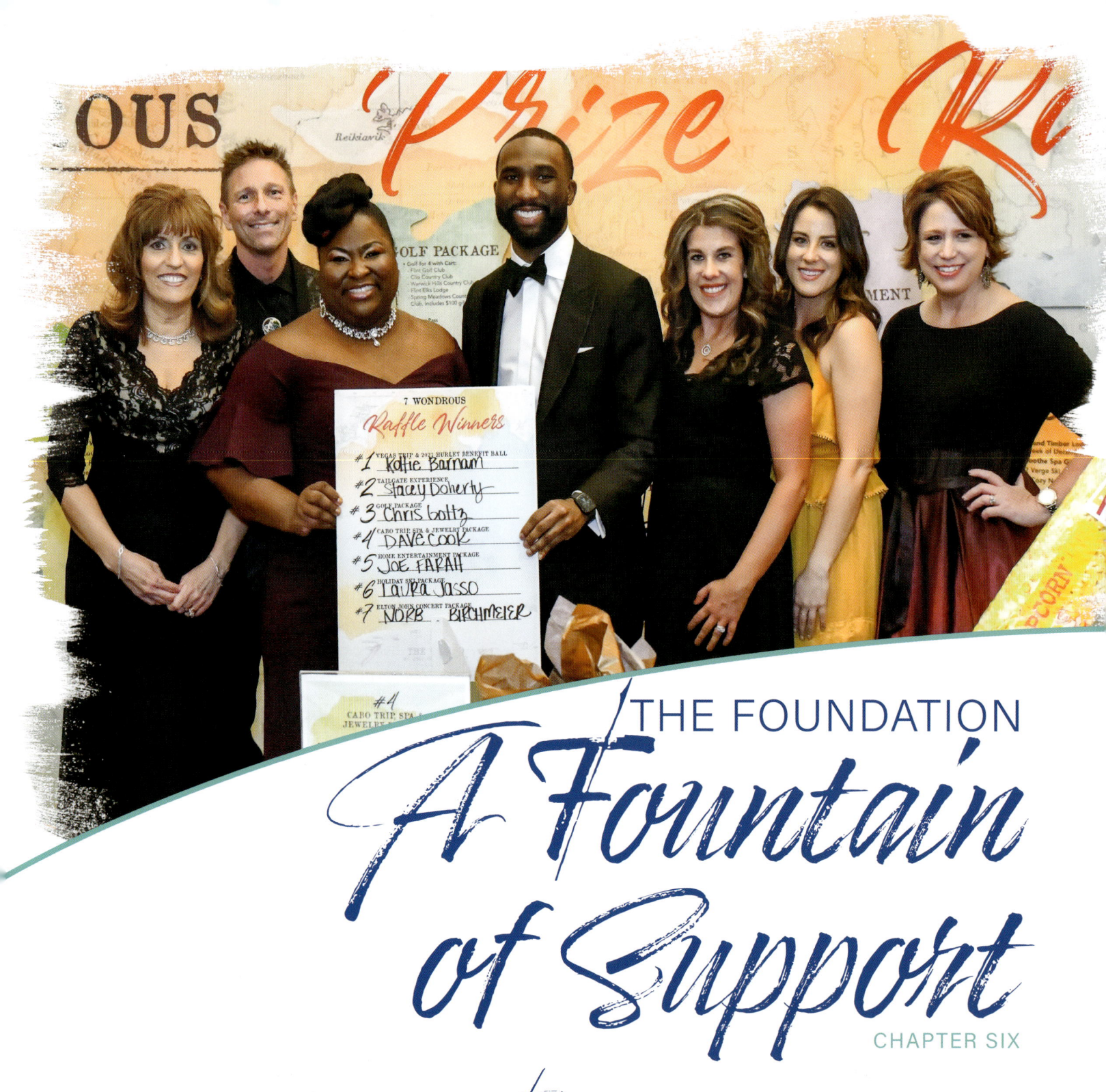

THE FOUNDATION
A Fountain of Support
CHAPTER SIX

Hurley Benefit Ball, 2020 (left to right): Melany Gavulic, RN, MSN, president, and CEO; Mike Burnett, Hurley Foundation president; Mattie Pearson, MSN, RN, Service Line administrator, Women and Children's; Omari Young, MD; Elizabeth Wenstrom-Williams, Hurley Foundation, senior managing director; Jordan Brown, Hurley Foundation director of Volunteer and Community Engagement; and Patricia Creighton, Special Events coordinator.

The Hurley Foundation, a 501(c)(3) nonprofit organization, was incorporated in 1993 to operate for the advancement of medical sciences, education, medical care, and the delivery thereof for the benefit of the residents of the greater metropolitan Flint area.

The first foundation president was Richard Warmbold, PhD. The foundation was the result of an administrative brainstorming session held in the late 1980s, facilitated by former HMC president

Phillip Dutcher; his vision was to appoint a person to develop and nurture the new foundation. The founding Hurley Foundation Board of Directors included Phillip Dutcher, Vivian Lewis, MD, and Arthur Turri, MD, among others. The foundation celebrated its 25th/silver anniversary in 2018.

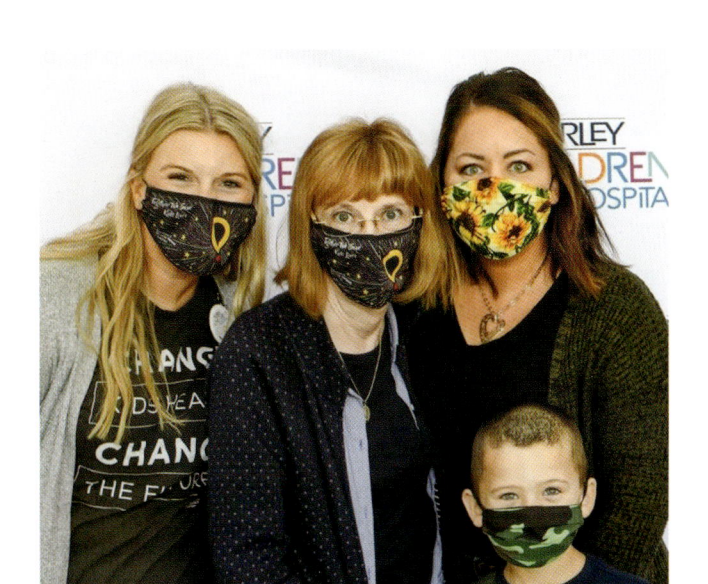

As HMC receives no city tax dollars and is an entirely self-supporting medical center, the focus of the foundation's fundraising is to host events and to seek out grants, which bring together local businesses and individuals who are committed to the hospital and its mission. Successful annual events include the Hurley

Left: Children's Miracle Network (CMN) Radiothon, 2020 (left to right): Brooklyn Sondgeroth, assistant director of CMN Programs, Linda Tracy-Stephens, CMN hospitals director, with Carsen Titus and his mom, Angela Titus.

Below: For 39 years, proceeds from the annual Hurley Benefit Ball have raised funds to support various hospital service areas. First held in March 1981, the annual ball has continued to be a significant fundraiser. The 39th annual Hurley Benefit Ball was held on March 7, 2020. The theme was "World Showcase," with proceeds in support of HMC's obstetrics services, including Labor and Delivery and Mother/Baby Units.

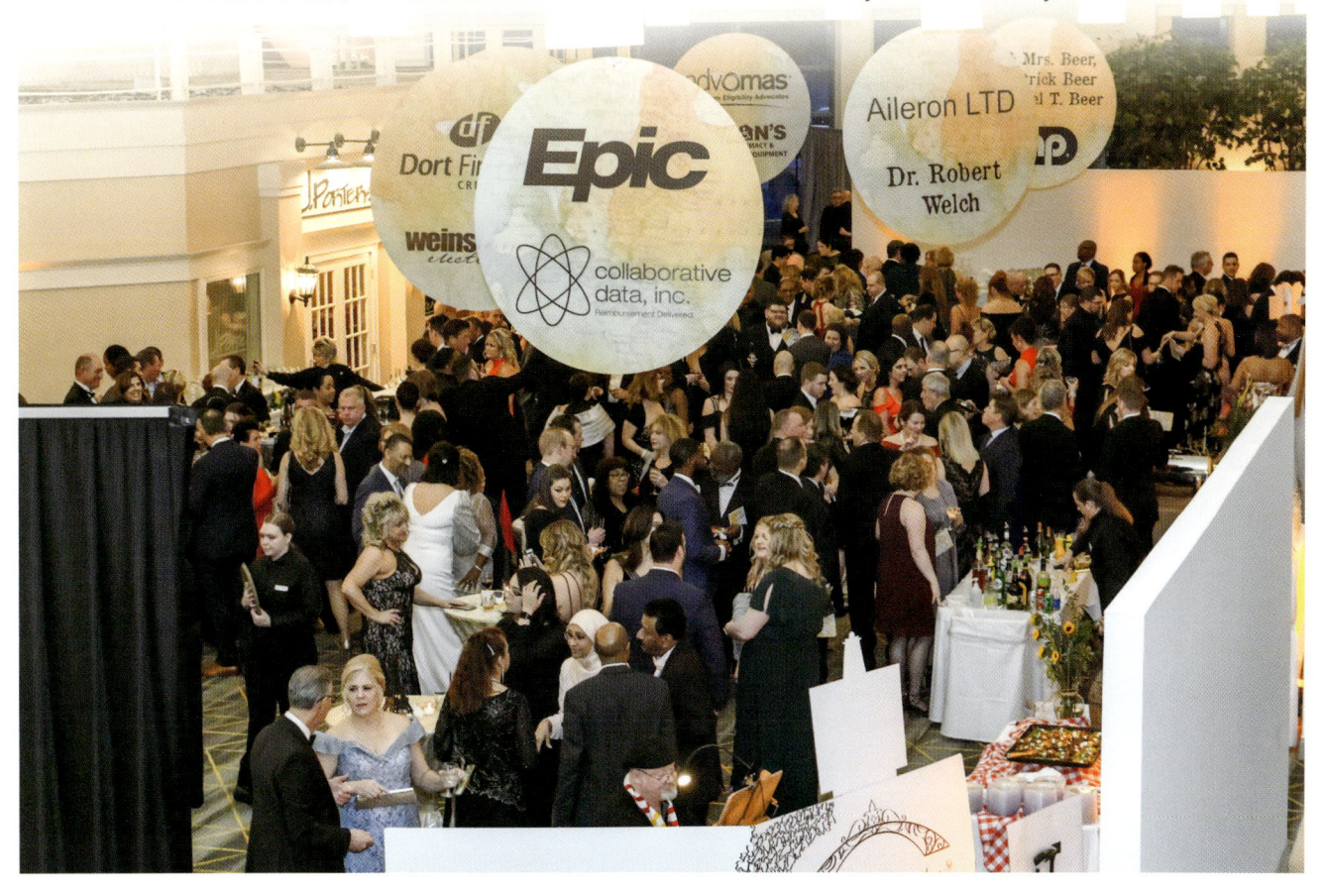

CHAPTER SIX THE FOUNDATION — A FOUNTAIN OF SUPPORT • 125

Richard Warmbold, Foundation President, 1991–2016

Rick Warmbold started working for HMC in August 1991 as director of Development, when he told the board and CEO Phil Dutcher that it would take three to five years to start a foundation to meet their objectives. Hurley was a city hospital that needed a mechanism to grow individual assets to benefit hospital programs and needs. Warmbold established the 501(c)(3) foundation in 1992 and began fundraising in 1993. "Hurley is a special place," Warmbold shares. "It's a premier public teaching hospital that takes care of everybody who comes through their doors. They have the opportunity to make a difference in people's lives, both children and adults. It can be very rewarding."[1]

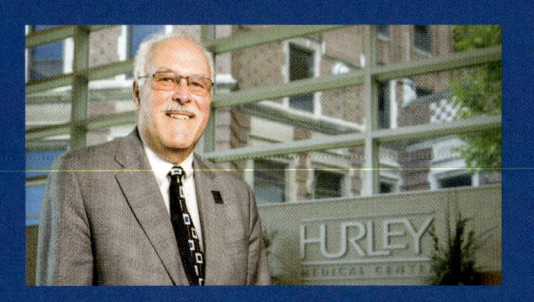

Immediately, Warmbold was drawn to the CMN hospital program. The first CMN telethon took place in June 1991, and the funds that were raised paid for the Hurley Child Life Program. "We became more involved in funding pediatric services as a way to pay for the high-expense medical unit," he said. "We turned toward bottom-line fundraising, establishing an endowment, and building our volunteer force by combining the volunteer programs into one program."[2] According to Warmbold, "Hurley is one of the few hospitals where former staff come back to volunteer; they are Hurley ambassadors out in the community."

Warmbold continues, "Looking back, there were so many great things—watching families grow together, seeing some of our kids [former HMC patients]—they'd hug me and talk to me. While out in the community, I'd hear stories of nurses who went above and beyond to make a family or patient comfortable. They will tell their stories . . . and hearing it from someone who has experienced it, rather than an employee, was motivating. You never know what the connection is, but there's always something that was done here at Hurley."

According to Warmbold, "If you treat someone with respect, while providing the best care possible, then you feel as if you have made a difference. One of the first things that Dr. Tuuri told me was, 'Don't get too close because the outcomes may not be what you want.' The hardest part of my job was attending a child's funeral; it's always tough to lose a child, whether several months old or 20 years old."

Warmbold attended all the Hurley fundraising events, such as the annual ball. "It's always fun to see people dressed up and having a good time," he says. "You get to see Hurley staff members, who are typically in scrubs, wearing tuxedos or fancy dresses." In the summer, he attended the annual golf outing, benefitting trauma services, and other events, including Pink Night Palooza, benefitting the Breast Navigator Fund, and CMN picnics and bowling nights for the "Miracle" children. "Each one is different, and they were always a pleasure to attend, even if I was working," he shares.

After 25 years, Warmbold left the Hurley Foundation knowing that he had helped put the medical center on solid footing. "I am most proud of developing a professional team that has the commitment and energy, the skills and talent to work together to make a difference," he says. "And seeing team members' eyes light up when they talk about their work. Teamwork makes a difference; I hope that's my legacy. The team not only lives up to James J. Hurley's initial vision—they internalize it. They continue to expand services to meet the needs of the communities they serve. That's the only reason why they're here. Looking back, I see that success takes a dedicated staff. The hospital and foundation staff were very stable, and if we lost someone, we were fortunate to replace them with people that brought something more to us. HMC has long-term employees, which is not a regular situation, but it shows the quality of the culture in that organization."

Benefit Ball, the Hurley Trauma Golf Classic, and Pink Night Palooza. The foundation also hosts three special CMN events annually: the Bowlathon, the Miracle Picnic, and the Radiothon. The funds that are raised go right back into the community, from the inner city to rural areas, providing financial assistance to patients, creating a learning center of excellence for medical professionals, and providing educational events for the community.

"The thing that makes Hurley Medical Center so different is that it is a hospital for the community. We are always talking with the community, with the people," said Mike Burnett, MBA, MSW, vice president of Service Line Development, and Hurley Foundation president.

"We are here to support Hurley and everything it stands by for all patients and their families, regardless of their ability to pay. Every dollar, every hour, and every item you donate stays here to benefit our community," said Elizabeth Wenstrom-Williams, senior managing director of the Hurley Foundation. Wenstrom-Williams urges people to get involved—as donors, as volunteers, or as both. "The foundation team is always looking for new ways to reach out to the community—to help, to educate and to innovate."[3]

"The special thing about Hurley is that you meet so many people in this community that have a Hurley story and are eager to tell you about their one of-a-kind experience," said Jordan Brown, MBA, director of Volunteer and Community Engagement. "It is easy to feel connected to this organization because you see the results of our services and initiatives in every corner of this community. Hurley already had an amazing group of dedicated volunteers; our vision is to find new and innovative ways for this diverse group of talented people to transcend the definition of volunteerism, both internally and to expand the reach of Hurley volunteers within the community—helping meet their goals as well. Hurley volunteers and employees are committed to Hurley's mission and to the care of patients and their families," adds Brown. "Whether they are high school students or have been serving this organization for over 50 years, Hurley volunteers serve with pride and tenacity, and enthusiastically look for new ways to serve."[4]

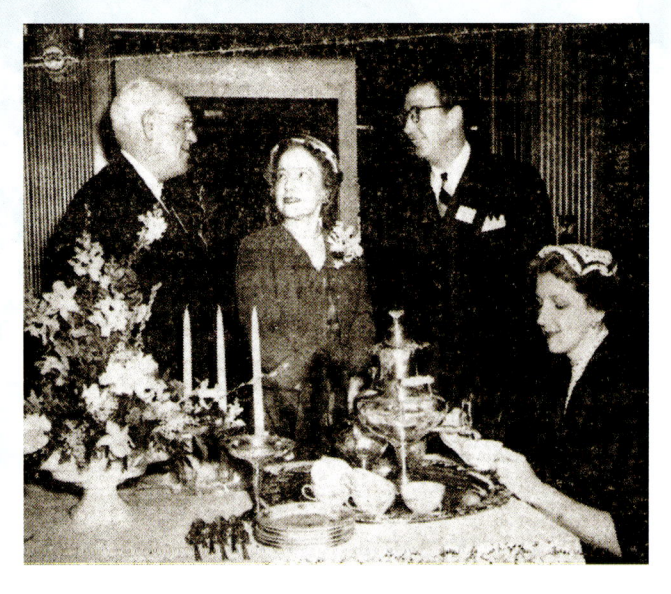

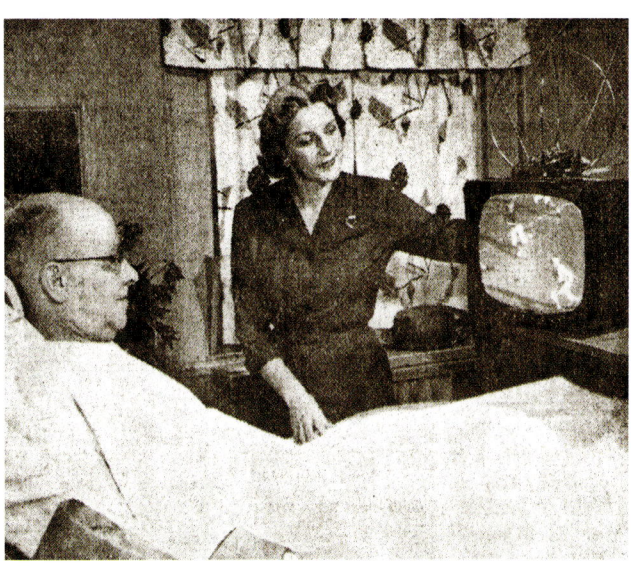

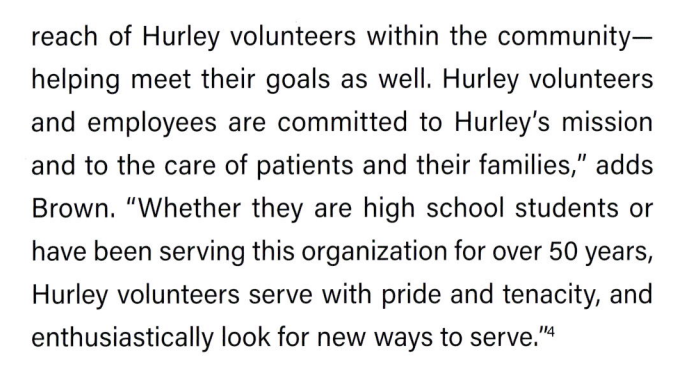

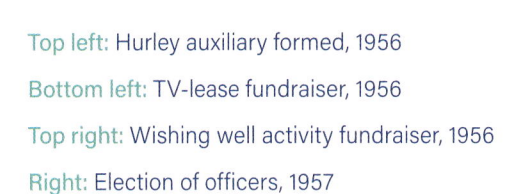

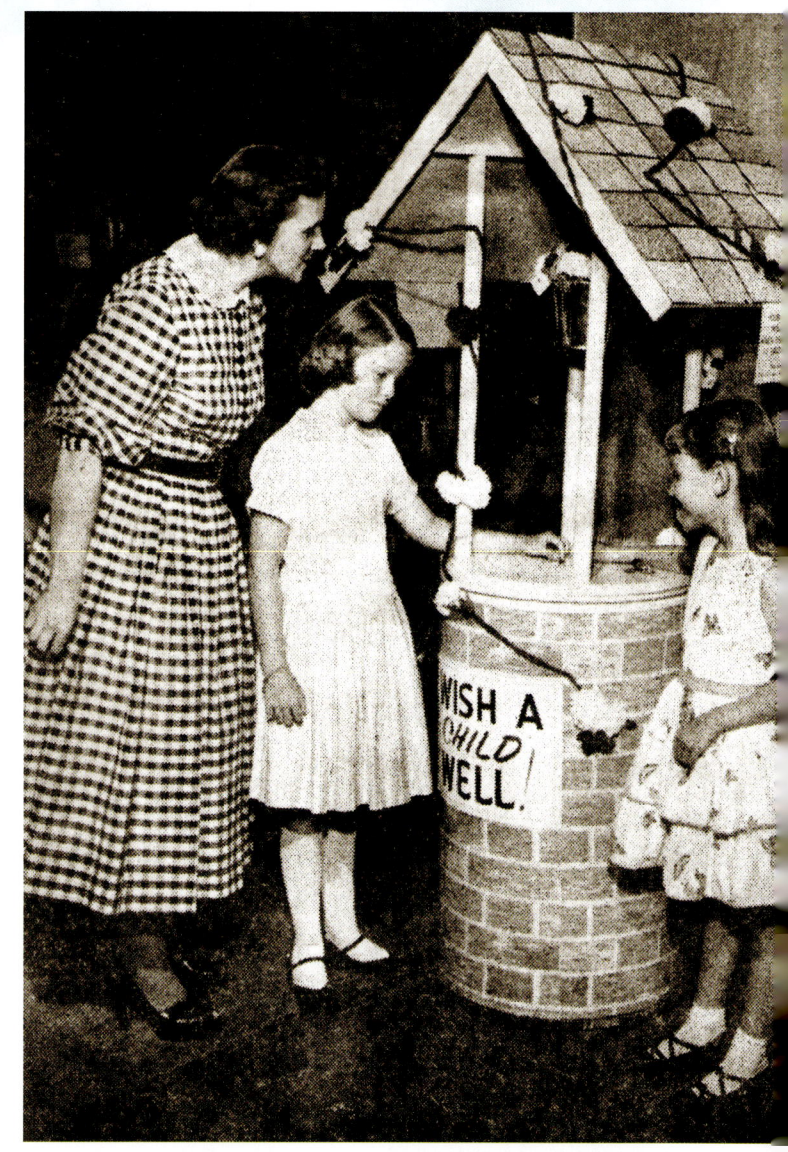

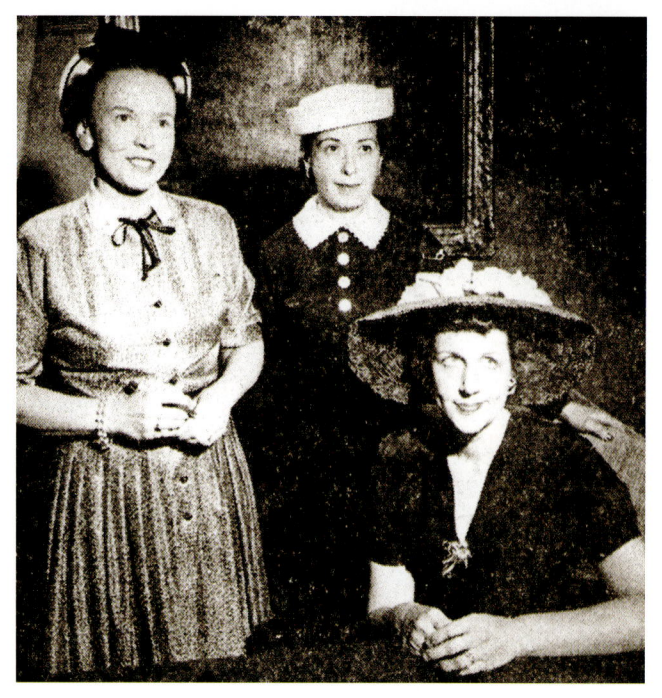

Top left: Hurley auxiliary formed, 1956

Bottom left: TV-lease fundraiser, 1956

Top right: Wishing well activity fundraiser, 1956

Right: Election of officers, 1957

128 • HURLEY MEDICAL CENTER

Foundation Leadership Remains Strong

Michael Burnett, Hurley Foundation President

THE HURLEY FOUNDATION BOARD OF DIRECTORS, 2019–2020

- Carl Bekofske
- Susan Steiner Bolhouse
- Lindsay Clark
- Cornelius "Kip" Darcy
- Alison Dedrick
- Donna Dodds Hamm
- William Moeller
- Marcus Randolph
- Philip Shaltz
- Andrew Suski
- Lynne Taft-Draper
- Gregory Viener
- Glenn Wilson
- Melany Gavulic, HMC President & CEO
- Phillip Dutcher, Founding Member Emeritus
- Richard Warmbold, Founding Member Emeritus

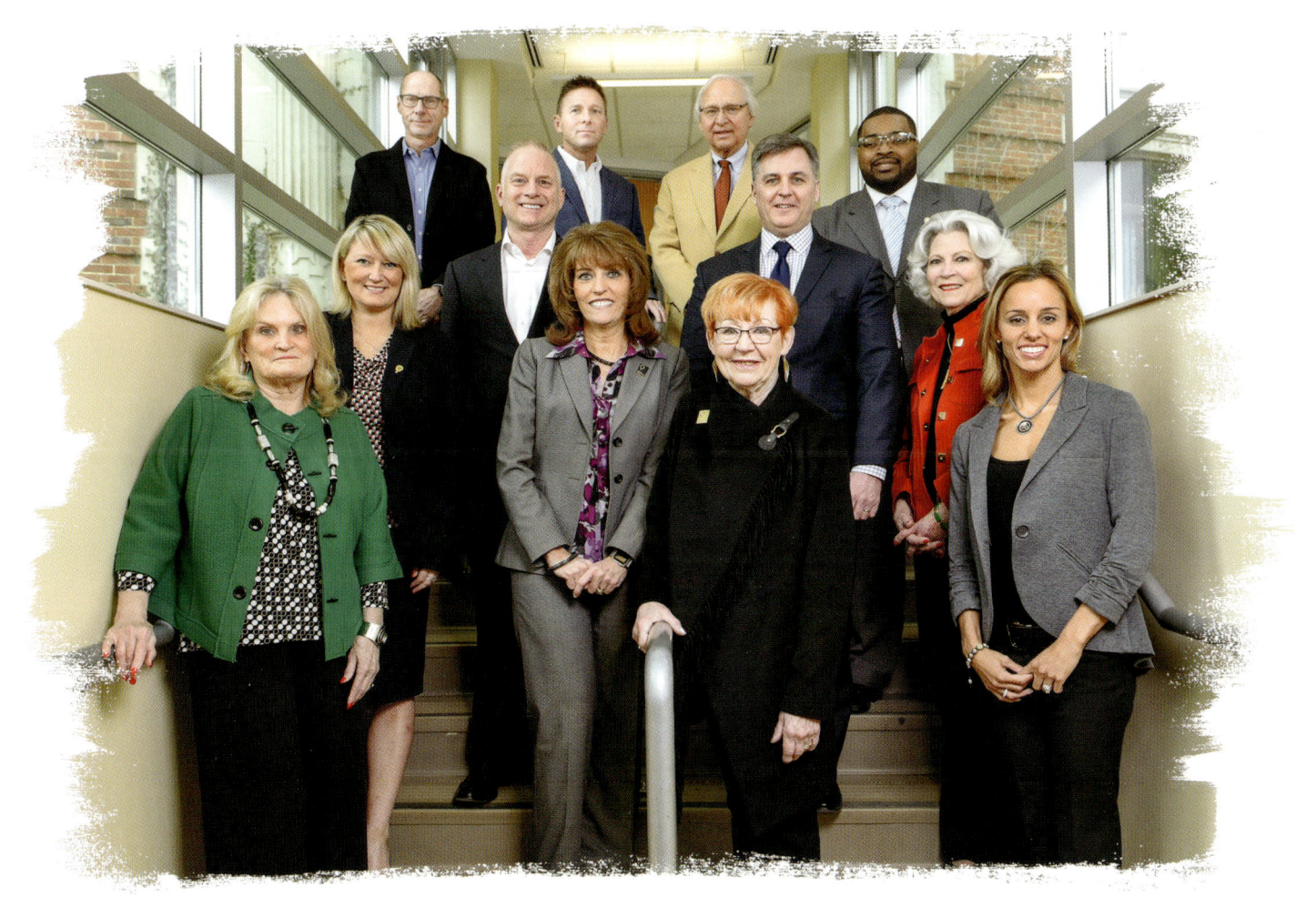

Hurley Foundation Board of Directors, 2017. Back row, left to right: Phil Shaltz, Mike Burnett, and Carl Bekofske; middle row: Angela Shook, Kip Darcy, Greg Viener, Glenn Wilson, and Susan Steiner Bolhouse; front row: Lynn Taft Draper, Melany Gavulic, Donna Dodds Hamm, and Lindsay Clark. Not pictured: William Moeller, Dr. Victor Rabinkov, Bryn Mickle, Marcus Randolph, Ira Rutherford III, Andrew Suski, Phillip Dutcher, and Richard Warmbold.

History of the Hurley Medical Center Auxiliary and Volunteer Corps

The Women's Auxiliary Hospital Board was established on November 15, 1907, after a group of local women raised $1,000 for a women's ward at the new hospital, which was under construction; they then set out to raise funds to purchase bed linen for the ward. After the task was accomplished, the group disbanded on October 18, 1912. The group briefly formed again in 1919 to supply the hospital with needed linen supplies.

It was 44 years before the auxiliary would formally reorganize again. The inception of the Hurley Hospital auxiliary occurred in 1955, when Mrs. Lorene Jermstad was looking for something to keep her busy after her husband, a Hurley pathologist, passed away. She started as a public relations worker, visiting patients; she then formulated an arts and crafts project to occupy the hospitalized children. The auxiliary program was formalized, and 115 regular and active members were enrolled. Mrs. Clyde Peterson was named chairman of Volunteer Services. Mrs. Paul Darnton was named president in February 1956. The organization set about an active fundraising role, along with providing volunteer services for the front desk and the lobby shop. The first

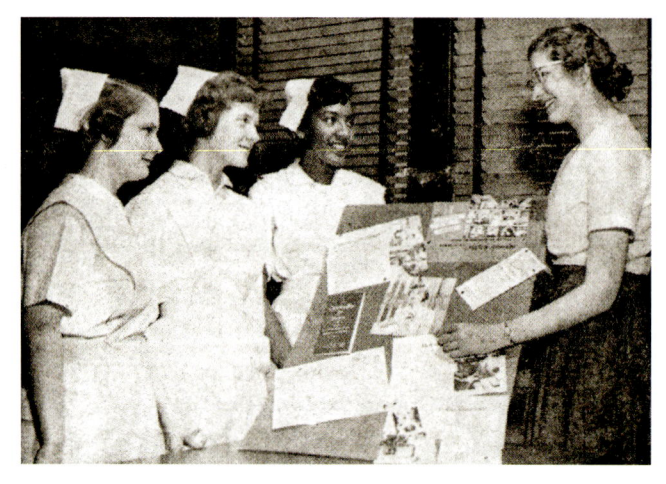

National Hospital Week display by the auxiliary, 1957. Looking at job opportunities at Hurley Hospital are (left to right) Nancy Winters, Ann Bishop, and Meredith Burns, all Central High School students. Cornelia Van Doorn is the sponsor of the Future Nurses Club.

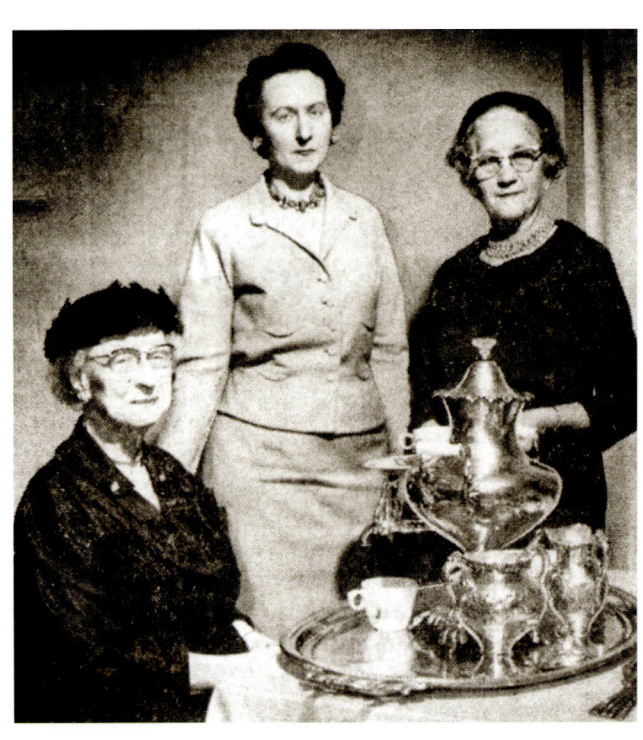

The auxiliary's second anniversary was in 1958, which coincided with Hurley Medical Center's 50th anniversary.

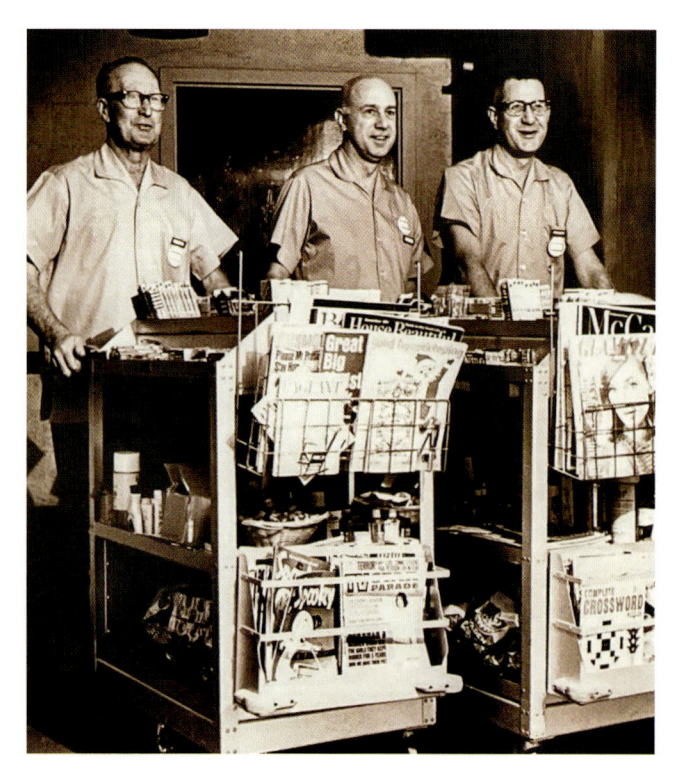

Men began volunteering with the auxiliary in 1959.

fundraising campaign was named "Wish a Child Well," an effort to raise funds for the children's ward. Wishing wells, designed and built by auxiliary members, were placed in the local Sears and Roebuck Co., Citizens National Bank, Genesee Bank, and Michigan National Banks for one month to raise funds. The group also intervened in political efforts by spurring citizens to vote for a successful $1.5 million hospital bond issue. They produced a film about Hurley Hospital called "The Need Exists-Regardless," narrated by Robert White's personnel director, which highlighted hospital overcrowding. The group became members of the National Association of Hospital Auxiliaries, and officers attended national conferences.

The auxiliary board continued to grow, and a small army of volunteers coordinated eight projects within the hospital. In 1957, the Alpha Iota Sorority handled hospitality carts by visiting patients and bringing sundry items, such as toothpaste, combs, candy, magazines, etc. Art teachers oversaw arts and crafts programs for children. Senior high school students in the Future Nurses Club fed patients and assisted with simple nursing duties.

Girl Scouts worked in the central supply department, wrapped dressings, prepared and packaged surgical gloves, and checked needles and packaged them for sterilization. Gray Ladies from the American Red Cross devoted time to helping patients by running errands, making phone calls, and distributing mail and stationery. A roster of volunteers staffed the front lobby reception desk. A "Selective Menu" team met with patients over meal choices and coordinated with hospital dieticians. The United Church Women assisted patients to and from Sunday chapel services.

At the end of the auxiliary's first year, volunteer membership had grown to 191 women. According to Byrnece Vivian, who started in the lobby shop just after the first anniversary, "I remember the old lobby shop didn't have walls; it was enclosed by folding doors, and our stock room was in the basement." After three weeks in operation, the lobby shop had brought in $660.

Men began joining the auxiliary in 1959. By the time the auxiliary celebrated its 50th anniversary in 1961,

Left: Auxiliary members, 1963 (left to right): Mrs. Philip Seven, Mrs. Benjamin Ring, and Mrs. John Wagner greet members and guests before the annual luncheon and fashion show.

Right: The Holiday Santa Workshop (seen here in 1959) was a multiyear tradition for the auxiliary. Several hundred holiday Santas were made and placed at each patient's bedside during the holidays.

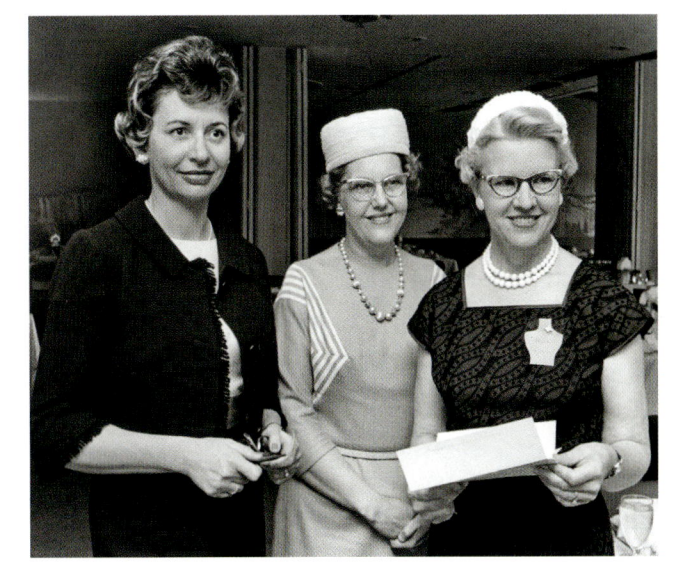

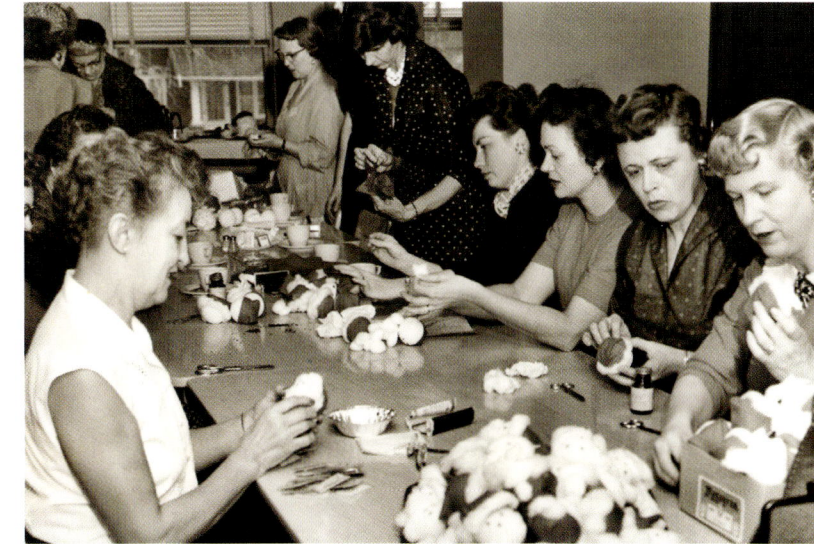

The fourth-floor surgical lounge, 2008

Right: the sixth-floor surgical lounge, 1965

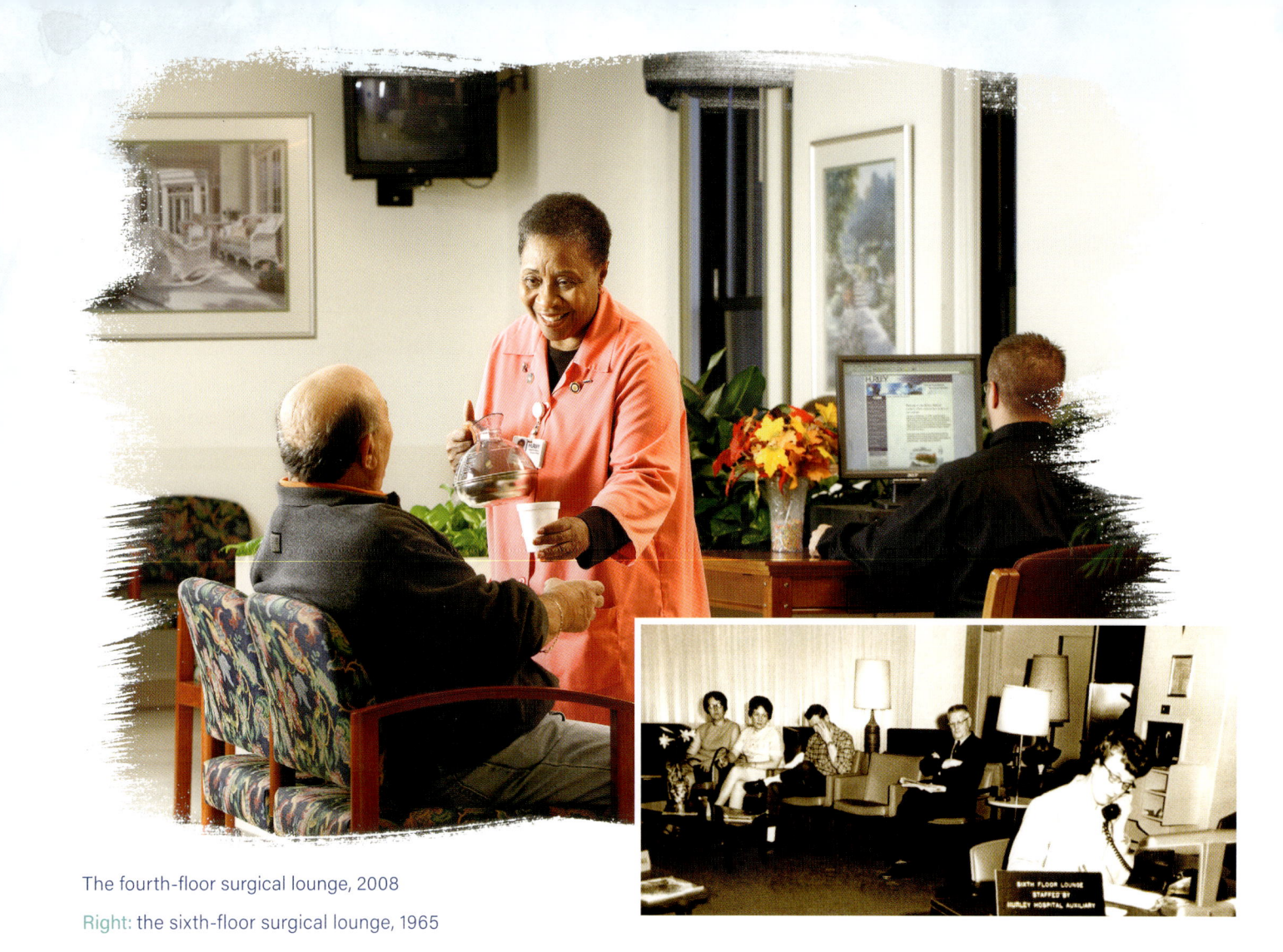

five volunteers had donated 500 hours of time, while 34 women had logged 100 hours or more in the year. The group had four main areas of activity: the income-producing lobby shop, the memorial fund, the youth recreation program, and the reception desk and carts.

President Vera Madden gave Jane Scott, Jeane Darnton, and Avery Mallison honorary lifetime memberships.

In early 1962, the auxiliary voted to purchase three isolettes for the premature nursery at a cost of $2,400, and they

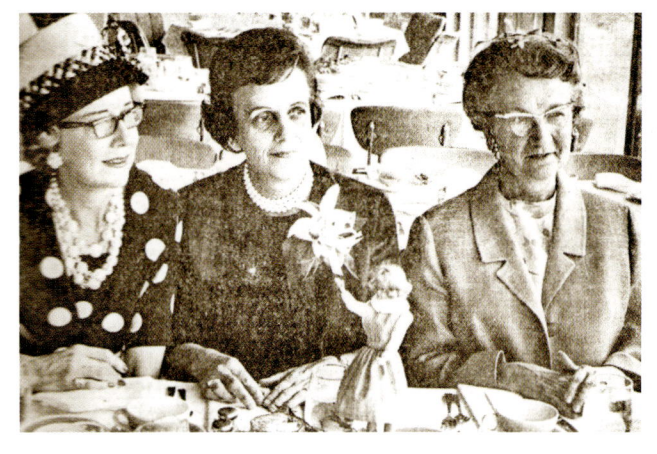

Auxiliary officers at the spring luncheon, 1964 (left to right): First VP Mrs. Robert Edwards, President Mrs. Martha Dimmick, and Mrs. Thorsten Johnson, a past president.

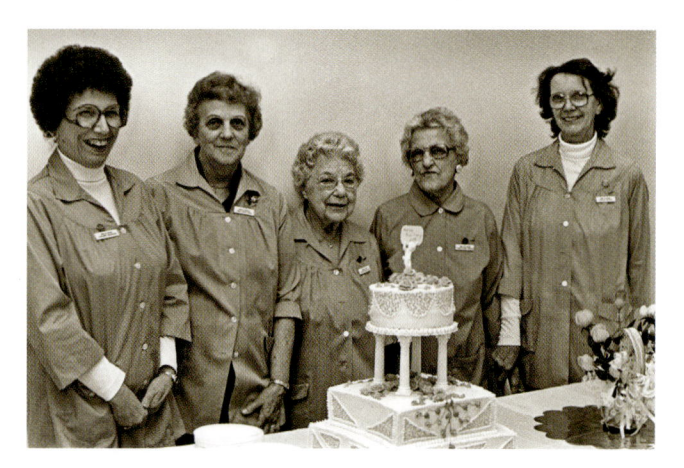

The auxiliary's 25th anniversary, 1981. Charter auxiliary members (left to right) Byrnece Vivian, Martha Dimmick, Bertha Gay, Rhonwin Chase, and Ida Dawson.

spent $200 to send a Hurley Hospital employee to serve for four months on the naval hospital ship SS *Hope*. In February 1962, at the sixth-anniversary luncheon, the total financial contributions to Hurley Hospital had reached $9,755.63. The auxiliary's link to the wider Flint community came with annual fashion shows, quarterly speaker luncheons, and occasional field trips to the GMI Institute, Hamady House, and the Stepping Stones program, which assisted girls in the skills of homemaking and effective living. By 1963, auxiliary funds had furnished and helped decorate the new sixth-floor surgical lounge. A newly formed TLC Corps (Tender, Loving, Care) was charged with feeding babies, reading and entertaining pre-school children, and, in the quiet time, mending pajamas.

From the September 27, 1965, Hurley newsletter: "The ladies in the gray and the pink uniforms, the teenagers in the yellow, and the candy stripes are all volunteers who are devoted to 'service to patients.' The Gray Ladies are Red Cross volunteers, girls and boys in yellow are from the Future Nurses Clubs in the high schools, and the Pink Ladies and the Candy Stripers are sponsored by the Hurley Hospital Auxiliary."

In 1975, the auxiliary changed its name to Hurley Medical Center Auxiliary, and Hurley Hospital became Hurley Medical Center. "The auxiliary's primary goal has been to promote goodwill for the hospital," added

Auxiliary installs officers

The Hurley Auxiliary installed new officers during a recent May luncheon. Sanita Petriella was installed as the new President. She is pictured at the right with first Auxiliary President Jeane Darnton (right). At the bottom Carolyn Tambling (left) is installed as Recording Secretary of the Auxiliary. She is congratulated by Evelyn Ward, new Assistant Membership Director, and Tom McWhirter.

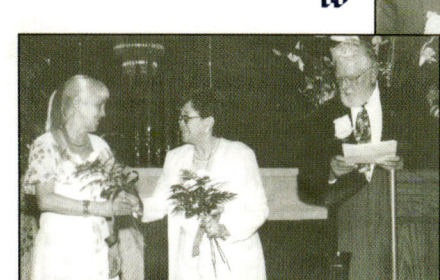

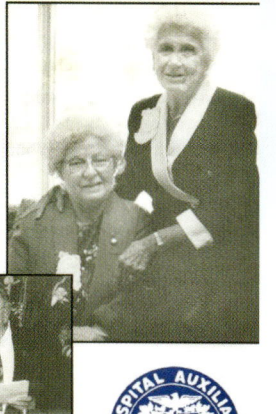

Auxiliary 41st anniversary, 1947

Vivian, who helped craft the group's constitution and bylaws. The Hurley auxiliary and the first auxiliary president, Jeane Darnton, shared a 40th anniversary in 1996 and commemorated the occasion by giving HMC a final check for the "People Helping People" campaign for recliner-sleeper chairs for the Pediatric Units, ventilators for the NICU, and a sculpture for the lobby, all totaling $195,000. "I am so proud of the auxiliary and what it has done over the years," said Darnton. "We've generated a tremendous amount of money and hours. We have been an active group, and the

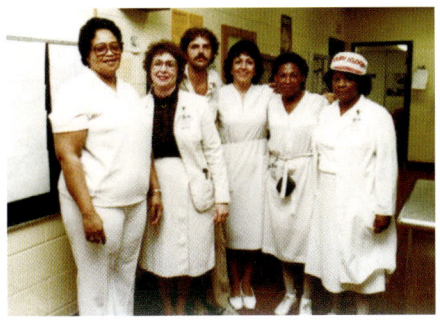

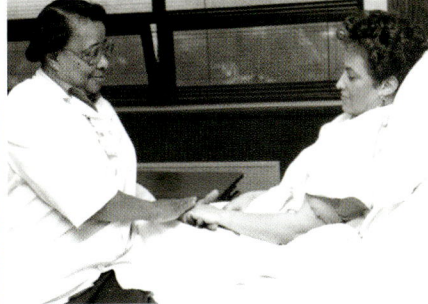

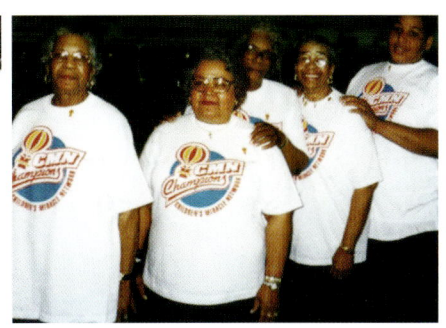

Left: Volunteers, 1983

Middle: Hurley's Action Cancer Team (ACT) volunteer Katherine Williams gives compassionate comfort to a cancer patient in 1989.

Right: Volunteers, 1998

CHAPTER SIX THE FOUNDATION — A FOUNTAIN OF SUPPORT • 133

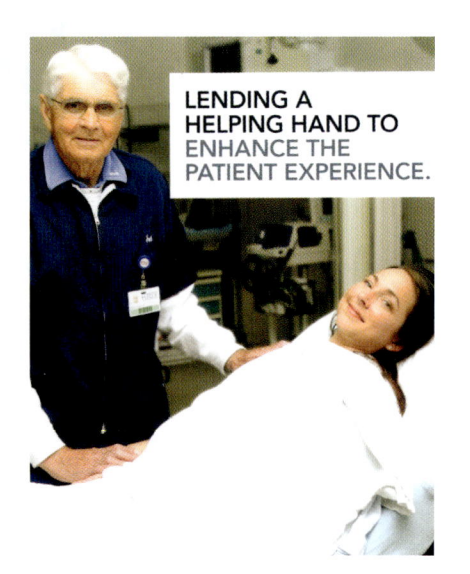

LENDING A HELPING HAND TO ENHANCE THE PATIENT EXPERIENCE.

Jack Burton, Auxiliary Volunteer

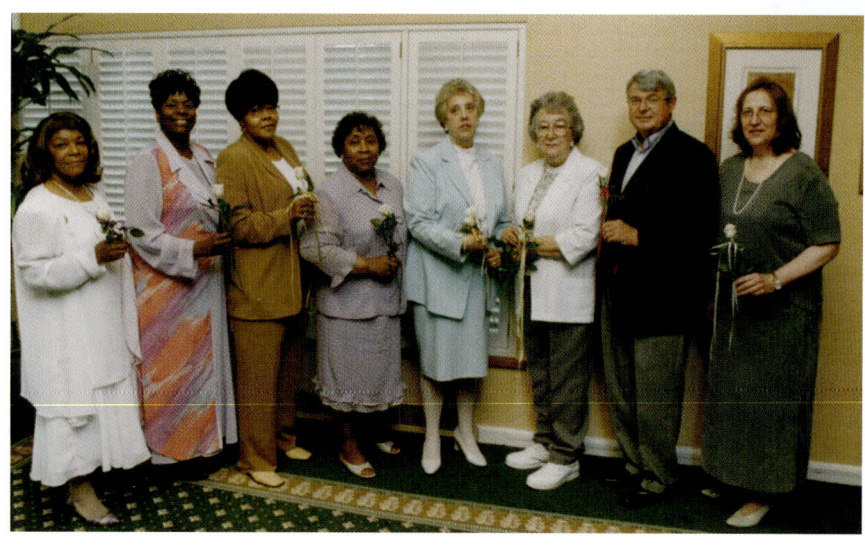

2003

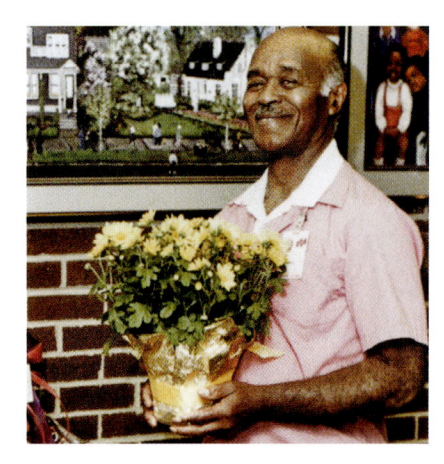

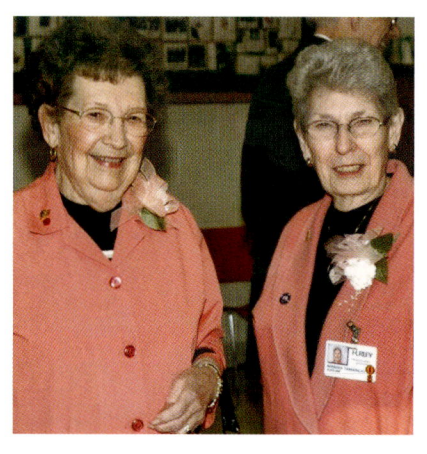

2006

2006

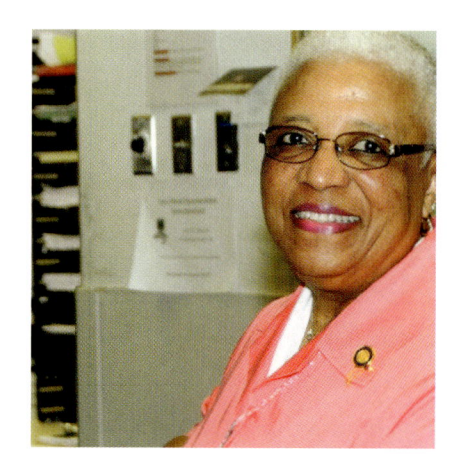

Thelma Watson, Auxiliary President, 2009–2010

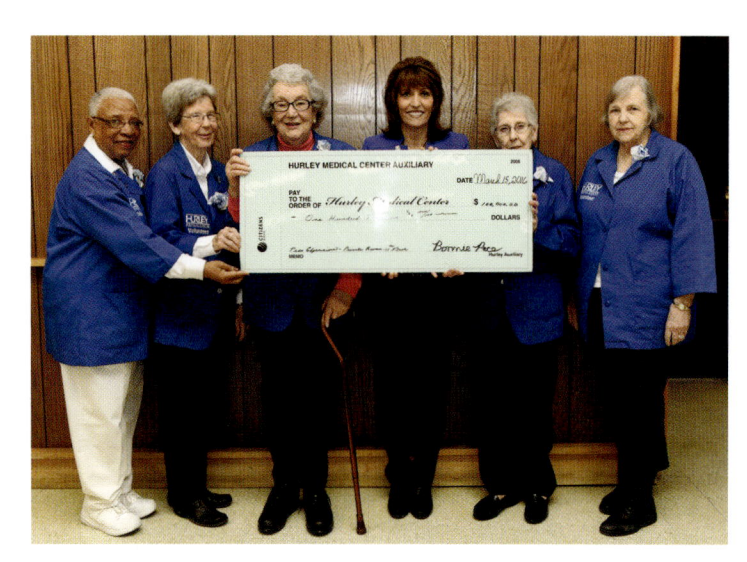

Auxiliary 60th anniversary, 2016

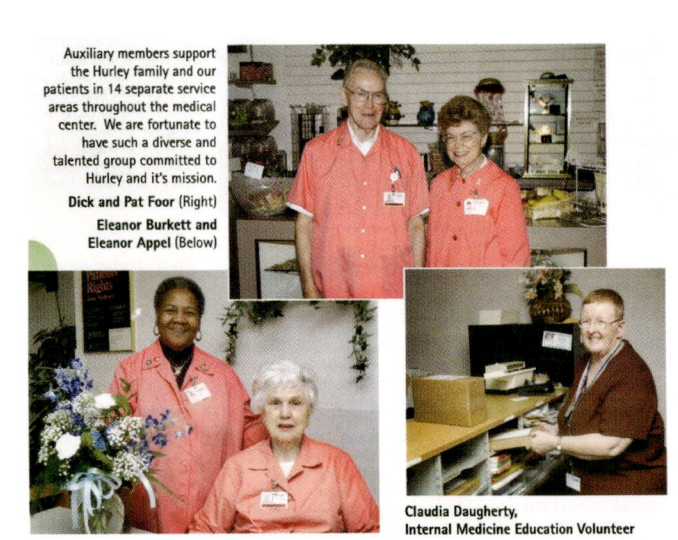

Auxiliary members support the Hurley family and our patients in 14 separate service areas throughout the medical center. We are fortunate to have such a diverse and talented group committed to Hurley and it's mission.

Dick and Pat Foor (Right)
Eleanor Burkett and Eleanor Appel (Below)

2006

Claudia Daugherty, Internal Medicine Education Volunteer

134 • HURLEY MEDICAL CENTER

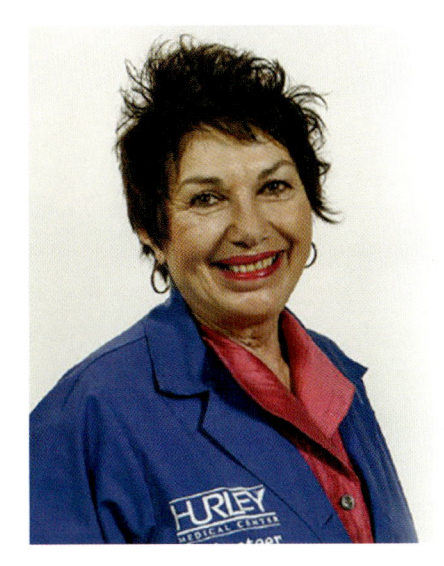

Annette Saseen

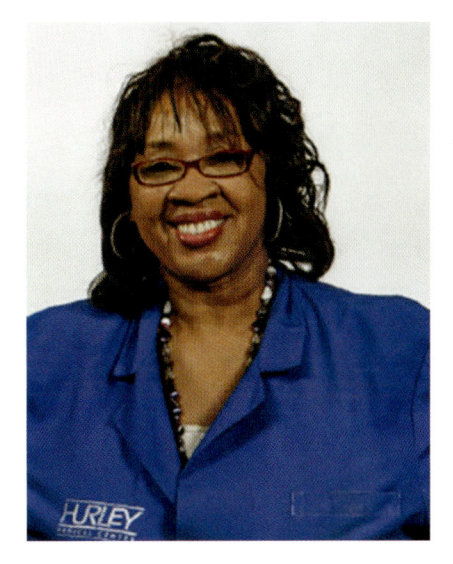

Dollie Starling

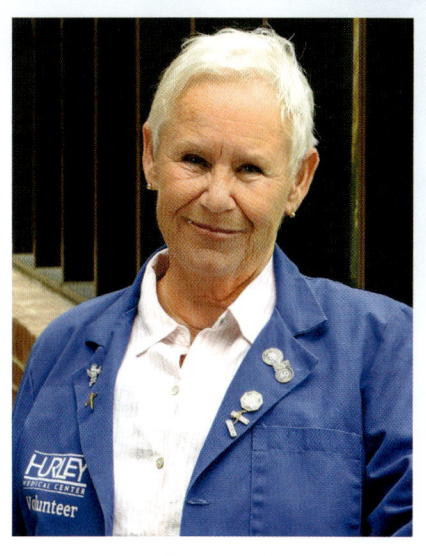

Alison Dedrick, first chair of the Volunteer Corps, 2018

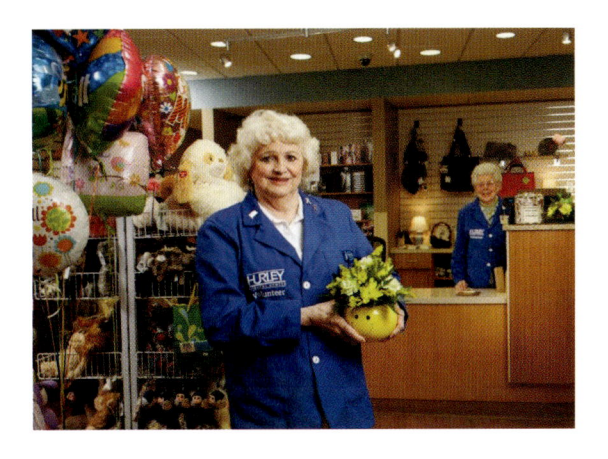

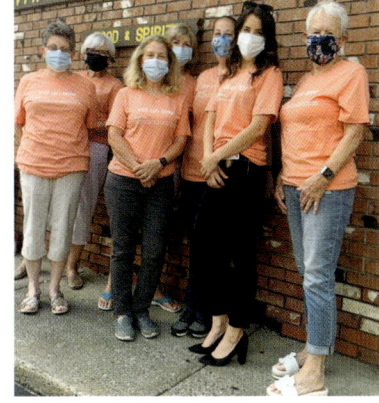

Left: Volunteers Bonnie Pace and Lucille Welker man Hurley's popular lobby shop.

Right: 2020 steering committee members Kathy Hayes, Sylvia Keeler, Kathleen Russell, Sandi Pattillo, Lauren Romankewiz, Jordan Brown, and Alison Dedrick

Making holiday ornaments with the Flint Junior Firebirds hockey team, 2019

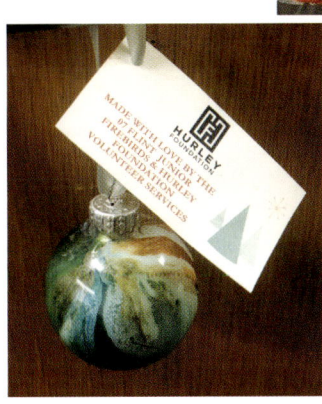

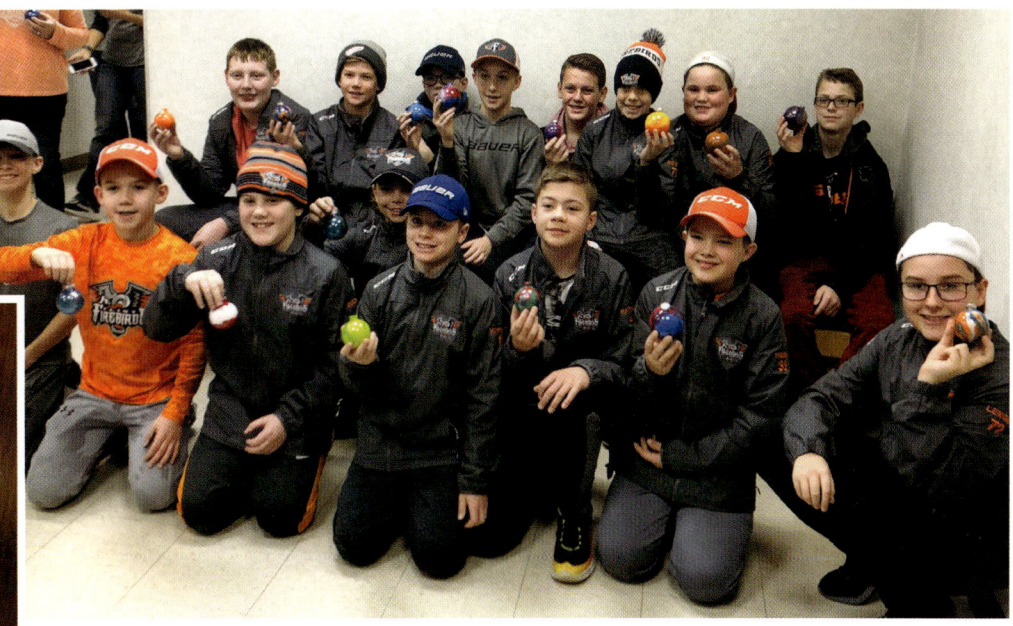

CHAPTER SIX THE FOUNDATION — A FOUNTAIN OF SUPPORT • 135

Auxiliary 45th anniversary, 2001

work was interesting. In 1996, there were 200 active members contributing 40,000 hours of service annually at the information desk, admitting office, ED, radiology, GI [gastrointestinal] lab, pediatrics, newborn nursery, and surgical lounge."

In February 2002, the auxiliary celebrated its 46th birthday with a donation of $75,000 to the hospital, also pledging another $200,000 to the NICU renovation campaign (2002–2006), which brought the total raised by the group to $3 million since 1956.

In 2018, the HMC Auxiliary was reborn as the Volunteer Corps. Alison Dedrick was named chair for the steering committee, which combined members of the disbanded auxiliary with the newly formed Volunteer Corps. Their goal was to increase the number of volunteers and to be inclusive of a larger range of age groups.

Debi Peters, Volunteer Services Coordinator and Eleanor Poole, Auxiliary President, accept a Service Excellence Award on behalf of all Hurley volunteers. The award was given at the August managers' meeting to recognize Hurley volunteers for consistently high scores on the patient satisfaction surveys.

"We are the face of the hospital," said Dedrick. "If we can provide a really good experience for patients and their families, they'll be more likely to come back." Volunteers serve in the surgical lounge, the cath lab, admitting, the GI lab and the lobby shop, among other areas. Some cuddle premature babies in the NICU, walk with patients, or give vital information as liaisons in the ED. "We can empathize with the patients' families. I don't think there's one of us who hasn't had someone in the hospital. We take pride in Hurley," she said.

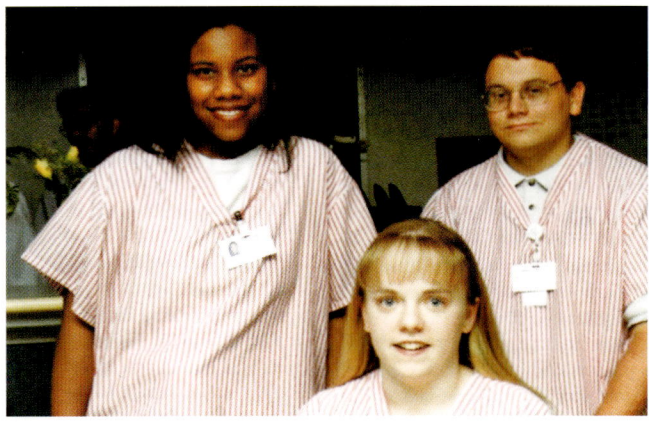

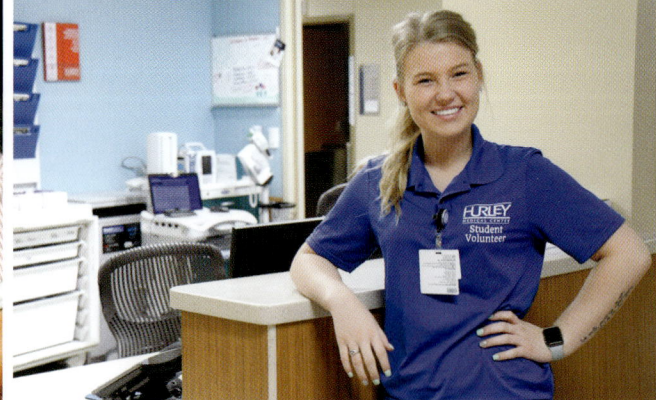

Youth Volunteer Program
Hurley's Youth Volunteer Program has provided a valuable service since 1956 in partnership with the Genesee County Medical Society Alliance. Thousands of young people have explored health careers and given back to their community in one of the only hospital programs in the region. Today, volunteers 16 years and older can volunteer in service areas across the hospital or attend the Healthcare Career Day (HCD) at HMC with their high school. Most students learn about HMC at Healthcare Career Day in their respective high schools. HCD offers on-site speakers, tours, mock clinics and local college representatives. Volunteer Services engages students in a pre-professional program that combines volunteer service with job shadowing tailored to their professional goals.

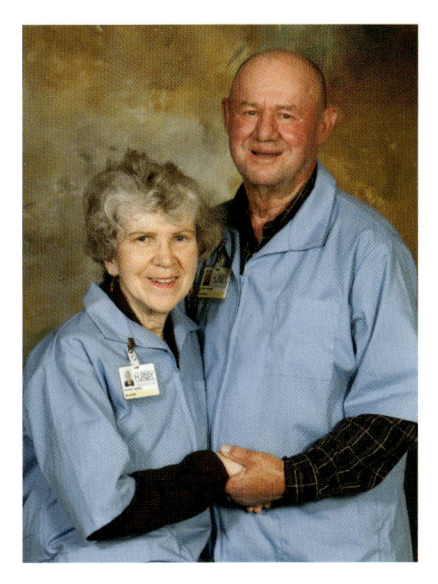

A Heroic Heart – A Volunteer's Story

Jeff Umphrey is an amazing volunteer. Over 30 years ago, he survived burns to 54 percent of his body. Now, he volunteers at Hurley's Burn Unit, giving inspiration and encouragement to families going through the same thing. On December 10, 1985, Umphrey, a body shop mechanic, was removing a gas tank from a car when gasoline spilled on Umphrey and a nearby light bulb; the gas ignited and lit him on fire. He spent six weeks in Hurley's burn unit, four weeks in a medically induced coma, and received multiple surgeries and skin grafts, followed by several months of rehabilitation, which changed his life. Today, he visits the Burn Unit each week, sometimes multiple times, talking with patients and their families, giving them encouragement to know that healing will come. "He shines when he's up there. He's a natural. He understands the emotional and spiritual healing that needs to go on and he can connect. I am so proud of him," says his wife, Kathryn, a volunteer chaplain in Hurley's Spiritual Care Program. Umphrey gives back and shows patients that they can heal from burns, anger, and pain. He is a true role model for all volunteers and former patients. Umphrey was selected as Hurley's trauma ambassador for the 2015 annual Hurley Trauma Center Fall Golf Classic.

Honoring Longtime Volunteers

Barb Arndt came from the Upper Peninsula to Flint in 1947 after graduating from high school, following in the footsteps of two sisters who had taken part in nursing training at Hurley. Arndt got involved as a Red Cross volunteer at the hospital and joined the auxiliary shortly thereafter. She began volunteering in radiology and also knitted hats and footies for babies, created heart-shaped pillows for breast cancer patients, and sold belts and bags for walkers. Through her 41 years volunteering at Hurley, Arndt said, "The surgical lounge is where I really love to work; there, we are the liaison between family and surgery."

"In the surgical lounge, we know it can be a difficult situation for visitors, so we try to help them the most we can and in any way we can," she said. Richard Warmbold, president of the Hurley Foundation, said Arndt takes pride in her volunteerism, having it on full display when she walks the halls in the surgical lounge. He said, "If you could write a description of the perfect volunteer, Barb would be it." In 2019, Barbara Arndt was honored for 50 years of volunteer service at Hurley.

Barbara Tankersly started volunteering at Hurley in 1979. She has volunteered in most all of the roles and departments. "I had a young son who was starting school, and thought that I would volunteer at Hurley with the extra time," said Tankersly. She recalls wearing a yellow smock during her 10 years volunteering on the 9 East Tower Cancer Unit. "It was a learning experience on how to deal with sickness and how to accept a patient's passing." Tankersly also served in the ED,

Barb Arndt, longtime volunteer

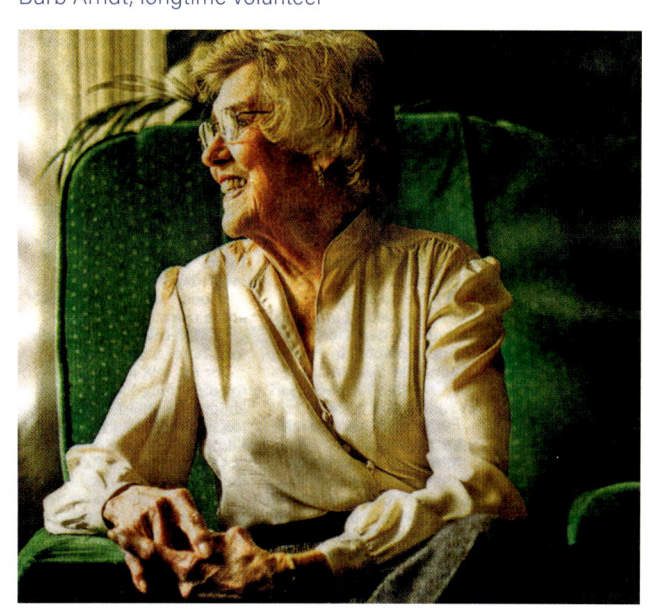

CHAPTER SIX THE FOUNDATION — A FOUNTAIN OF SUPPORT • 137

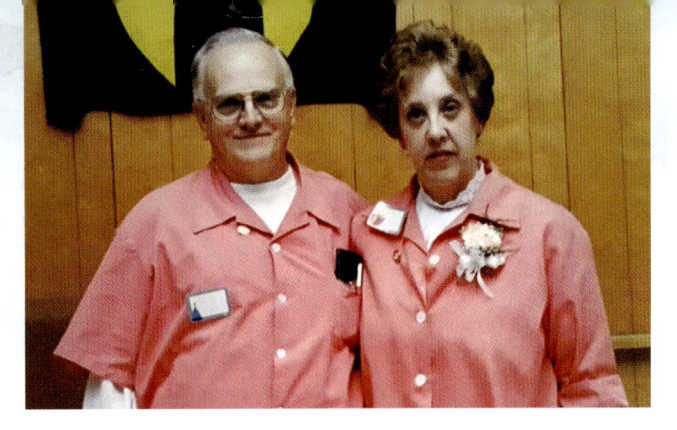

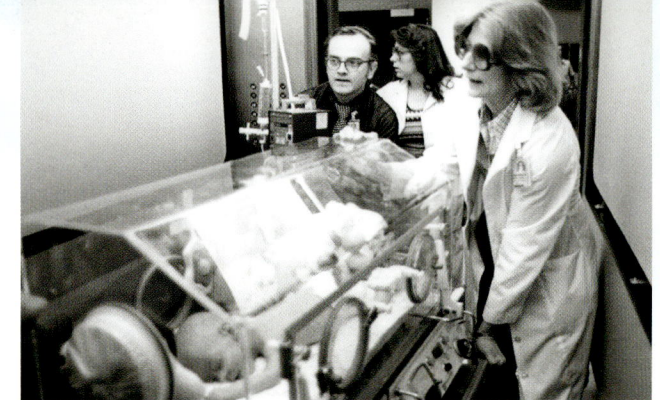

Garry Viele and Nancy (Tilson) Viele represent former HMC staff members who returned as volunteers.

X-ray, the information desk, and the lobby shop. For the last 25 years, she has volunteered several days a month in the lobby shop. At the end of 2017, Tankersly had volunteered for almost 40 years, including as a two-term auxiliary president, program chair, and fundraising chair over the years. "We held bake sales and flower sales as fundraisers, and everyone worked together," she said. "It was a good team and we had positive results. We could see that our hard work had paid off. I am proud to have helped out the community and made a lot of friends along the way. I still keep in touch with some, and we still get together for an occasional lunch."

Staff Who Return as Volunteers

As a Hurley family, some staff work outside of their regular work as volunteers—such as at the Food Bank of Eastern Michigan and the Crim Festival of Races—to support our community; Hurley is often looked to by other organizations to provide volunteers. Brown noted, "Hurley has also developed corporate volunteerism opportunities for our community partners that want to provide gifts or services to our patients while team building, which has become very beneficial to our community partners." Additionally, many former employees volunteer time at Hurley.

Flo Greer, RN, worked at Hurley for almost 29 years and then volunteered for another 14 years. Greer started in 1975 as a CCU nurse, remaining until 1984, when she moved to staff development until she retired in 2003. "After my retirement, I went into the GI lab for a colonoscopy and ran into the most dedicated volunteer, Dale Burris. It was he who talked me into being a volunteer," recalls Greer. "In the end, I don't think that I did anything outstanding. I did what I did because it helped other people."

Pama Holmblade, RN, worked at HMC for 40 years in the Adult Medical, Surgical, and Critical Care Units, as well as in the Nursing Education Department. Soon after retiring, she joined the auxiliary as a way to stay connected to the hospital and her many friends. "I don't miss the work, but I do miss the people I worked with," said Holmblade. "I volunteer in the lobby shop, where I see many familiar faces and can keep up with their news."

Garry Viele, RN, and Nancy (Tilson) Viele met in the 1960s while working at HMC for 25 years, before retiring. Garry started as an orderly, worked his way through nursing school, and served as acting director of Nursing before becoming program director for CISCO Computer System Installation. Nancy began in 1967 as an administrative secretary for the directors of Nursing, where she also supervised clerks in the Nursing office. Both enjoyed the business of working in a large city hospital, where the high level of service was given to both the affluent and poor patients alike. Garry shared a Hurley memory: "One winter, during a massive blizzard, the local sheriff deputies had to drive nurses to work on skidoos." After retirement, they have each volunteered for another 25 years. Garry volunteered at the goodie cart, the lobby shop, and the information desk, and he also served as the auxiliary's president, counselor, and co-editor of their newsletter. Nancy volunteered in the lobby shop and also served as auxiliary president, treasurer, and other roles. Both held leadership roles in state-level volunteer organizations as well. "Hurley has been very good to me over the years," said Garry. Both said they "wanted to return some of the benefits that they had received through the years."

Denise Barrett has been a volunteer for the past four years after being employed by HMC for 15 years as a cardiac ultrasound technician. "I always said I was going to volunteer after I retired," said Barrett. "I was going to hold and rock babies in NICU but went to the lobby shop two weeks after retirement and that's where I've been since." Barrett loved working for HMC and especially with her fellow staff members. As part of her volunteer duties, Barrett goes to the Farmers' Market to purchase fruit to be sold at HMC. She also

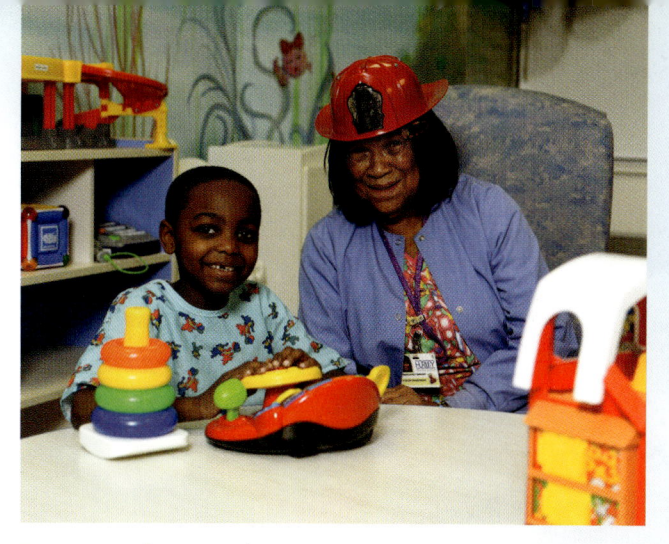

Foster-grandparent volunteer Margaret Wright steps in to help children have a happier stay.

has made good use of her embroidery skills by spearheading the selling of embroidered jackets in the lobby shop. "We used to sell hoodies in the shop until I found a nicer-style jacket to sell," said Barrett. "It was a hit … we have sold over 1,000 jackets."

Fundraising and the Community at Large

The first community education and fund development programs were started in the mid-1970s under the leadership of CEO Schripsema, who tasked Frankie Perry, assistant to the medical center director, to develop the public relations and fund development programs to include annual giving, deferred giving, grant writing, and the annual Hurley Ball, all in support of the $6.7 million capital campaign. Since the establishment of the Hurley Foundation, many of the programs have continued to evolve.

Today, Hurley and the Hurley Foundation have several partnerships with local nonprofits in the area. Examples of these are the YMCA of Greater Flint, Voices for Children, and Whaley Children's Center. "Our partnership with the YMCA of Greater Flint circles around the health of our community," said Wenstrom-Williams. "We work together alongside the Flint Farmers' Market to promote healthy eating—we have staff active on their boards, and Hurley partners with YMCA Camp Copneconic to offer two specialty camps: Camp Move It and Camp Easy Breathers."

Bikin' for Burns

The first Bikin' for Burns was held in 2001 and attracted more than 1,000 motorcyclists from around the state, raising $21,689 for Hurley's Burn Unit. Hosted by the American Bikers Aiming Toward Education (ABATE) of Michigan, Region 20, and the Genesee County Fire Chiefs Association, a Grand Blanc fire engine escorted motorcyclists on the 30-mile ride.

BIKING FOR BURNS

Biking for Burns, a bike-a-thon, involves eight communities in Michigan and Ohio through the Great Lakes Biking for Burns organization. Flint's bike-a-thon group established funds, beginning in 1985, to raise money for the Franklin V. Wade Regional Burn Unit and the Bicycle Coordination Council; 90 percent of the funds were deposited into an endowment fund to guarantee perpetual support for the Burn Unit. The remaining 10 percent was deposited into an account for grants that outline a need for program equipment that positively impacts burn patients' quality of life and care.

Breast Health Nurse Navigator

Hurley's breast cancer program, certified by the National Accreditation Program Breast Centers (NAPBC) of the American College of Surgeons' Commission on Cancer, consistently provides the highest level of clinical breast cancer care and compassion for patients and their families at Hurley. This is the highest accreditation awarded, and HMC is the first and only medical center in Genesee County (and one of only a few statewide) to offer this program.

In 2008, with the support of Raouf Mikhail, MD, FACS, FRCS, Hurley created a Breast Health Nurse Navigator program to provide education, support, and coordination of care for men and women diagnosed with breast cancer. Marsha Schmit, RN, BSN, CBCN, was hired for the navigator role. "When someone gets a breast cancer diagnosis, it can be overwhelming. My role is to step in and help them make sense of what they hear, know, and understand, as well as what treatments will be required. Many times after patients hear the word 'cancer,' very little is absorbed." Schmit continues, "I explain their diagnosis in simple terms and give them a road map to follow to ensure success. Because I too have been a patient with breast cancer, I feel as though I have credibility. I think that women and men identify by knowing that I have personally experienced what they are going through and can rely on me to share what I know and to provide hope. In addition to the clinical aspect, during cancer treatments, many patients or their family members incur great loss, including their job, home, spouse, self-esteem, and more. Patients need an advocate. My greatest joy is to get to know each person and find the areas that are the most challenging. It is an honor to walk alongside each patient, helping them find their way. Most times, it's about getting this experience in their rearview mirror, where they can reflect on how far they have come from diagnosis to recovery, and sometimes, it's end-of-life support. In all cases, I believe it's the connection that has been established that allows the best experience possible."

Schmit has led support groups for more than 10 years to aid women and men in learning to cope with the diagnosis, treatment, and post-recovery phases of their lives. She has mentored nursing students, and she also speaks to church groups and various organizations in the community to help raise awareness and improve breast health.

According to Schmit, "I keep the lines of communication open so that patients can call and dialogue about anything that might be weighing on their minds. I make sure our patients have access to resources, and when times get tough financially, I work with the Hurley Foundation and Hurley's marketing team to find financial resources for patients to tap into, such as the Breast Cancer Navigation Fund. Hurley strives to offer programs that make our patients' lives better, thus improving the health of our community."

Pink Night Palooza – Raising Funds and Awareness for Breast Cancer Navigation Fund

Since 2008, this fun and highly entertaining event has been sponsored by the Hurley Foundation and Financial Plus Credit Union in support of Hurley's Breast Cancer Navigation Fund for breast cancer

Pink Night Palooza, 2019 and 2020

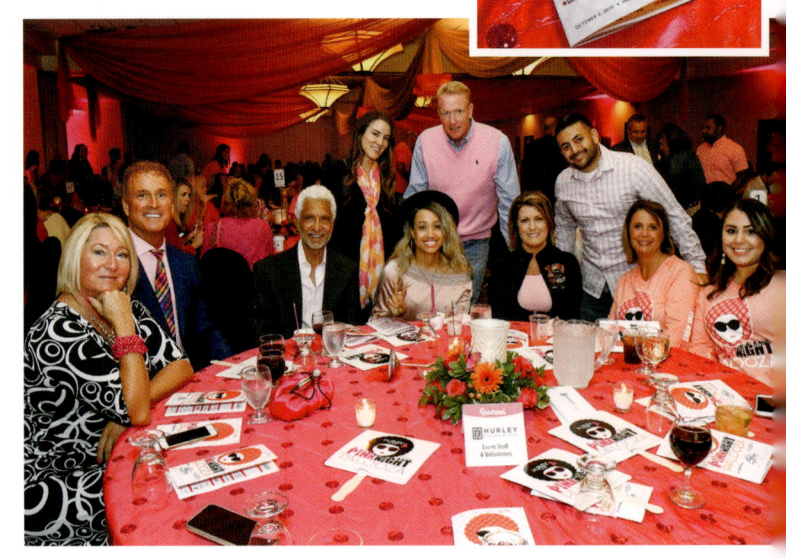

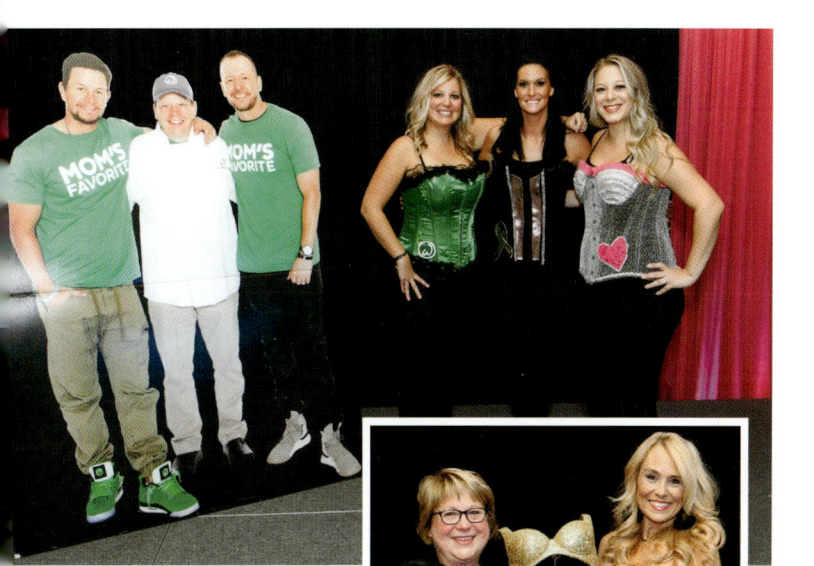

Pink Night Palooza, 2019 and 2020

patients going through testing, treatment, and recovery. Funds for the Breast Cancer Navigation Fund are raised through many community partnerships, including (in alphabetical order): American House GB, Biggby Coffee, Cops & Robbers, Edible Arrangements, Fick Landscape Supplies, Financial Plus Credit Union, Grand Blanc Huntsman's Club, Halo Burger, Hurley employee bake sales, Instalube, Jazzercize, Chandra Jones, Serendipity, and Texas Roadhouse, culminating with the annual Pink Night Palooza event every October. The main highlight of Pink Night Palooza is the bra fashion show, which includes celebrity-signed bras (Kid Rock and Mark Wahlberg, for example) that are tastefully decorated, modeled by breast cancer survivors, and auctioned. Bras have fetched from $200 up to $12,500 at the auctions. In addition to the celebration of survivors, the games and good food make it a top fundraiser. In 2020, the event was held virtually due to the Covid pandemic, and it raised a record-breaking $191,864.12.

DID YOU KNOW | . . . Volunteer service hours were valued at $1.3 million in 2018–2019: sixty-one as NICU cuddlers, 28 in the surgical lounge, 31 in the lobby shop, and 113 throughout HMC.

Annual Hurley Trauma Center Fall Golf Classic

The Hurley Foundation has hosted an annual golf competition to benefit Hurley's Level I Trauma Center and Burn Unit since 1984. In 2019, HMC celebrated the 35th annual event. The total amount raised in 2019 was $175,000.

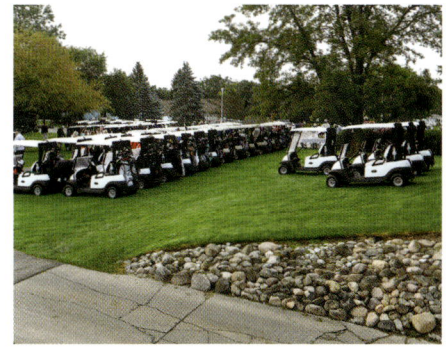

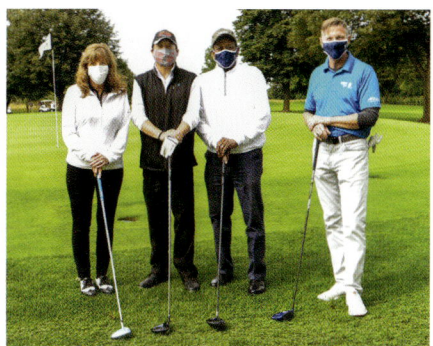

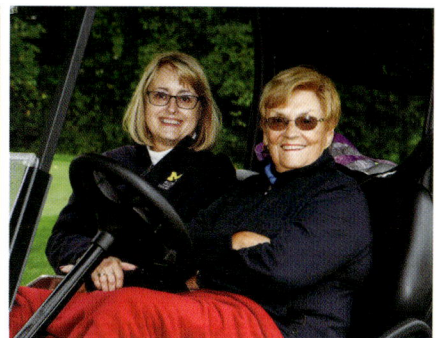

Middle: Golf classic, 2020 (left to right): Melany Gavulic, HMC CEO; Flint mayor Sheldon Neeley; Khalid Ahmed, MD; and Michael Burnett, Hurley Foundation president.

Right: Volunteers Dawn Bentley (left) and Carol Hartley at the 2018 Trauma Center Fall Golf Classic at Flint Golf Club

The James J. Hurley Society

Even though James J. Hurley had the amazing foresight to bequeath his gift and ensure his legacy, he could not possibly have imagined what Hurley has become today. If only he could come back and see all the good done in his name, he would be amazed. The Hurley Foundation is the steward of his vision. The James J. Hurley Society, a planned gift program offering an important element to Hurley's sustainability, is a way for others to bequeath a specific gift in their will or list the Hurley Foundation as a beneficiary via a life insurance policy. Some have named Hurley as beneficiary of their pension plan or IRA, or have given a gift of real estate or an annuity to the Hurley Foundation Endowment Fund. "You have to meet people, establish relationships, and seek their donations so that they can play a significant role," said Richard Warmbold, former Hurley Foundation president.

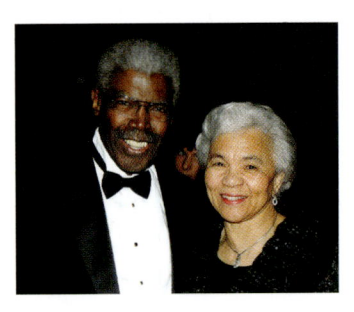

Dr. Samuel and Jan Dismond

In the early 1960s, Flint provided Samuel Dismond Jr., MD, the setting to begin his professional career. "I have received many blessings from my Hurley Family and my patients. It is a privilege to be a contributing member of the James J. Hurley Society and to keep alive the mission of Hurley Medical Center," said Dr. Dismond. Hurley has also touched Jan Dismond's life, with Hurley School of Nursing being instrumental in the completion of her professional training as a registered nurse.

Bill and Kitty Moeller

Bill Moeller has served on the Hurley Foundation Board of Directors since 2002; for 15 of those years, he has served as treasurer. He manages the foundation's funds to be in line with HMC's mission: keeping financial reporting as transparent as possible to both the hospital and the donors. "It's always been important to me that the donors know where their funds are being used," said Moeller. Bill and his wife, Kitty, have had a lifetime relationship with HMC, and they are

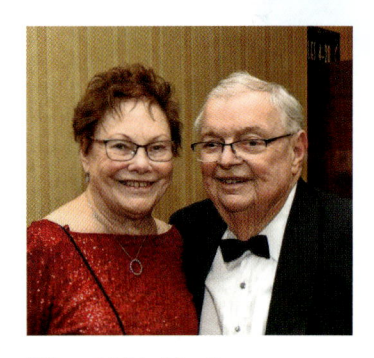

Bill and Kitty Moeller

continuing this connection with a legacy to the James J. Hurley Society. "There are many people, just like us, who have been forever impacted by the medical support we received from Hurley," said Moeller. "In many ways, we still have a son because of Hurley," said Kitty. "When he was 18 months old, his lungs shut down. He needed a tracheotomy, but they didn't have equipment small enough back then. Dr. Tuuri, Dr. Dwyer, and Dr. VanDuyne tirelessly worked around the clock until our son made it through," said Moeller. "Today, he is a healthy man with his own kids and grandkids." Last year, it was Moeller who needed medical help. "I was impressed with Hurley before, but after being a Hurley patient, my wife and I didn't run across one employee who wasn't totally dedicated; the entire staff was amazing! Every individual that I encountered was courteous and helpful. I can't say enough about how impressed I was about everything that we encountered. As a patient, and as a volunteer, it was very impressive." Bill and Kitty have taken their appreciation to action by leaving a legacy gift to the Hurley Foundation. "It's a more generous gift than we could give while we are alive," said Moeller. "I can't help but think of all of the families out there with great feelings about Hurley because of what Hurley has done to save one of their family members. They may not have the wherewithal now, but I think it's important for them to consider leaving a legacy to honor that experience, and to thank those who worked to make them well."

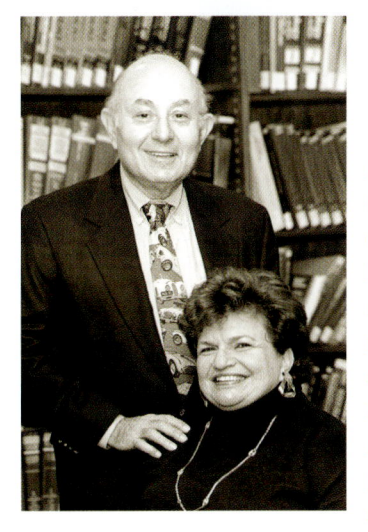

During a 40-year career at HMC and in Genesee County, oral surgeon Arnold Schaffer, DDS, was internationally known, widely published, and an adjunct faculty member at both Michigan State University and the University of Michigan School of Dentistry. Dr. Schaffer was a tireless advocate for oral cancer education in the community. In 1962, Dr. Schaffer and his wife, Miriam Schaffer, a social worker, lost their son Bruce to cancer. To honor his memory, the Schaffers and the Hurley Foundation created the Bruce Alan Schaffer Endowment Fund to promote professional education for social workers who work with terminally ill children and their families.

The Barnett Family

As a founding member of the James J. Hurley Society, Rick Barnett has been involved with Hurley for over two decades. Rick and his wife, Leah, were familiar with HMC's services because Leah was a surgical nurse in Hurley's Labor and Delivery Unit for 10 years. Little did they know that they would require those same services when their children were born prematurely. Hurley's expert team was there to care for them the minute they were born.

"At birth, you look at them laying there, with lines going into each extremity, and a breathing tube just to keep them alive. You wonder if they will survive, and if they did, what kind of life they would have," said Barnett. "Now, at 16 and 14, they are both tall and strong. I look back and think, with extreme gratitude, what tremendous work the NICU team did. I remember the empathy and compassion the Hurley team provided, knowing we were one of many parents going through the same thing. The doctors and nurses gave us great peace and confidence that our boys would be okay. It was a stressful time, but we felt at ease knowing they were receiving excellent care. They have had zero problems associated with their early birth, and for that we are thankful. Thankful for all that Hurley has done for us with our boys, and over the years for our family. To this day, I proudly serve as one of the founding members of the Hurley Foundation and give back to others at every chance." Barnett also notes that the James J. Hurley Society is a wonderful foundation in our community. "Flint and Genesee County would not be the same place without Hurley. All of the essential services, including NICU, are vital for Hurley's continuation and growth. Hurley continues to add services and specialties, which make it the 'go to' hospital. Contributing to the James J. Hurley Society not only means continuity, but also continual expansion for our area's needs," says Barnett. Barnett's company has conducted financial education workshops for Hurley employees since 1993. They participate on the Hurley Benefit Ball Committee, the annual Hurley golf outing, and as a major contributor to Hurley Children's Clinic in Downtown Flint.

Rick Barnett

NOTES
1. Allison Rosbury, *My City Magazine*, January 1, 2017.
2. Ibid.
3. *Kudos Magazine* Vol. 4 (Issue 2, 2018), p. 27.
4. Ibid.

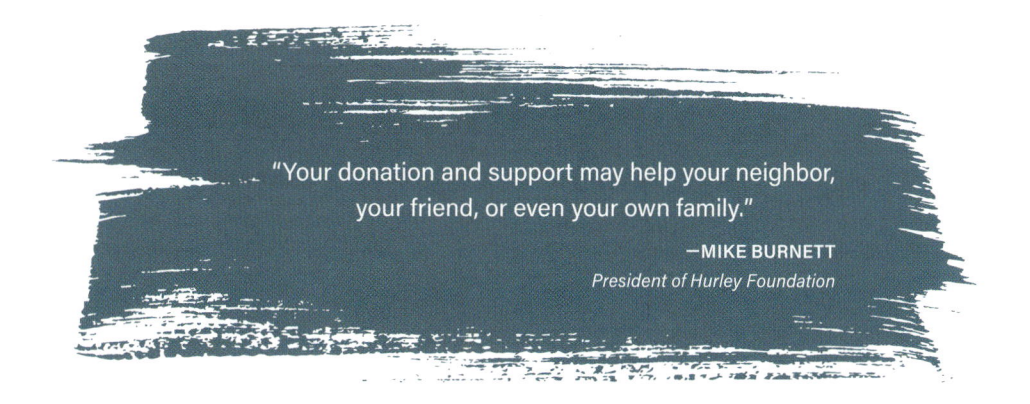

"Your donation and support may help your neighbor, your friend, or even your own family."

—MIKE BURNETT
President of Hurley Foundation

TRANSFORMING Health

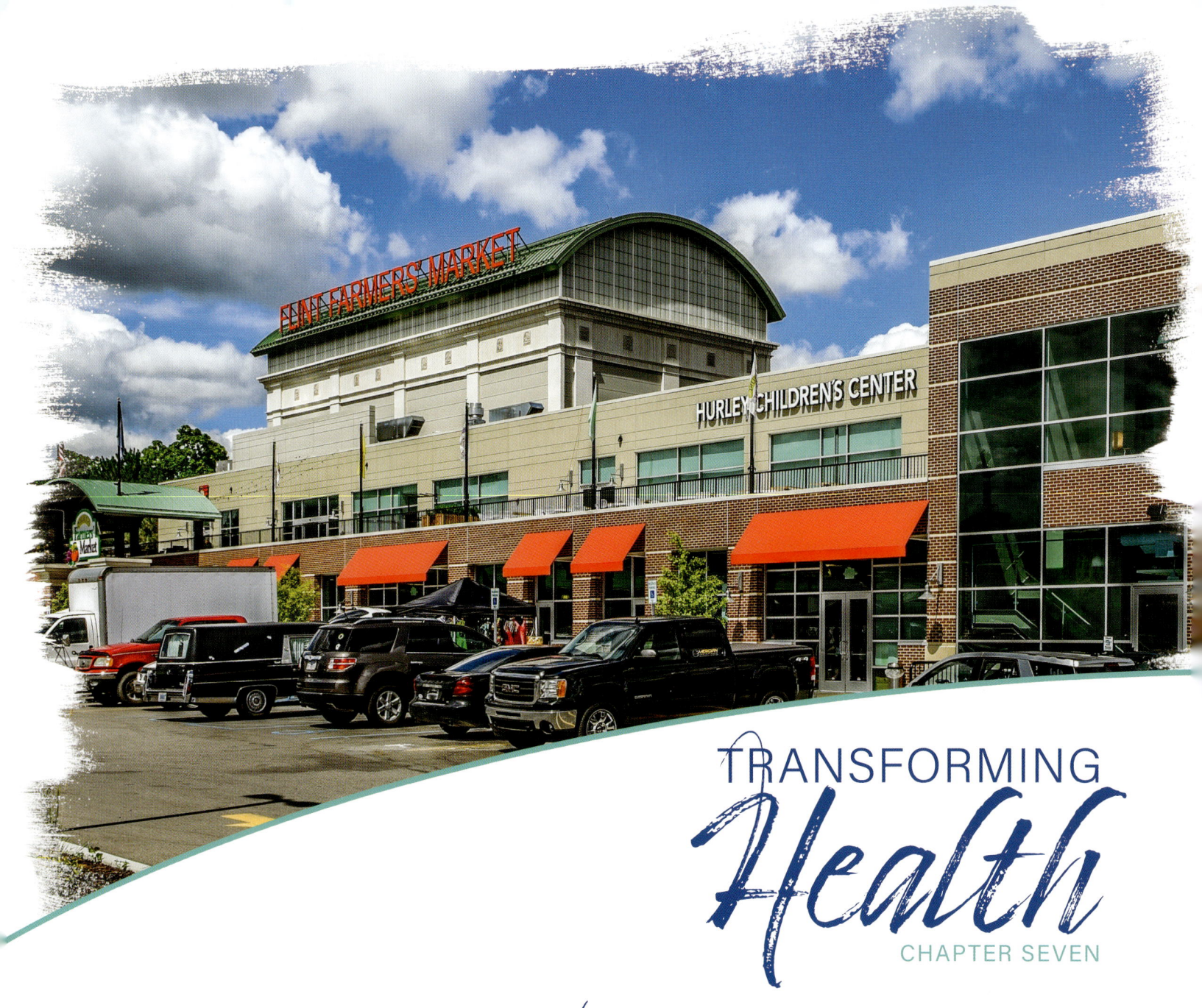

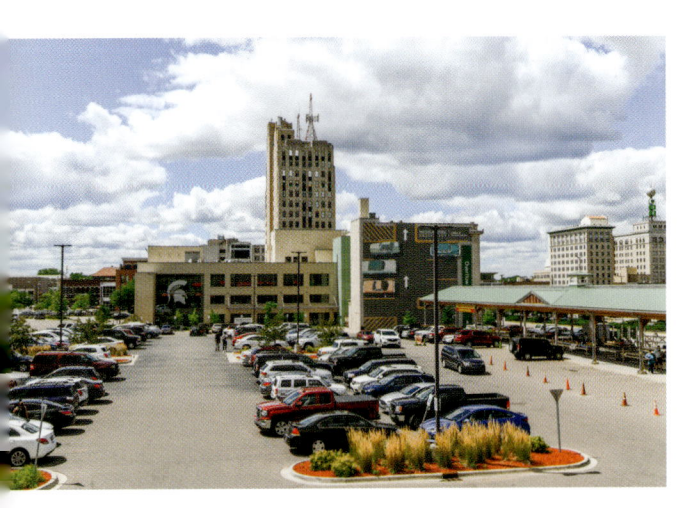

CHAPTER SEVEN

Hurley Children's Clinic, located in the downtown Farmers' Market complex across from Flint's main bus station

The present-day vision for Hurley Medical Center is to transform the overall health of residents of Genesee County through academic and clinical excellence, and by expanding access to innovative care; although, one can easily see that this has been part of our historical actions since 1908. The move toward building service locations within patient populations, followed by wellness hubs offering programs and services with long-lasting health benefits, has been taking place for decades.

Reaching into Neighboring Communities

What was once a city hospital has become a regional network of health clinics and services located in the communities that need it most. In 1991, the Hurley Health and Fitness Center opened (as the

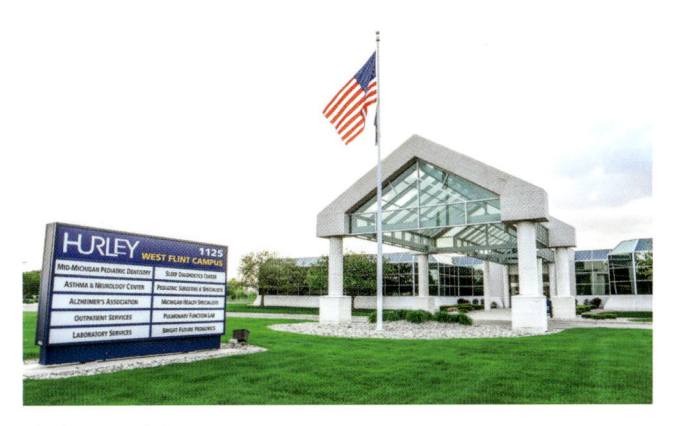

Linden Road Campus

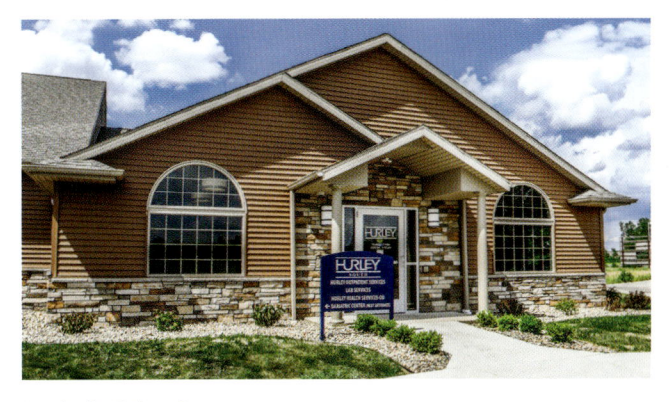

Rochelle Drive Campus

service area's only hospital-affiliated fitness center) in an effort to address wellness. Concern for the community at large remained at the forefront, and in 1996, HMC established a new entity called Hurley Health Services, which expanded Hurley's primary care network to include community-based clinics with the opening of Hurley Children and Family Health Center on Linden Road. The 43,000-square-foot medical arts complex offered patients who lived in Flint and surrounding counties access to specialized and general treatments that were previously only offered at the hospital location. HMC provides various hospital-based pediatric subspecialists, ensuring that patients and families continue to receive the most comprehensive and state-of-the-art pediatric care in both the inpatient and outpatient settings.

Hurley was the first major health care provider in Genesee County to operate on Flint's northwestern side. In July 1996, HMC began treating patients at North Pointe Community Health and Education Center. Providing comprehensive, primary care in a facility located within the community was the start of a decades-long strategy. According to Glenn Fosdick, HMC president and CEO at the time, "The community has a strong need for this type of facility. We will offer a high-quality program that is efficient and effective . . . going beyond a simple medical clinic concept to provide a comprehensive program that combines care, education and prevention."[1] The clinic relocated to the Hurley Campus in 2016.

In 1999, the Hurley Center for Comprehensive Weight Loss opened its doors and celebrated a milestone in 2000, when the first Roux-en-Y gastric bypass surgery for the treatment of clinically severe obesity was performed. Hurley Diabetes Center, a comprehensive program offering full diabetes services for outpatient customers, opened at the Hurley Eastside Campus in 2000.

In 2001, ground-breaking ceremonies were held for the Genesys Hurley Cancer Institute, offering 49,000 square feet of space dedicated to the most comprehensive cancer prevention programs, early detection services, all-encompassing care from diagnosis to treatment to survivorship, and effective, compassionate follow-up care for cancer patients and their

Genesys Hurley Cancer Institute

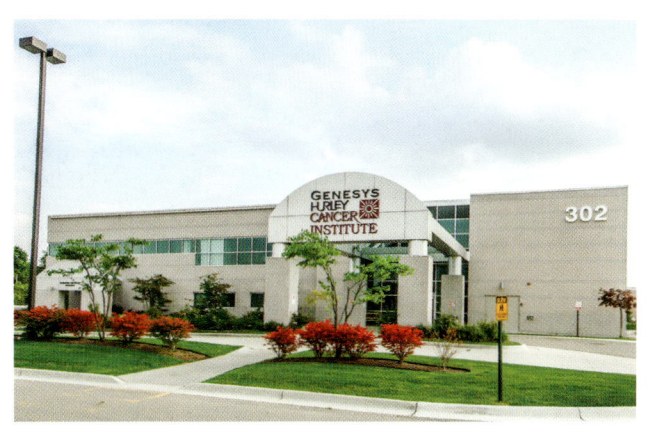

families. This highly innovative collaboration between Hurley Medical Center and Genesys Hospital offers specialization in the most advanced treatments. Patients benefit from an array of support services, including financial counseling, transportation services, free classes and support groups for both patients and caregivers, an on-site social worker, and a registered dietician, as well as access to a myriad of clinical trials. The institute provides physicians with a wide range of complex cancer-fighting options and is the only center in Michigan to offer Accuboost, a noninvasive, innovative, evolutionary brachytherapy approach used exclusively for the treatment of breast cancer. The institute is a member of the Michigan Radiation Oncology Quality Consortium, a collaborative group of specialists across the state working on quality improvement projects to impact radiation treatments. The institute is accredited by the American College of Radiology, recognized as the gold standard in medical imaging and therapeutic radiation accreditation, which ensures that patients receive the safest and best care possible.

In 2001, grand-opening ceremonies were held for the Hurley Northwest Kidney Center, a dialysis and educational center with 14 high-tech dialysis chairs, located in northwestern Flint to better serve those in the community.

In 2006, the Hurley Foundation received a grant from the C. S. Mott Foundation for a master-facilities plan for neighborhood redevelopment and greenbelt projects. This grant enabled the new ED expansion, but also kept in mind how HMC's central campus could be more integrated with the surrounding community. The ground breaking for the new ED on April 27, 2010, through its completion in January 2012, was seen as an opportunity to shift access to Hurley's buildings—effectively moving main public entrances to face Fifth Avenue and rerouting emergency vehicles to the back of the building off of Mackin Road. This had the

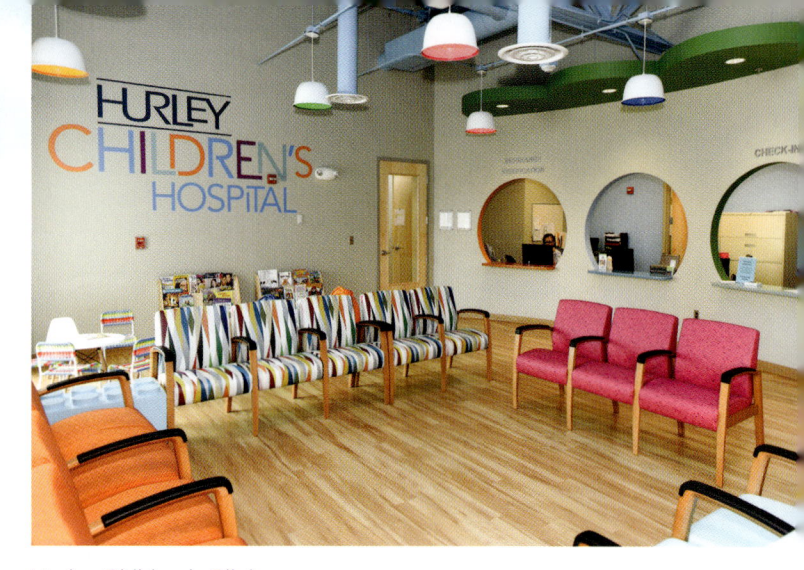

Hurley Children's Clinic

double benefit of improving traffic flow and embracing a more direct connection to Fifth Avenue and the revitalization of Downtown Flint.

One of the most significant urban revitalization projects in Hurley's history launched in August 2015 at a ribbon-cutting ceremony for the Sumathi Mukkamala Hurley Children's Center. The Children's Clinic, which had been housed at Mott Children's Health Center across from Hurley, moved into the Flint Farmers' Market. The clinic's design incorporates physician/provider areas to accommodate team-based care. The center is located in the heart of Downtown Flint within the new Health and Wellness Corridor and across the street from Flint's bus station—potentially eliminating transportation issues for many patients. Placing a pediatric center in a Farmers' Market was a novel concept that sought to change the culture of health in the Flint community by opening up opportunities for families to live healthier lives and for HMC to build a healthier community.

In 2016, a grant-funded program began at Hurley Children's Clinic: the "Take One Apple Twice a Day Program." At each appointment, patients six months and older receive a five-dollar gift card to the Flint Farmers' Market (located below the clinic) to purchase fresh produce. At following appointments, patients are asked about their fruit and vegetable consumption, which is recorded as a vital sign in their medical record. Good nutrition and a healthy diet are especially important for children in order to support healthy development throughout childhood and into adolescence. Each patient receives age-appropriate nutritional education, handouts, recipes, and local resources, such as Double-Up Food Bucks, Flint MTA Ride to Groceries, and cooking demonstrations. Families may use their Double-Up Food Bucks at the Farmers' Market. Additionally, Supplemental Nutrition Assistance Program (SNAP) beneficiaries may use Double-Up Food Bucks for a one-to-one match to purchase healthy, locally grown fruits and vegetables. A registered dietician provides individual

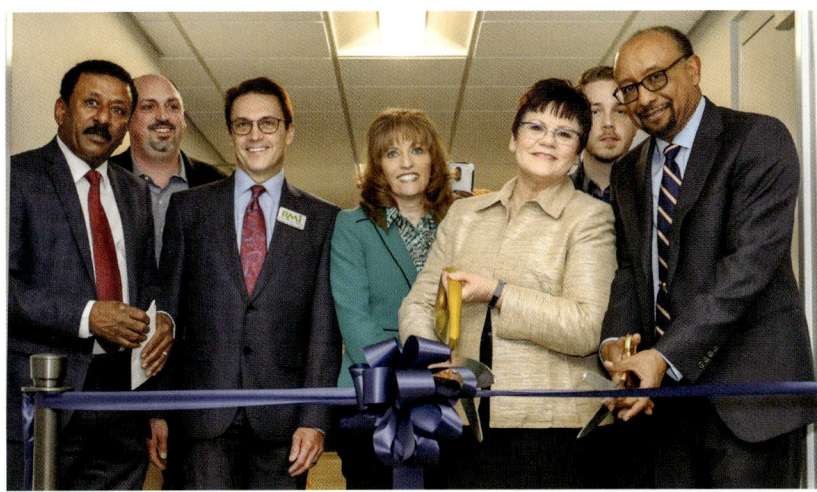

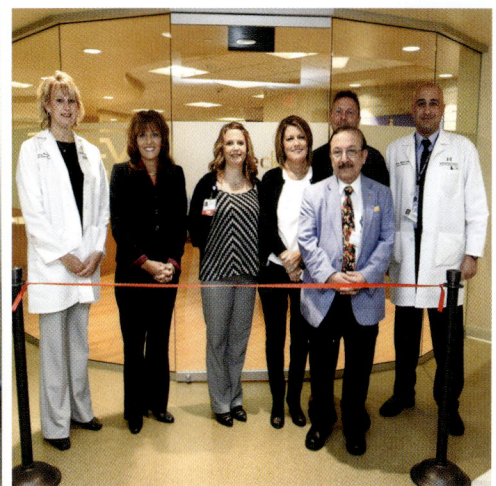

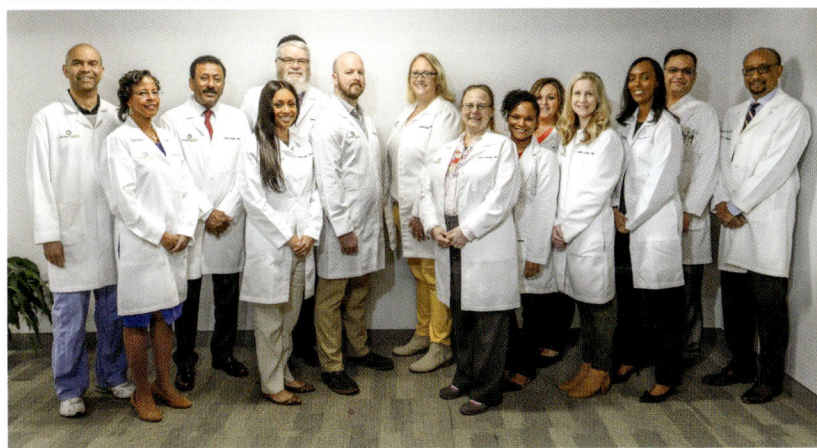

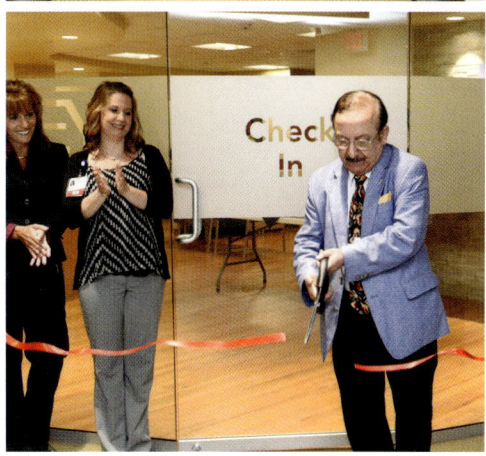

Clockwise from top left:

Urgent Care in Burton opened in 2019 and was immediately dubbed a "wellness hub." In addition to the off-site Urgent Care, Diabetes Center, and Food FARMacy, it also houses Michigan Health Specialists, Pointe Pharmacy, Regional Medical Imaging, and the Holistic Health Center, offering support from food insecurity to wellness. Left to right: Khalid M. Ahmed, MD, MRCP, FACP; Pete Clinton, View Newspaper Group; Randy Hicks, MD, RMI; HMC CEO Melany Gavulic, RN, MBA; Paula Zelenko, former mayor of Burton; Steven Elkins, Genesee County Chamber of Commerce; and Seif M. Saeed, MD.

Amy Benko, PharmD; Gavulic; Bachman; Annette Napier, RN, MPA; Towfiq; Mike Burnett, MSW, MBA; and Firas Amed, MD. Outpatient services include the internal medicine, orthopedic, and surgical clinics, along with the complex care clinic, the infusion clinic, MRI, occupational health, outpatient lab, urgent care, and wound care.

Melany Gavulic, CEO, and Melissa Bachman, RN, watch Basim Towfiq, MD, cut the ribbon to open the remodeled outpatient services in September 2015.

Michigan Health Specialists Group serving the Burton location when it opened in April 2019

and group education and produces tours of the market.[2] Children with a health care provider referral receive healthy food for themselves and their entire household for up to six visits.

Food FARMacy

According to the Community Health Needs Assessment Report in 2019, many residents in the city of Flint lacked convenient access to a full-service grocery store and were effectively living in a food desert; this lack of access prohibits healthy food choices. Many patients, especially low-income minority groups, are highly likely to experience nutritional insufficiencies, which lead to poorer health outcomes and can have a number of repercussions on disease management, prevention, and treatment strategies. Families with food insecurity may forgo up to 100 meals a month, and 74 percent must decide upon paying for medicine or food.

Food FARMacy and staff in 2018 (left to right): Kadira Sahic, volunteer; Susanne Gunsorek, RD; Sheryl Deutsch; and Alisa Stewart.

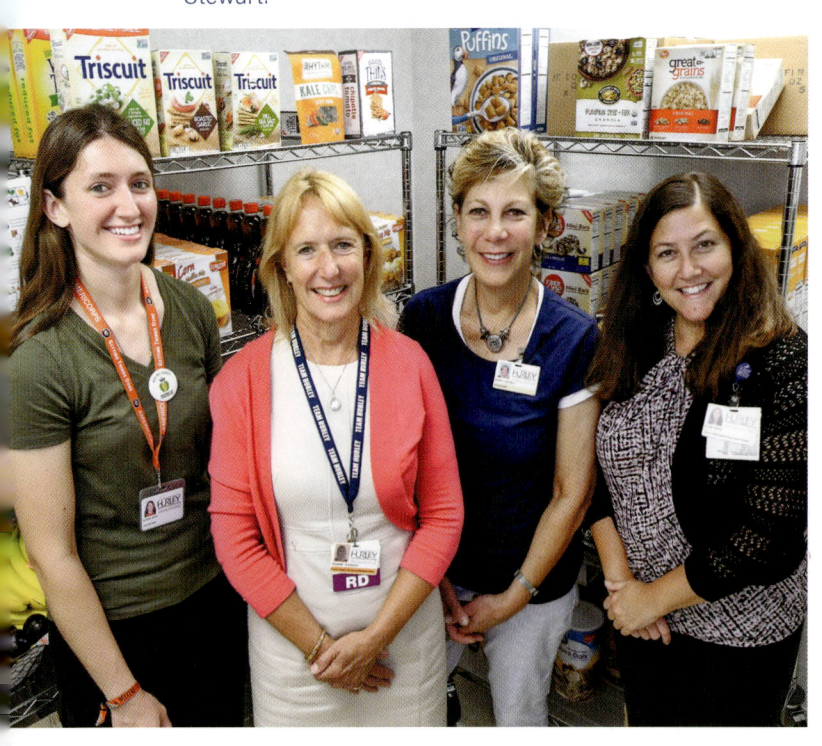

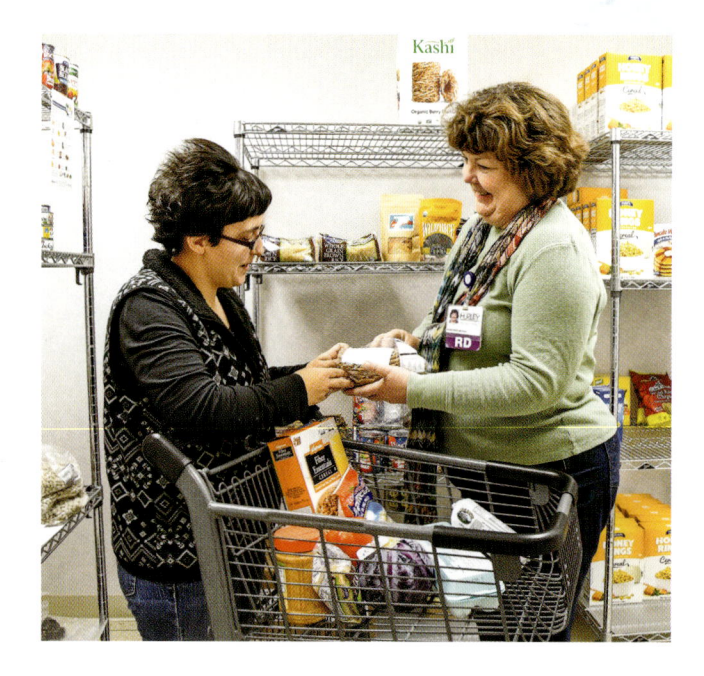

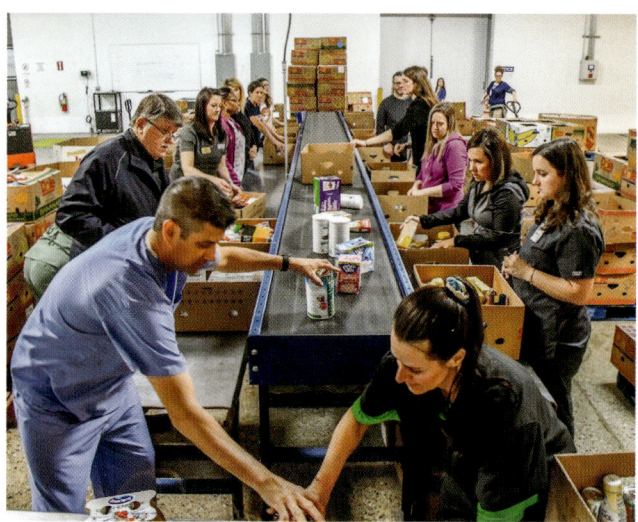

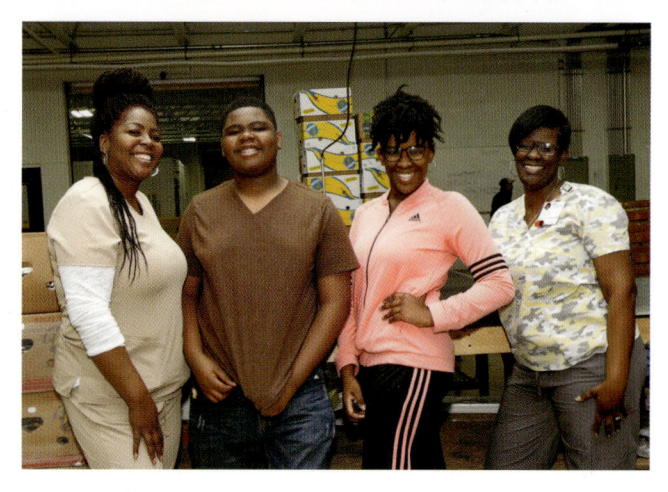

Hurley staff members volunteer for Food FARMacy

Hurley once again took a leadership role in providing and educating the community and helping to further mitigate community food insecurity. HMC launched the Food FARMacy program in 2017 with a vision to be a one-stop shop, addressing a patient's many needs, along with the root causes. According to Alisa Stewart, former administrator for Wellness and Population Health, "This initiative couldn't have come at a better time for our community."

Partnering with Habitat for Humanity (HFH) helped develop the Food FARMacy into a designated Financial Opportunity Center (FOC). HFH has on-site office hours so that patients can make one trip to the Food FARMacy for food, meet with a registered dietician to help with nutrition, and also receive financial coaching offered by HFH. The results have been life changing for clients like Beverly Johnson, who first attended the FOC orientation in January 2019 and decided to participate. Her coaching sessions were tailored to her top priorities of finding employment and learning how to identify quality job leads, update her resume, and write cover letters. She met with her coach every few weeks and via e-mail between sessions. By mid-February, she had accepted a job at Church's Chicken. "We consider our successes one person at a time; for instance, moving from being food insecure to receiving financial coaching and then finding employment. Now, she doesn't need the Food FARMacy anymore," said Stewart.

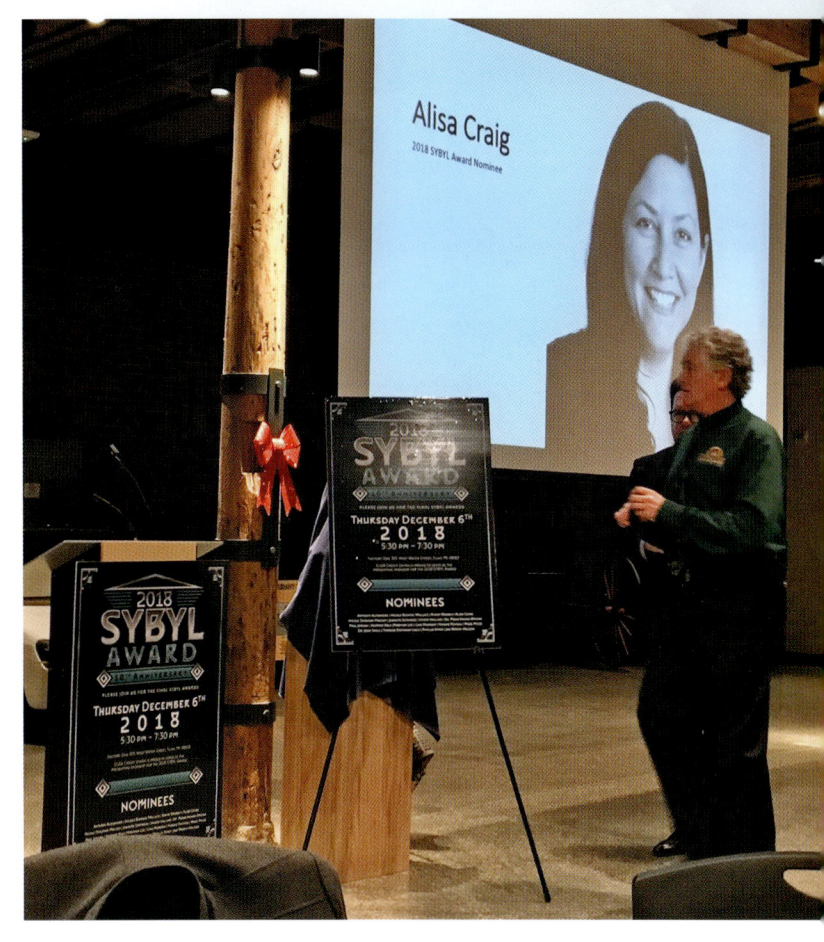

Alisa Stewart received the Sybyl Award in December 2018 for her dedication in making the communities of Flint and Genesee County healthier through managing the Diabetes Center and Food FARMacy, and by creating community engagement in multiple wellness initiatives: Farmers' Market vendors to HMC each week, securing a grant for 30 scholarships to Camp Move It, and obtaining a grant to provide 118 cooking demonstrations to thousands of residents.

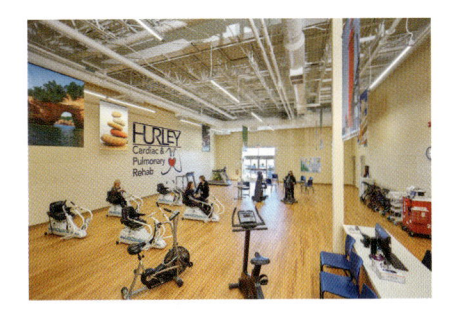

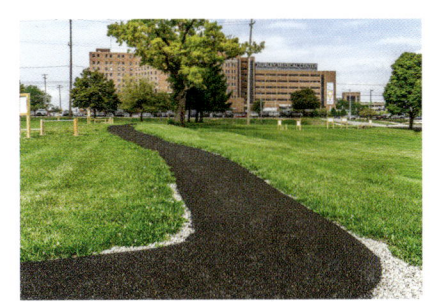

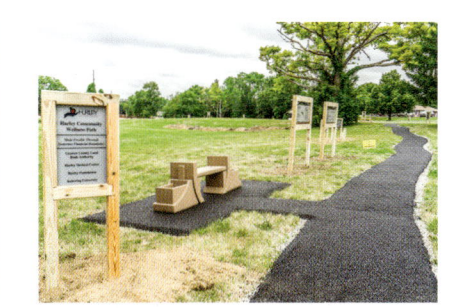

Left: HMC Cardiac Rehabilitation Center

Middle and right: Inspired by and dedicated to the late Alisa Stewart, former administrator for Wellness and Population Health, the Hurley Community Wellness Path opened in September 2020 along West Fifth Avenue, with 10 fitness stations. The outdoor path is close enough so that HMC staff can utilize it during their breaks.

CHAPTER SEVEN TRANSFORMING HEALTH • 149

In 2018, Stewart accompanied CEO Melany Gavulic to Washington, DC, for a policy briefing on food insecurity. Invited by the America's Essential Hospitals organization, they shed light on the grim reality faced by many Genesee County families who do not have the means or access to buy healthy food. They provided an overview of HMC's initiatives to combat food insecurity, including the grant-funded Food FARMacy. "Eventually, I envision health plans partnering with us," said Stewart at the Senate Finance Committee hearing. "With the cost of hunger at roughly $42,400 per US citizen over a lifetime, providing resources for the food insecure makes economic and moral sense to improve our community's health outlook."[3]

Senior Services

For decades, HMC staff have been designing programs to support the senior population. Much like the special consideration HMC gives to their pediatric population, the senior population is an equally fragile group, and it is important to tailor care to their specific needs. Thanks to a $38,500 grant from the Flint Area Health Foundation, in March 1980, an innovative program, the Flint Senior Nutrition Aide Program, was designed to promote nutrition awareness among senior citizens using a peers-teaching-peers concept. Twenty senior nutrition aides took a 12-week training course, which included human relations and understanding the aging process. They then conducted presentations at local senior centers and made in-home visits. According to Charlotte Gibson, program coordinator, "People in all economic brackets suffer from diabetes and heart disease, needing special diet and nutrition advice. Inflation keeps seniors from following proper diets, and foods with essential nutrients can be priced out of reach for those on fixed incomes." The program was a

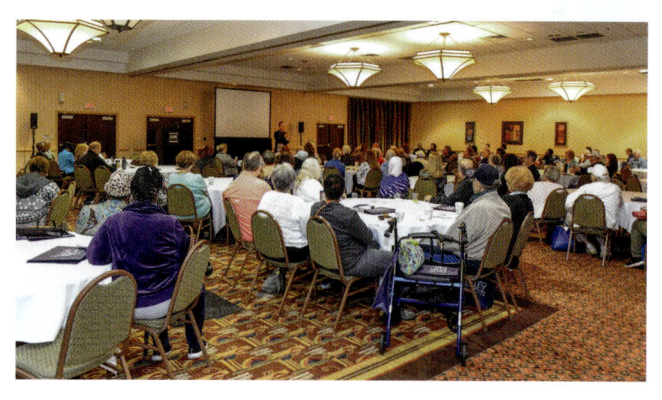

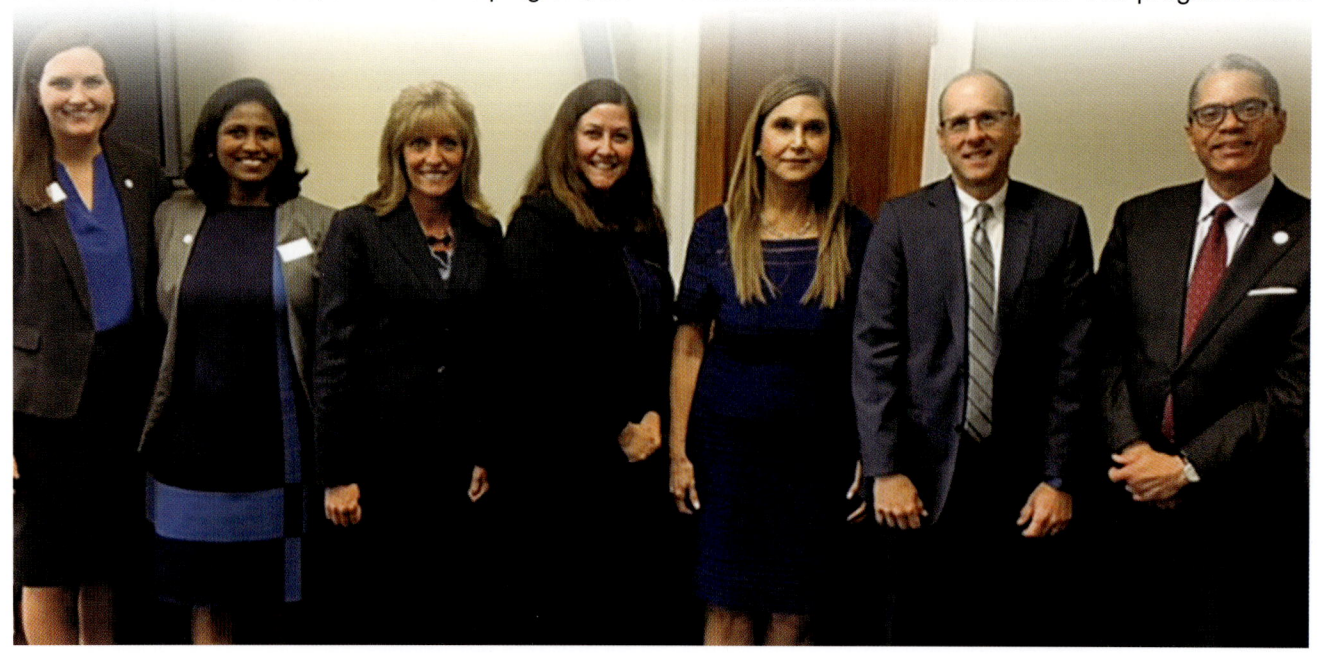

Senior and Caregiver Workshop, September 2019

Hurley CEO Melany Gavulic and Alisa Stewart during a Congressional briefing in Washington, DC, in 2018

result of Hurley's Project Nutrition, which was started in the fall of 1979, to target nutrition services to especially high-risk groups, including the elderly.

Later in 1980, Hurley's Home Care Program was established for geriatric patients over 60 years of age to help with cleaning and laundry assistance, personal needs such as skin care, bathing, and bandage- and wound-dressing changes, and home-delivered meals in partnership with Valley Area Agency on Aging and the Genesee County Community Action Agency. By September 1981, the program was expanded to include a hospice program.

The Hurley Senior Care Center, designed to provide a broad range of services to the senior adult population, became a reality in 1997. The North Pointe Senior Care Center opened in 1998 at the North Pointe Health and Education Center. In early 1999, the West Flint Senior Care Center and the Eastside Senior Care Center opened. All three centers provided comprehensive cognitive, social, and emotional care, along with medical needs, including lab and X-ray capabilities to facilitate on-site health screenings and diagnostic procedures. Geriatric-trained physicians provided primary care, wellness and preventative care, and referrals for the treatment of acute illnesses and injuries, along with a pharmacist and social worker to provide case management and community resource connections. According to Ghassan Bachuwa, MD, medical director of Hurley Senior Services and 1996 Hurley Pinnacle Award recipient, "You must listen to all of a patient's health concerns and their emotional concerns, especially as we age. At the Senior Care Centers, we take the time to get to know the patient. This enables us to treat the whole person."

Elder abuse can be a legitimate concern for seniors. Many times, it goes unreported because oftentimes, the caregiver is the abuser. In 2005, Dr. Bachuwa received a one-year grant to increase clinician awareness and to inform resident physicians and other health care providers on how to recognize and better manage elder abuse.

Between May 2018 and 2019, the volunteer-led Hospital Elder Life Program (HELP) served 342 older patients, providing over 349 hours of extra patient care.

HMC is the service area's only Senior Center of Excellence and one of only five hospitals in the state with exemplar status from Nurses Improving Care for Healthsystem Elders (NICHE), a geriatric nursing distinction that provides excellence in caring for patients 65 and older. HMC is also the only hospital in the area to offer a free, comprehensive program designed to prevent delirium in hospitalized seniors.

In 2019, the Michigan Health Endowment Fund awarded HMC a $78,538 grant to focus on increasing Food FARMacy use by seniors who may not have enough food, but who are less likely to reach out for help. The program has served more than 1,600 patients and provided healthy food and resources to more than 5,000 households.[4] Geriatric nurse specialists provide food bags to all patients aged 65 or older as they are discharged from HMC. The bags contain a Food FARMacy referral, recipes, and food to make meals specifically for those with diabetes, congestive heart failure, and hypertension, the most common ailments for seniors. Transportation passes to the Food FARMacy, along with follow-up calls by staff members, are provided to determine if a patient needs more support; food delivery is also offered to homebound patients.

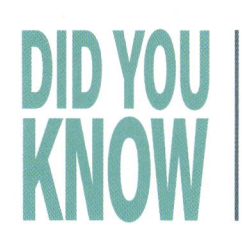

DID YOU KNOW | . . . the Food FARMacy was honored as a noteworthy project for the Gage Award in Public Health at the national conference VITAL2019. HMC also won the America's Essential Hospitals' "We are Essential" Twitter campaign.

In March 2019, HMC received $8,500 from the Martha Merkley Charitable Trust to provide professional haircut and styling services for 210 hospitalized patients 65 years and older. "This grant makes a big difference in improving the morale of our elderly patients. It increases patient satisfaction and provides a sense of connection during what can be a stressful time away from home," said Cathy Metz, PT, MBA, Geriatric Service Line administrator.

In 2020, HMC was honored with a Level III GEDA-accredited Geriatric Emergency Department for its Fast-track Emergency Room for seniors. "Hurley continues to receive recognition for the many layers of services and medical excellence for our patients 65 and older," said Metz. "From admission to discharge, Hurley cares for seniors."

Palliative Care and Hospice

The goal of Hurley's palliative care services is to relieve suffering and improve the quality of life of patients and their families. The palliative care staff members work with physicians, nurses, medical social workers, and chaplains to provide coordinated care that serves the whole patient and ensures that families are active participants in the treatment and decision-making processes to define and clarify the most important goals of care for the patient.

"The most challenging work is communicating with families. Discussing a prognosis is a very psychosocial and emotional journey, especially with the symptoms the patient is physically going through. When you educate a family on a poor prognosis and the family thanks you, that is very rewarding. Families, for the most part, are very appreciative when we talk honestly and don't beat around the bush," noted Diane Welker, RN, nurse practitioner for Pain and Palliative Care. "The goal of palliative care is to alleviate their symptoms. I can have as many as six family meetings a day; meeting with multiple doctors and specialists to identify the whole person has an impact on care."

HMC's palliative care team works toward pain and symptom management, offers emotional support to both patients and families, and, if the patient has a terminal illness and is no longer seeking curative treatment, recommends hospice care, whether in the patient's home or in a residential setting. Hospice care focuses on relieving symptoms and supporting patients who have a life-limiting prognosis. The palliative care team also works with patients to help complete their advance directives.

HMC Awarded Gold Plus by the American Heart Association

In July 2020, Hurley Medical Center received the American Heart Association/American Stroke Association's (AHA/ASA) Get with the Guidelines Stroke Gold Plus achievement award. This award ensures that stroke patients receive the most up-to-date, evidence-based treatment guidelines, which improve patient care and outcomes in our community. To receive the gold award, HMC maintained their stellar performance level for at least two consecutive years. HMC also qualified to be recognized as AHA/ASA's Target: Stroke Elite Honor Roll Award.

Behavioral Medicine

Patients with mental health and substance abuse disorders are considered behavioral medicine patients; patients with developmental disabilities, learning disorders, dementia, or other cognitive limitations are not. That distinction was not fully understood in the era when Hurley Hospital was founded. The definition of mental illness and its treatment has dramatically changed, not only by a differing understanding of what mental illness is, but also by changing national policy and consumer attitudes. In the 1880s, inpatient care, in which patients lived in hospitals and were treated by professional staff, was considered to be most efficient at the time and was also welcomed by families and communities struggling to care for mentally ill relatives.[5] Statistics from 1945 to 1946 indicate that Hurley Hospital accommodations totaled 484 beds, which included 28 beds in the Psychopathic Hospital section of Hurley. By the mid-1950s, there was a push to deinstitutionalize, along with outpatient treatment, accompanied by a variety of new antipsychotic drugs.

According to Millie Evans, RN, former nurse manager of the Psychiatry Unit, "The department name was changed to Behavioral Medicine Department in an effort to get away from the negative stigma." From 1986 to 1990, which was a time of growth, "Hurley treated involuntary [persistent, chronically ill] and voluntary patients separately, into two units—those cared for by private psychiatrists and patients being cared for by psychiatrists who worked for Community Mental Health," said Evans.

As the health care system changed, the Behavioral Medicine Department was downsized. "We saw a decrease in the use of seclusion and restraints, due to training, de-escalation skills, and more individual, one-to-one contact with the patients. We took the holistic approach in treating this population, by stabilizing the patient, focusing on the behavior that led to them being hospitalized, including any contributing medical issues, and their spiritual needs," noted Evans. Staffing changed over the years, with more nurse practitioners added to assist the psychiatrists in the daily care and evaluation of the patients. "It takes a special person to work with patients dealing with a mental health crisis. I loved every minute with my patients, and would do it all over again," Evans shared.

Most of today's behavioral medicine patients are encountered in the ED-based Behavioral Health Unit (BHU). A BHU does not exist in all hospital EDs, so this innovative approach makes HMC uniquely equipped to provide for both the safety and emotional needs of these patients. Many voluntary and involuntary patients are recommended for a short-term stay of inpatient treatment to stabilize the acute psychiatric symptoms and to identify on-going treatment. Hurley also offers a consultation liaison, who supports the assessment, medications management, and discharge needs related to their mental health treatment.

Outpatient mental health care is provided through Hurley Mental Health Associates (HMHA), which has

---

HMC Wins 2019 and 2020 "My City" Wellness Awards

As sponsored by *My City Magazine*, Hurley was named Hospital of the Year and Emergency Facility of the Year in both 2019 and 2020.

one of the largest outpatient mental health clinics in Michigan, offering a group of highly skilled psychiatrists, psychologists, social workers, nurses, nurse practitioners, and physician assistants to help understand all emotional and behavioral issues. HMHA is also licensed to provide outpatient substance abuse treatment. The Advanced Neuropsychology and Pediatric Psychology Services (ANPPS) is another outpatient service for the community that provides specialized psychological testing and assessment for both adults and children. These clinics provide both a meaningful resource within the community and support for patients discharged from inpatient care.

Hurley Wellness Services – Community Programs

Determined to be more than just a hospital, HMC has been a longtime partner of the community, giving families the resources they need to make healthier choices to improve their own health. HMC's Wellness Program reaches out to adults and children through diabetes education and prevention programs, injury prevention, healthy-living seminars, smoking-cessation classes, and geriatric programs for seniors. The focus on nutrition, heart health, wellness, and many other issues that affect a person's well-being is helping to transform the overall health of our community.

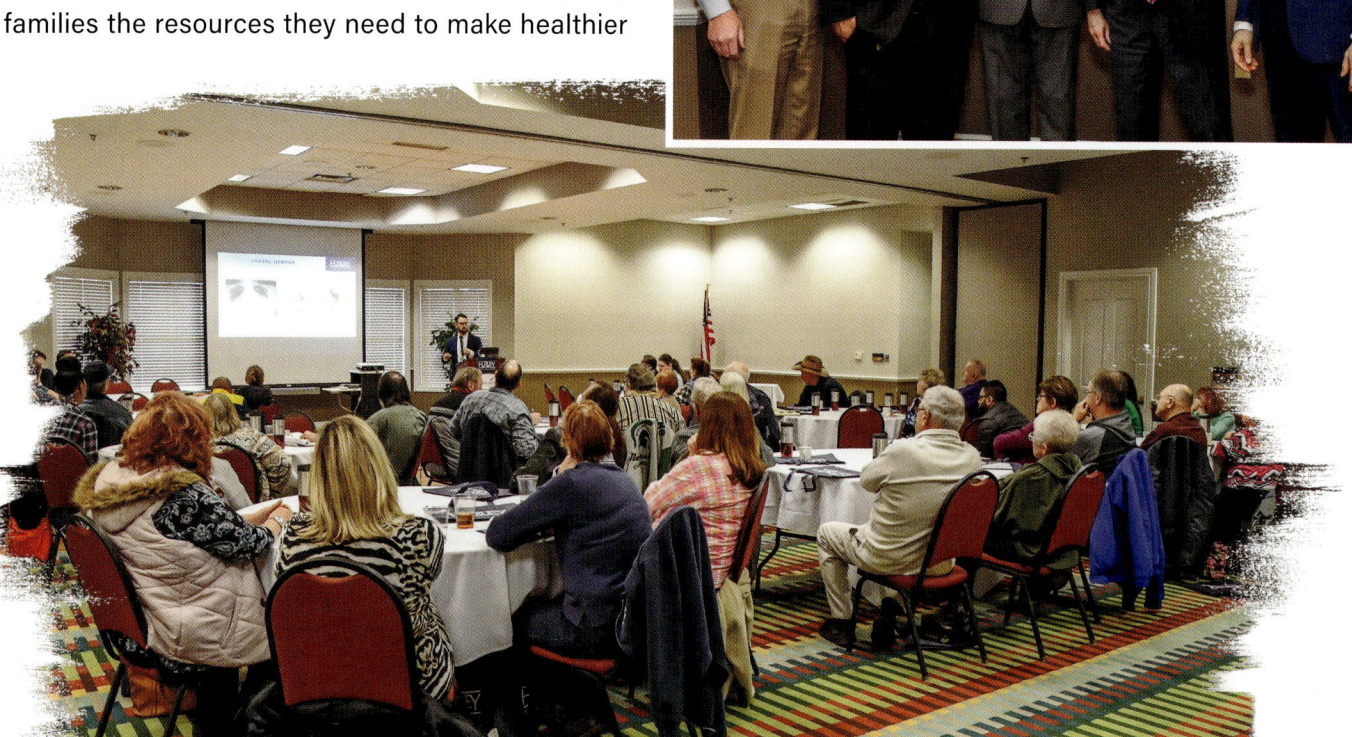

"Minimally Invasive Options to Treat Hernias" is part of the Hurley Healthy Living Series, which further enhances HMC's community role with health literacy, engagement, education, and awareness. Left to right: John Stewart; Kristoffer Wong, DO; Gul Sachwani-Daswani, DO; Leo Mercer, MD; and Dean Kristl, MD.

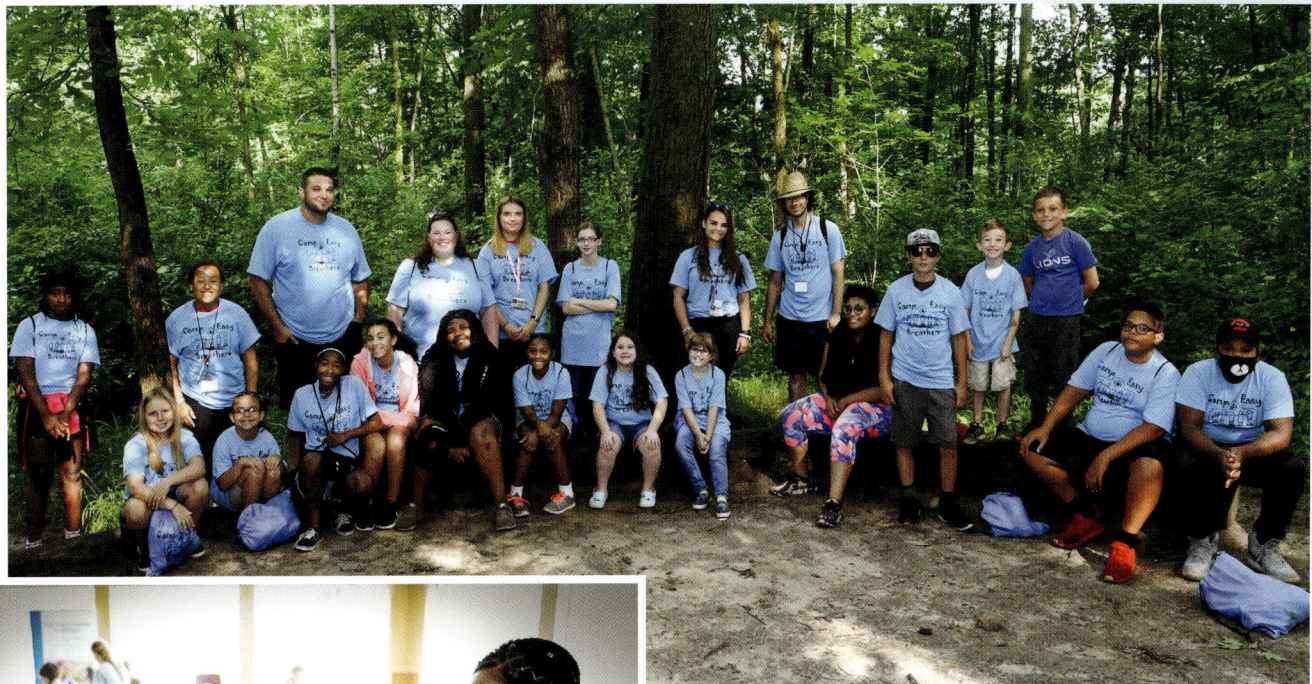

Camp Easy Breathers and Camp Move It

Partnering with YMCA of Greater Flint – Camp Copneconic

Camp Easy Breathers

Kids ages eight to 14 with asthma can participate in four days of adventure at Camp Copneconic, complete with swimming, canoeing, archery, climbing, hiking, arts and crafts, and other fun activities in the great outdoors. Kids have the benefit of an on-site wellness center equipped with treatment and exam rooms, a pharmacy, and other details to ensure quick medical care if their asthma is triggered. If treatment is necessary, their camp adventure can continue safely afterwards.

Camp Move It

Kids in third to sixth grade can build healthy life habits and reduce health risks associated with being overweight at this annual overnight camp involving fun, physical activity, healthy eating, and cooking. The experience these children enjoy by being a part of summer camp allows for a more interactive learning opportunity for teaching healthy lifestyle choices.

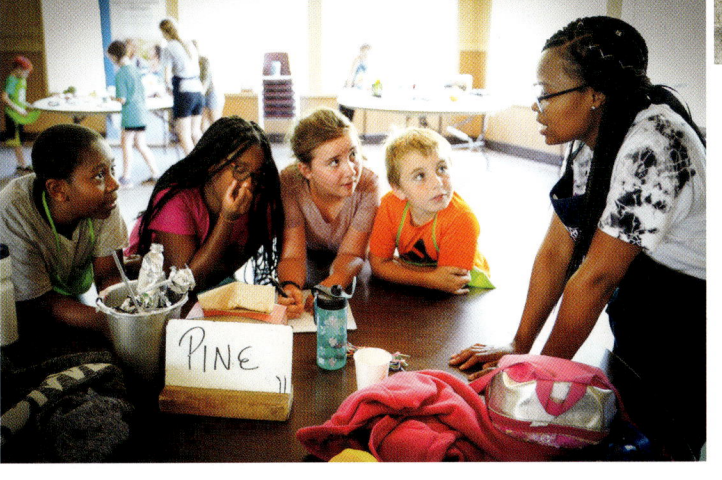

Asthma Disease Management Programs

A state leader in pediatric asthma care, HMC has the only home-based Asthma Disease Management Program in the region that teaches children and adults how to control their asthma. Asthma disease managers go to health fairs, schools, churches and synagogues, doctors' offices, and community centers to conduct asthma screening tests, show how to reduce asthma triggers, and demonstrate what to do during an asthma attack.

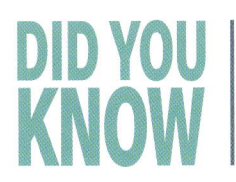

DID YOU KNOW | . . . Hurley staff provided all the local sports programs with concussion training at Flint and area schools.

CHAPTER SEVEN TRANSFORMING HEALTH • 155

Diabetes Education Programs

HMC's diabetes program is the largest in Genesee County, with classes recognized by the American Diabetes Association and certified by the Michigan Department of Health and Human Services. Diabetes educators help patients control diabetes through self-management. Trained nurses and dietitians offer education and support towards lower risks for serious health problems through a lifetime commitment. There are diabetes education programs for pediatrics, adults, and women during pregnancy.

National Diabetes Prevention Program

This yearlong wellness program, facilitated through the National Diabetes Prevention Program, is aimed at people with pre-diabetes, providing information and support to reduce the risk for developing type 2 diabetes, which can be avoided or delayed through moderate weight loss and regular physical activity by 58 percent.

Kohl's Healthy Kids

The Hurley Children's Hospital and the Kohl's Cares program provide ongoing activities in schools and other community settings to engage children to eat healthier, limit sugar-sweetened drinks, limit computer and/or TV screen time, and be physically active.

Injury Prevention and Youth Safety Outreach

The goal of the Injury Prevention and Safe Kids of Greater Flint programs is to reduce traumatic injuries in Genesee County and surrounding areas by taking lifesaving information out into the community in partnership with schools, police departments, fire departments, community groups, car dealerships, and countless local businesses. In 2019, Hurley's Injury Prevention coordinator, Nicole Matthews, RN, along with other members of the Region III Trauma

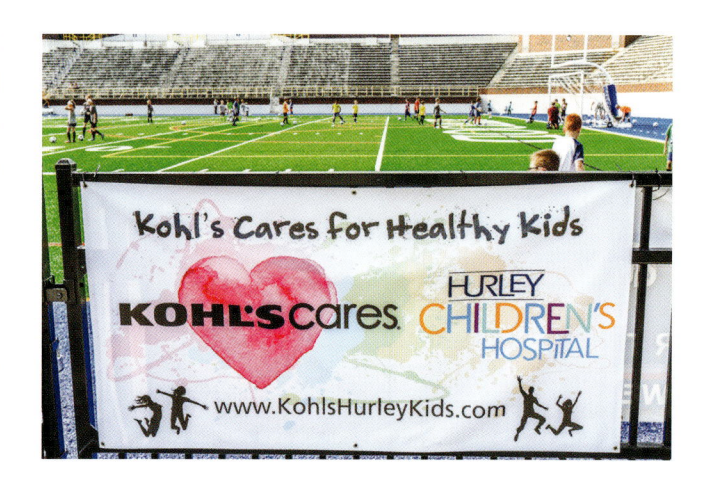

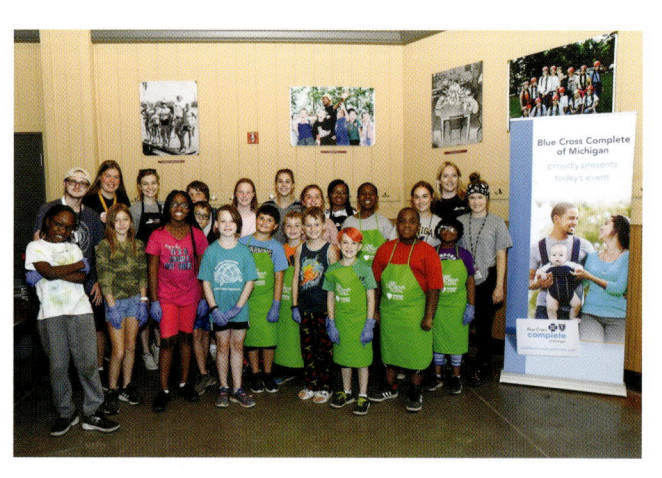

Kohl's Healthy Kids Program
Kohl's has been a Hurley Children's Hospital partner since 2006. As of September 2020, Kohl's has provided a total of $1,726,276 in grants to Hurley for a variety of children's health initiatives. Past events have included a free soccer clinic for kids with the Flint City Bucks at Atwood Stadium, free days at the Flint Children's Museum, and school assemblies focused on physical activity and healthy eating.

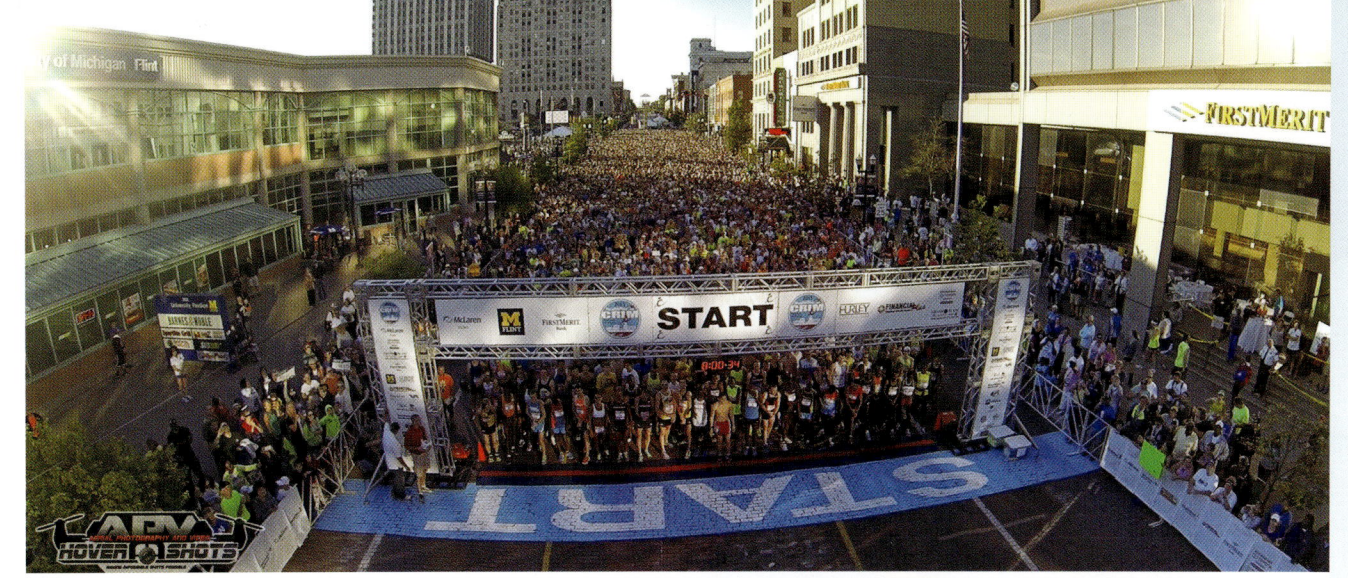

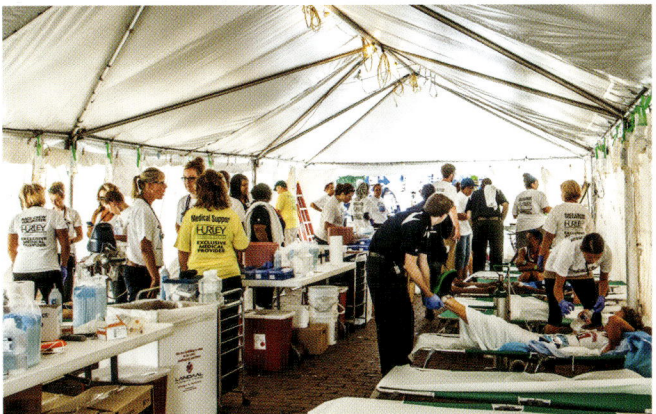

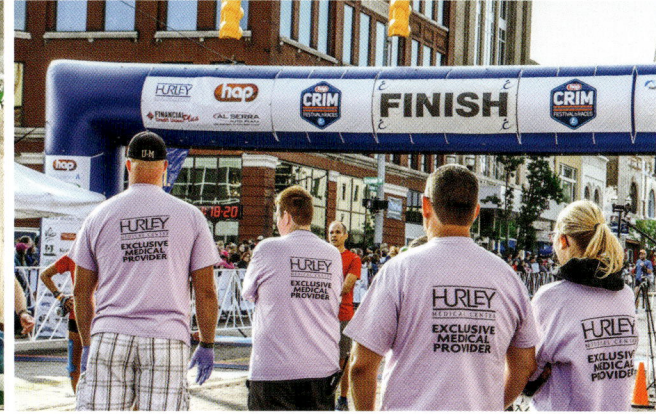

Crim Festival of Races, 2015
The annual Crim Festival of Races has been an important local event in Flint since 1977. HMC proudly serves as the exclusive medical provider for the event. This world-class festival of road races is held annually on the fourth Saturday in August and attracts athletes from all over the world.

Network, presented a distracted driving demonstration to 250 teens at Deckerville High School. The "Fatal Vision" hands-on simulator demonstrates the dangers of texting while driving or operating a vehicle with an altered mental capacity. "Fatal Vision" is also used in HMC's Trauma Drama and Rescue 911 annual safety programs for local middle school kids. Research shows that interactive programs help teens understand the choices they make in a more personal and direct way.

HMC volunteers also offer their skills as part of the Great Start Head Start Preschool Car Seat Program. Parents and expectant parents are taught how to correctly install car seats and booster seats. During the 2019 event, more than 30 car seats were inspected, many of which were found to be unsafe and were replaced with grant-funded seats from the Michigan Office of Highway Safety Planning through the Michigan State Police.

As part of the Injury Prevention program, HMC staff members team up with school nurses and the Genesee Intermediate School District to provide the highest level of safety training: medical emergency response team (MERT). MERT teams are composed of non-health care volunteers who receive advanced medical emergency training to provide immediate,

Teddy Bear Trot at Crim Festival of Races, 1999

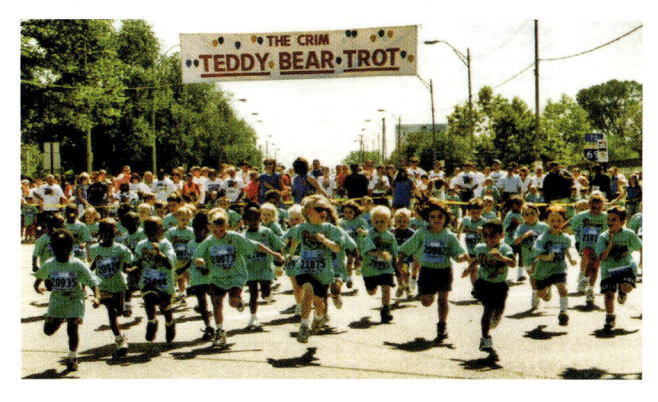

CHAPTER SEVEN TRANSFORMING HEALTH • 157

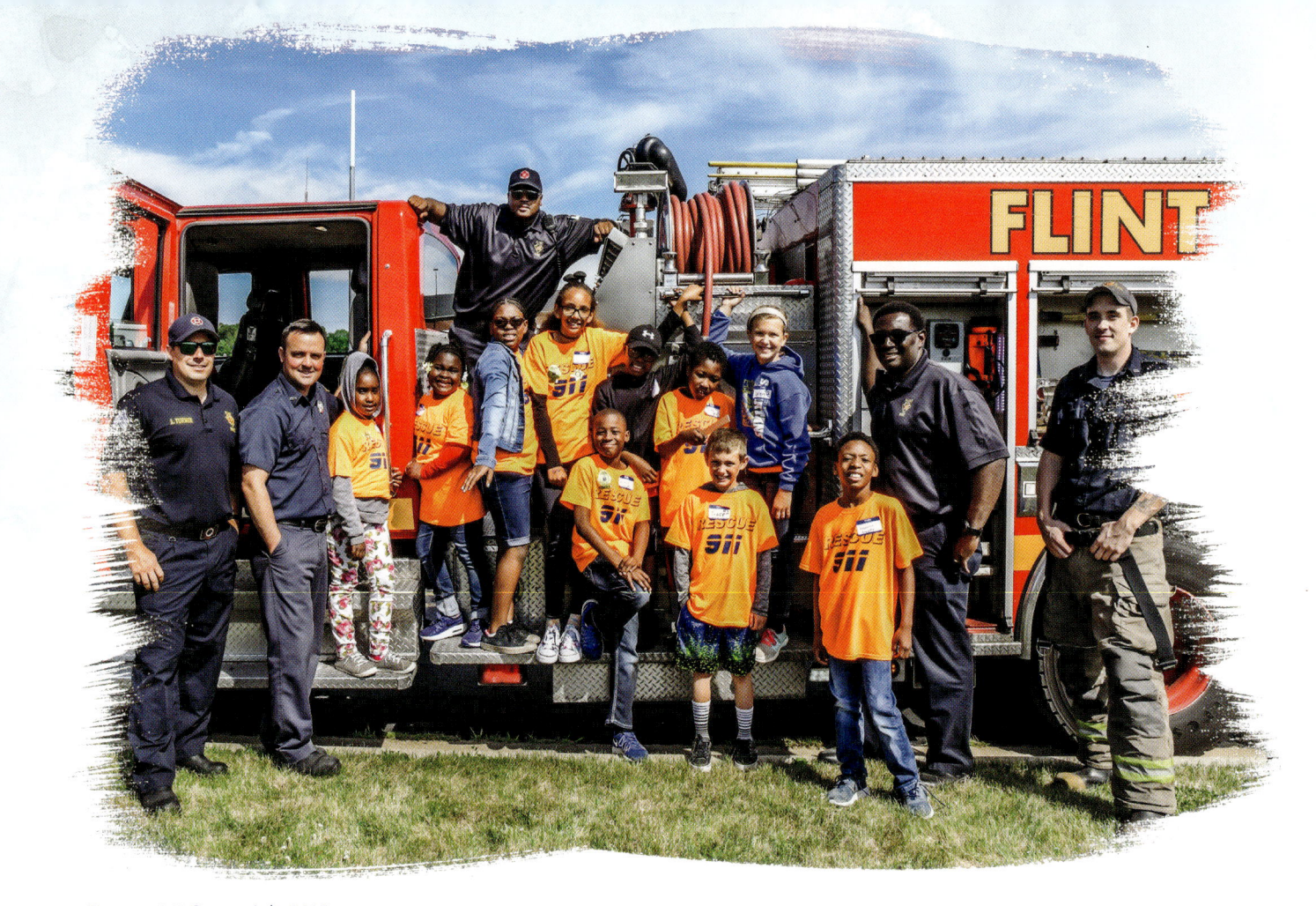

Rescue 911 Camp, July 2019

temporary care to seriously ill or injured persons. There are 3,000 MERT personnel in the local school districts, including office staff, coaches, and teachers who have agreed to take on this leadership role.

Teen Heart Health Check

In 2011, Tom Smith returned home from high school football practice, collapsed from an unknown heart ailment (sudden cardiac arrest, or SCA), and died at age 17. If victims of SCA do not get help (cardiopulmonary resuscitation/automated external defibrillator) to start the heart, it will lead to sudden cardiac death (SCD). Over 7,000 young people die in the United States each year from SCA. Tom's parents, Mary and Jonathan Smith, created the Thomas Smith Memorial Foundation in hopes of preventing all families from suffering the loss of a child by providing early detection and education for teenage heart ailments. The foundation partners with Hurley to provide free heart screenings to teenagers. Clinical experts and nonclinical volunteers are provided by Hurley at each screening. To date, over 3,552 teenagers have received free heart screenings (electrocardiogram/echocardiogram). Medical issues were discovered in 154 of those students, and 35 teens' lives were saved when severe heart ailments were discovered during their Teen Heart Health Check. Patricia Uhde, who has volunteered at every screening, remembers a woman from Detroit that had heard about the screening on the radio. Concerned because cardiac issues ran in her family, she drove six teenagers up from Detroit to be checked; three of the six kids had undiagnosed cardiac concerns.

Rescue 911 Camp

An annual summer kick-off, kids ages eight to 12 have fun while learning about safety. They enjoy police-, EMS-, and fire-vehicle tours, demonstrations about bike/helmet safety, ways that kids can combat bullying, and nutrition/wellness information, games, and lunch. Community partners include STAT EMS, HMC

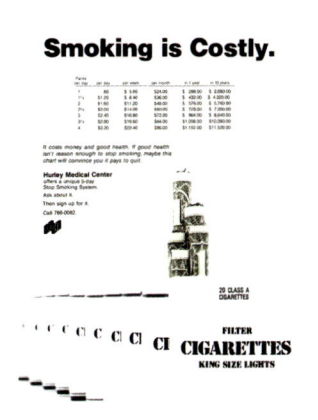

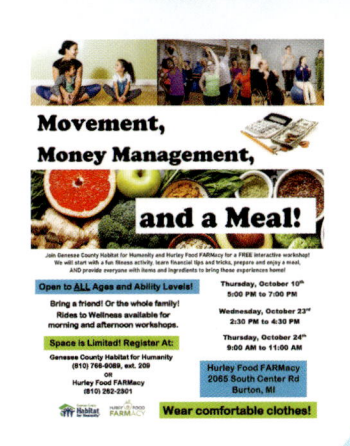

Hurley flyer educating about the cost of smoking, circa 1960, and a Hurley flyer educating about movement and money management, 2019

trauma nurses, UM-Flint nursing, Fenton City Police, Fenton 911, Fenton Fire Department, Genesee County Sheriff K-9 and Sheriff Paramedics, CN Railroad, and Hurley Health and Wellness.

Hopeful Hearts Methadone Clinic

HMC is addressing the opioid crisis by offering a best-practice program to other hospitals. The program provides educational meetings/support groups for pregnant women with a drug addiction. A team of social workers, doctors, and nurses provides patients on an individualized basis with what to expect in the NICU when their babies experience drug withdrawal shortly after delivery due to opioid exposure in the womb, whether it be heroin, prescription painkillers, or even medication-assisted treatment.

* * *

By increasing its presence within the community, away from its main campus, and reinforcing its role as the service area's premier public health care provider, Hurley fulfills its mission of "Clinical Excellence—Service to People"—the hallmark of service offered to every person who walks through the doors of any Hurley facility.

Burton Race Series

Since 2015, HMC has sponsored the Burton Race Series that includes the Burton/Kiwanis Hot Fudge 5K Run & Walk, the Race2Grace 5K Run/Walk, 1 Mile Run/Walk and Kid's Fun Run, the City of Burton Memorial Day 5K Run & Walk, and the Burton Veterans Honor Run, an 11K Run and 5K Run/Walk. Race proceeds benefit the City of Burton Parks and Recreation Department and the Disabled American Veterans organization.

NOTES

1. Hurley Foundation, *Inside Report* Vol. 4 (1996), p. 15.
2. Hurley Medical Center, *News You Can Use* Vol. 8 (Issue 3, March 2016), p. 3.
3. Hurley Foundation, *Inside Report* (2017–2018), p. 24.
4. Ibid., (2018-2019), p. 34.
5. M. Knapp, J. Beecham, D. McDaid, T. Matosevic, and M. Smith, "The economic consequences of deinstitutionalization of mental health services: lessons from a systematic review of European experience," *Health and Social Care in the Community*, Vol. 19 (No. 2, 2111), pp. 113–125.

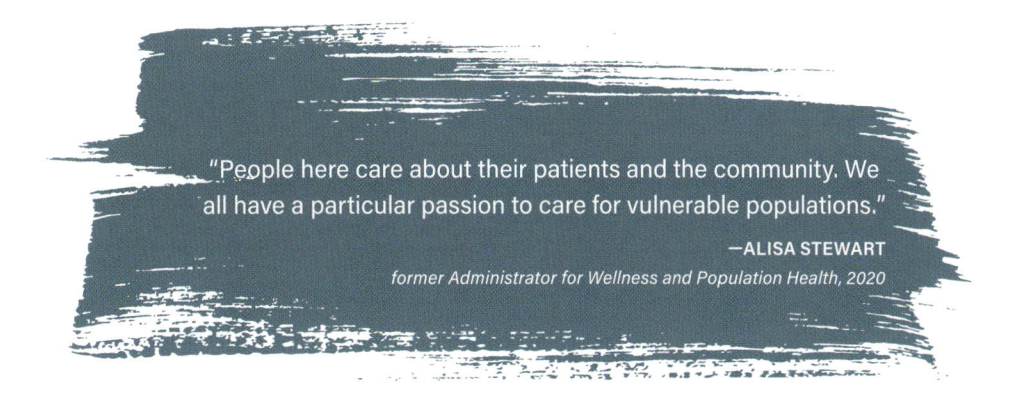

"People here care about their patients and the community. We all have a particular passion to care for vulnerable populations."

—ALISA STEWART
former Administrator for Wellness and Population Health, 2020

HMC Benchmarks of Excellence as of 2020

MEMBERSHIPS
- American Hospital Association
- America's Essential Hospitals
- Michigan Health and Hospital Association
- National Association of Children's Hospitals

LICENSES
- Centers for Medicare and Medicaid Services (CMS)
- Michigan Department of Community Health, Bureau of Health Systems

ACCREDITATIONS
- Accreditation Council for Graduate Medical Education (ACGME)
- Accreditation from the Hartford Institute of Geriatric Nursing at New York University
- ACEP Geriatric Emergency Department Accreditation Program (GEDA)
- American College of Emergency Physicians Accredited Geriatric Emergency Department Bronze Seal
- Michigan State Medical Society and Accreditations Council for Continuing Education (ACCME)
- Nurses Improving Care for Healthsystem Elders (NICHE)
- The Joint Commission (TJC) Hospital, Lab, Medication Compounding and Primary Stroke

AFFILIATIONS AND PARTNERSHIPS
- American Diabetes Association (ADA for Diabetes Self-Management Education Program Recognition Status
- CDC for the National Diabetes Prevention Program Recognition Status
- Children's Miracle Network Hospitals
- Detroit Children's Hospital
- FBI Emergency Medical Support Program
- Henry Ford Health System
- Michigan State University, College of Human Medicine
- Mott Children's Health Center
- University of Michigan-Flint
- University of Michigan Health Systems
- University of Michigan Mott Children's Hospital
- University of Michigan School of Dentistry
- U.S. Military Special Operations Medics

VERIFICATIONS
- Blue Cross Blue Shield Center of Excellence for Hip and Knee Replacement
- Blue Cross Blue Shield Center of Michigan Designated Blue Distinction Center + Maternity Care
- CDC Recognition for Diabetes Prevention Program
- Institute for Healthcare Improvement (IHI) as an Age-Friendly Health System Committed to Care Excellence for Older Adults
- The American Academy of Pediatrics and the American College of Obstetricians and Gynecologists as a Level III Neonatal Intensive Care Unit
- The American College of Surgeons as a Bariatric Surgery Center of Excellence
- The American College of Surgeons as a Level I Trauma Center and Level II Pediatric Trauma Center
- The American College of Surgeons Commission on Cancer for the Community Hospital Comprehensive Cancer Program
- National Accreditation Program for Breast Centers (NAPBC) for Hurley Breast Cancer Program
- The Joint Commission Certified Primary Stroke Center

Letter dated March 18, 1970:

My husband will be interning at Hurley Hospital beginning June 1, 1970. I am wondering if Hurley Hospital has a hospital systems study group or uses a computer in any way. If so, I would like to be considered for a position as a computer programmer. Would you please let me know to whom I should apply for this? If there is no computer at Hurley, is there a library in the complex large enough to employ a library assistant?"

Reply letter dated March 26, 1970:

In regard to computer programming, we might suggest that she make application to the following: General Motors Institution, Buick Motor Division, A C Spark Plug Division, Chevrolet Motor Division, Fisher Body Division. [addresses included for all]

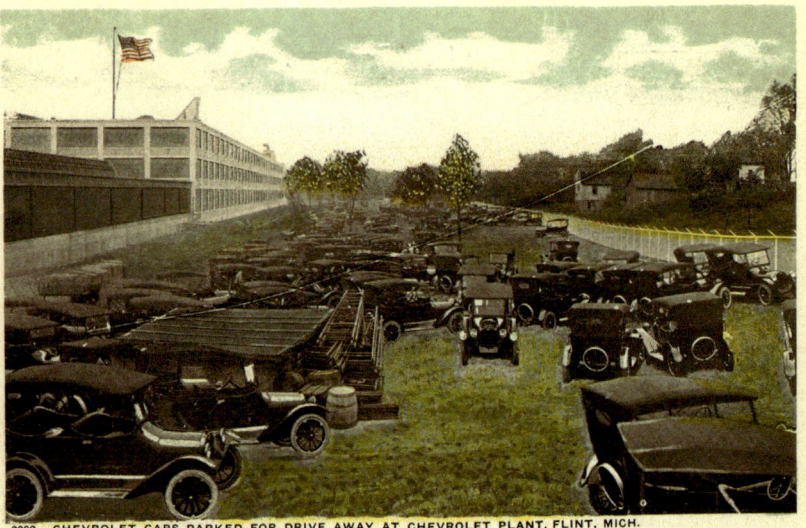

Letter to Lt. Conrad Reinhard, MC, USNR, dated October 10, 1966:

I am sure I speak for Doctor Collins and the other members of the Ob-Gyn Department in saying that we would be most happy to accept you as a first-year Ob-Gyn resident when you leave the service. We will be accepting applications for 1968 in October or November of 1967. In your case, letters of reference will not be necessary, but I would advise you to obtain a Michigan license. Our present group of 22 interns seem to be enjoying their year, and applications have shown that Internships and Residencies are better than ever, but I can't say for sure what the situation will become next March.

Letter dated August 17, 1978:

Currently, we have nine physicians from the University of Saskatchewan in our flexible internship program.

Letter dated December 18, 1967:

An independent survey of Michigan hospitals conducted by one of the medical schools, Hurley was picked as the top community hospital with the best teaching program. There have also been several other improvements, such as a catheterization lab, a raise in pay for the house staff and a tightening up of some of our teaching programs.

2202. CHEVROLET CARS PARKED FOR DRIVE AWAY AT CHEVROLET PLANT, FLINT, MICH.
New Assembly Plant at Left.

Letter dated April 6, 1966:

We have just completed our housing arrangements for the 1966-1967 Intern staff. 1011 Patrick Street, Apartment #12. This is a **two-bedroom apartment** on the ground floor of the Intern Apartment Building, located across the street from the rear entrance of the hospital. The apartment is furnished, with the exception of linens, dishes, pots and pans, and silver. The rental for your apartment, including heat, is $95 per month; however, since you will receive a housing allowance of $45 per month, your cost will actually be only $50, plus a utility charge for electricity. You will also be responsible for your telephone bill. You might also like to know that the apartment has a double bed and two twin beds, so you will know the type of bed linens to bring.

Radiology: D.R. Limbach, M.D.

Letter dated May 14, 1973:

In previous years, we have ordered skirts, blouses and short coats for female interns. However, the Administration has no objection to pant suits, and the other female intern that we will have this year would prefer pants rather than skirts. Please specify your preference.

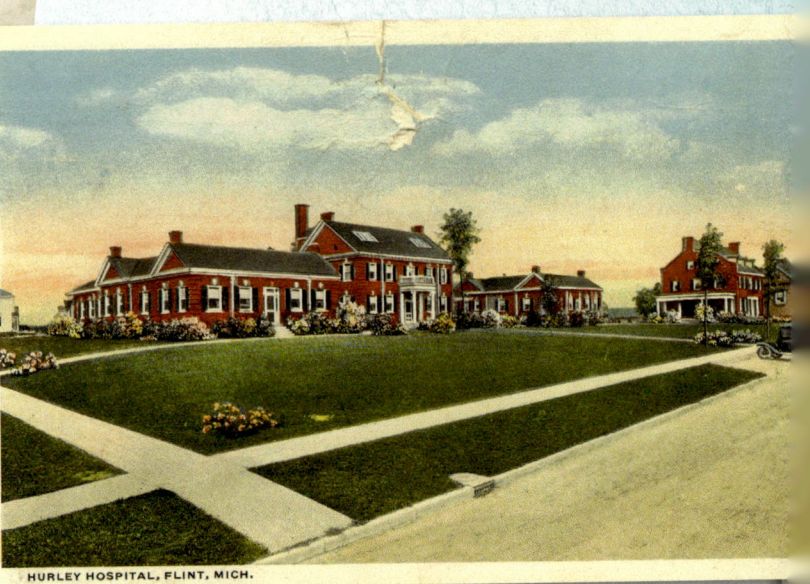

Letter dated March 9, 1972:

This is to confirm that Dr. Byron Schoolfield is presently a third year resident in Internal Medicine at Hurley Hospital. He receives a stipend of $9900.00 per year, plus full maintenance (housing and meals while on duty), except telephone. The hospital also pays for Blue Cross Insurance for him and his family, but not Blue Shield.

HURLEY HOSPITAL, FLINT, MICH.